Practical Neonatology

Practical Neonatology

Editor: Talia Atkins

AMERICAN
MEDICAL PUBLISHERS
www.americanmedicalpublishers.com

AMERICAN
MEDICAL PUBLISHERS
www.americanmedicalpublishers.com

Cataloging-in-Publication Data

Practical neonatology / edited by Talia Atkins.
p. cm.
Includes bibliographical references and index.
ISBN 978-1-63927-431-4
1. Neonatology. 2. Perinatology. 3. Newborn infants--Diseases. 4. Newborn infants--Care. I. Atkins, Talia.
RJ251 .P73 2022
618.920 1--dc23

American Medical Publishers,
41 Flatbush Avenue,
1st Floor, New York,
NY 11217, USA

ISBN 978-1-63927-431-4 (Hardback)

Contents

Preface

Neonatology is a field in pediatrics which is concerned with the medical care of newborn infants, in particular, infants who are ill or born premature. Infants may be born with low birth weight, congenital malformations, pulmonary hypoplasia, birth asphyxia, intrauterine growth restriction or sepsis. The infant in the neonatal period also adapts to extrauterine life and develops its physiological systems. The medical care for such infants is provided in neonatal intensive care units. The development of mechanical ventilation and pulmonary surfactant replacement therapy in recent decades has improved the survival of premature infants. This book unravels the recent researches in the field of neurodegeneration. It presents studies performed by experts across the globe. This book attempts to assist those with a goal of delving into the field of neonatology.

This book unites the global concepts and researches in an organized manner for a comprehensive understanding of the subject. It is a ripe text for all researchers, students, scientists or anyone else who is interested in acquiring a better knowledge of this dynamic field.

I extend my sincere thanks to the contributors for such eloquent research chapters. Finally, I thank my family for being a source of support and help.

Editor

1

Foot length, chest and head circumference measurements in detection of Low birth weight neonates in Mekelle, Ethiopia

Marta Yemane Hadush[1*], Amanuel Hadgu Berhe[1] and Araya Abrha Medhanyie[2]

Abstract

Background: Low birth weight (Birth weight < 2500 g) is a leading cause of prenatal and neonatal deaths. The early identification of Low birth weight (LBW) neonates is essential for any comprehensive initiative to improve their chance of survival. However, a large proportion of births in developing countries take place at home and birth weight statistics are not available. Therefore, there is a need to develop simple, inexpensive and practical methods to identify low birth weight (LBW) neonates soon after birth.

Methods: This is a hospital based cross sectional study. Four hundred twenty two (422) live born neonates were included and anthropometric measurements were carried out within 24 h of birth by three trained nurses. Birth weight was measured by digital scale. Head and chest circumference were measured by using non extendable measuring tape and foot length with hard transparent plastic ruler. Data was entered into SPSS version 20 for analysis. Characteristics of study participants were analyzed using descriptive statistics such as frequency and percentage for categorical data and mean and standard deviation for continuous data. Correlation with birth weight using Pearson's correlation coefficient and linear regression were used to identify the association between dependent and independent variables. Receiver operating characteristic (ROC) curve was used to evaluate accuracy of the anthropometric measurements to predict LBW.

Results: The prevalence of low birth weight was found to be 27%. All anthropometric measurements had a positive correlation with birth weight, chest circumference attaining the highest correlation with birth weight ($r = 0.85$) and foot length had the weakest correlation ($r = 0.74$). Head circumference had the highest predictive value for birth weight (AUC = 0.93) followed by Chest circumference (AUC = 0.91). A cut off point of chest circumference 30.15 cm had 84.2% sensitivity, 85.4% specificity and diagnostic accuracy ($P < 0.001$). A cut off point of head circumference 33.25 had the highest positive predictive value (77%).

Conclusion: Chest circumference and head circumference were found to be better surrogate measurements to identify low birth weight neonates.

Keywords: Low birth weight, Anthropometry, Chest circumference, Head circumference, Foot length, Surrogate

* Correspondence: marsec112@yahoo.com
[1]School of Medicine, Mekelle Univesity, College of Health Sciences, Mekelle, Ethiopia
Full list of author information is available at the end of the article

Background

According to the World Health Organization (WHO) definition, neonates with birth weights of less than 2500g are classified as low birth weight (LBW) regardless of gestational age. Subcategories include Very low birth weight, which is less than 1500 g and extremely low birth weight, which is less than 1000 g [1].

A significant progress has been made in the reduction of child mortality in the past decades worldwide. Though the under five mortality rate has decreased globally by about 50% (from 90 to 48 deaths per 1000 live births) in the year 1990 and 2012 respectively, the neonatal mortality rate decreased only 36%, from 33 deaths/1000 live births to 21 deaths/1000 live births over the same period [2]. Globally one sixth of neonates are born low birth weight (LBW, <2500 g), which is an underlying factor for 60 to 80% of neonatal deaths [3].

The WHO country cooperation strategy 2008–2011 showed that the prevalence of low birth weight in Ethiopia was estimated to be 14%. It is one of the highest in the world [1]. Previous studies done in Ethiopia show that there is a decline in mean birth weight and that there is an increasing trend in LBW from 1970 to 1990's. For example in south western part of the country among health institutional deliveries the incidence of LBW is 22.5% [4].

LBW is a leading cause of perinatal deaths and remains a worldwide issue and one of the most important public health problems particularly in developing countries [5].

The risk of death increases as the birth weight is lower; neonates born with weight between 2000 and 2499g are 4 times more likely to die during their first 28 days of life than neonates born with weight between 2500 and 2999g, and 10 times more likely to die than those weighing 3000–3499g [6]. Thus early identification of the LBW neonates is essential for any intervention to improve their chances of survival. Despite most of the worlds' LBW neonates are born in developing countries, birth weight statistics are not available because significant proportion of births takes place at home. According to Ethiopian Demographic and Health Survey 2000, 2005, and 2011 the trend on neonatal mortality were 49, 39, and 37 respectively. But having this, Ethiopia has limited birth weight estimates as there are home deliveries, inaccurate weighing scales and poor documentation of birth weights [7].

Weighing scale was, is and will be the appropriate, accurate and standard for detection of neonates' birth weight. In this study finding a surrogate is particularly intended targeting the disadvantaged communities where the access to health facilities might be difficult and where neonates are not weighed routinely due to paucity of a suitable weighing scale at the health facilities. These surrogates will help in the detection of LBW neonates and bring them to medical attention. The measurements can be done by health extension worker whose responsibilities are to do home visits and detect health problems in the community and get the people come to medical attention.

Though the baseline population in Ethiopia is similar with WHO standard (uses WHO growth charts), for the aforementioned reasons there is a need to develop simple to use and carry, inexpensive and practical methods to identify LBW neonates soon after birth. This will be useful in early identification and prompt referral. Efforts should be made to find an effective method for identification of these high-risk neonates in the community.

A number of alternative anthropometric measurements have been proposed as surrogate for birth-weight. These include the circumferences of the neonates' head, chest, and mid arm [8–14]. In most studies done so far chest circumference has the highest sensitivity followed by head circumference, mid upper arm circumference (MUAC) and foot length [10] on identifying LBW.

Chest and head circumference were used to identify LBW preterm neonates in Ethiopia, and the cut-off points with the best sensitivity and specificity identified were 30 cm and 31 cm for chest and head circumference respectively [11].

Though in most of the previous studies chest circumference has a good sensitivity, the cut off points varies among the studies. This study aims to find a better surrogate anthropometric measurement to detect LBW neonates and will be a supplement to the previously done studies.

Methods

Study setting

The study was conducted in Ayder Referral hospital (ARH), which is located in Mekelle city, Tigray region, north Ethiopia which is found at 783 km from Addis Ababa, the capital city of Ethiopia. The Hospital provides a broad range of medical services to both in and out patients of all age groups. It stands as the second largest hospital in the nation with a total capacity of about 500 inpatient beds in four major departments and other specialty units. Pediatrics and child health is one of the departments in the hospital, care for neonates being one of the services it provides. There is fairly equipped neonatal intensive care unit (NICU) and provides a tertiary level of care. About 40% of the admissions to NICU are from other health facilities in the region and the remainder 60% being from obstetrics ward in the hospital which was also the second study area. The annual rate of delivery in the hospital is 2800.

Ethical clearance was obtained from the Ethical Review Board of Mekelle University, College of Health Science. Letter of permission was presented to Ayder referral hospital. Verbal informed consent was obtained from mothers/guardian of the newborns after the purpose of the study is explained. Verbal informed consent was done for most of the participants were illiterates.

Study design, data collection and analysis

This was a hospital based quantitative cross sectional study design. Data was collected by using data collection format by nurses who work at the NICU after being given one day training on how to measure the neonates' head and chest circumferences by using non extendable measuring tape, with a width of 1.0 cm and subdivisions of 0.1 cm and foot length using hard transparent plastic ruler. Reliability of measurements was checked by doing repeat measurements for each test intermittently by the supervisor.

Four hundred twenty two (422) live born babies were included which was calculated using single population proportion formula. Anthropometric measurements were carried out within 24 h of birth by the trained nurses. Head circumference (HC) was measured between glabellas anteriorly and along the occipital prominence posteriorly. Chest circumference (CC) was measured at the level of nipple at the end phase of expiration. Foot length was measured from the heel to tip of the big toe using hard transparent plastic ruler. Babies were weighed naked on digital weighing scale. Weight scale was calibrated before every measurement using a material of standard weight of 1000g (bag of 1000 ml IV fluid). Gestational age of the newborns was taken from mothers' medical record.

After the collected data was edited and checked for completeness and consistency; it was directly entered into SPSS version 20. Characteristics of study participants were analyzed using descriptive statistics such as frequency and percentage for categorical data and mean and standard deviation (SD) for continuous data.

Pearson's correlation coefficient and linear regression analyses were done to examine linear relationship between two or more continuous variables.

Using the chi square analyses, the accuracy of all the variables in identifying LBW neonates were compared. Statistical significance was declared at probability (P) value of < 0.05 and 95% confidence interval (CI) was used to show the strength of association between independent and dependent variables.

Non-parametric receiver operating characteristic (ROC) curve analysis was carried out to calculate 95% confidence intervals of areas under the curve (AUC) that is to determine the overall accuracy and the sensitivity of the cut off points to identify best surrogate anthropometric measurement. Finally the predictive performances of the cut off points were calculated.

Table 1 Sex distribution of the neonates based on weight categories

Weight(gm)	Male's frequency (%)	Female's frequency (%)	Total frequency (%)
>2500	163(53.27%)	143(46.73%)	306(100%)
<2500	48(42.1%)	66(57.9%)	114(100%)
Total	211(50.24%)	209(49.76%)	420(100%)

Table 2 Gestational age distribution of the neonates based on weight categories

Weight (gm)	Gestational age(weeks)			Total
	>42	37 – 42	<37	
>2500	2(0.66%)	293(96.38%)	9(2.96%)	304(100%)
<2500	0	47(41.23%)	67(58.77%)	114(100%)
Total	2(0.48%)	340(81.34%)	76(18.18%)	418(100%)

Result

Characteristics of study population

The total number of study participants enrolled in this study was 422, of which 50.24% of them were males (Table 1). The birth weights of the subjects ranged from 770 g to 4760 g, with a mean birth weight of 2807 ± 691.82 g. Using the World health assembly cut-off value of <2500 g, a total of 114 neonates (27%) were LBW. As Table 1 shows the proportion of LBW among females is found to be higher than males (57.9% vs. 42.1%).

Table 2 demonstrates the distribution of neonates in weight and gestational age categories. It shows that 58.77% of those with LBW (<2500g) are preterm and 41.23% are term. The rate of prematurity is 18.18%.

Anthropometric parameters for different weight categories

Table 3 outlines the mean values of the anthropometric variables for the different weight categories. Overall the mean for each of the measurements for LBW neonates were; 31.21 ± 2.48 for HC, 27.27 ± 3.2 cm for CC and 6.8 ± 0.85 cm for FL.

Table 4 shows the results of the analysis of variance with respect to the three measurements; there was a statistically significant difference among the two weight categories for all three measurements. It indicates that all the anthropometric variables had significant, linear, positive correlation with birth weight ($p < 0.001$). CC attained

Table 3 Mean values of anthropometric variables for the different weight categories

Parameters	Weight (gm)	Number	Mean	Std. Deviation
Head circumference of the neonate (HC)	>2500	308	35.2977	1.67445
	<2500	114	31.2132	2.48067
Chest circumference of the neonate (CC)	>2500	308	32.3712	2.01901
	<2500	114	27.2789	3.22091
Foot length of the neonate (FL)	>2500	308	7.9340	.45403
	<2500	114	6.8097	.85747

Table 4 Pearson correlation coefficient of anthropometric variables

Anthropometric Variables	Pearson Correlation Coefficient (r)	R^2	*P*-Value
Chest circumference (CC)	0.85	0.722	<0.0001
Head circumference (HC)	0.825	0.680	<0.0001
Foot length (FL)	0.746	0.557	<0.0001

the highest correlation with birth weight ($r = 0.85$) while FL attained the lowest ($r = 0.746$).

Linear regression analysis

Three linear regression models for CC, HC and FL as independent variables and birth weight as dependent variable were created. The highest coefficient of correlation (R) and coefficient of determination (R^2) were associated with CC followed by head circumferences and then foot length. All the correlations were significant at $p < 0.001$. CC had the lowest standard error of the estimate (SEE) and it had a higher coefficient of determination (R^2) when compared with HC (0.722 vs. 0.680). FL gave a coefficient of determination (R^2) of 0.557 which is the least.

Three scatter plot graphs were created, each representing CC, HC, and FL for the newborns (Fig. 1a–c). The positive gradients of the scatter plot diagrams show that there is a linear and positive relationship between all the anthropometric measurements and birth weight with the highest coefficient of determination (R^2) being associated with CC.

Receiver operating characteristic (ROC) curve analysis for cut-off point determination

The corresponding ROC curves for CC, HC and FL as surrogates for birth weight less than 2500 g are shown in Fig. 2a–c. ROC analysis to test how well the different measures predict LBW showed that HC and CC have comparable area under the curve (AUC) 0.933 and 0.912 respectively (Table 5). For three of the anthropometric

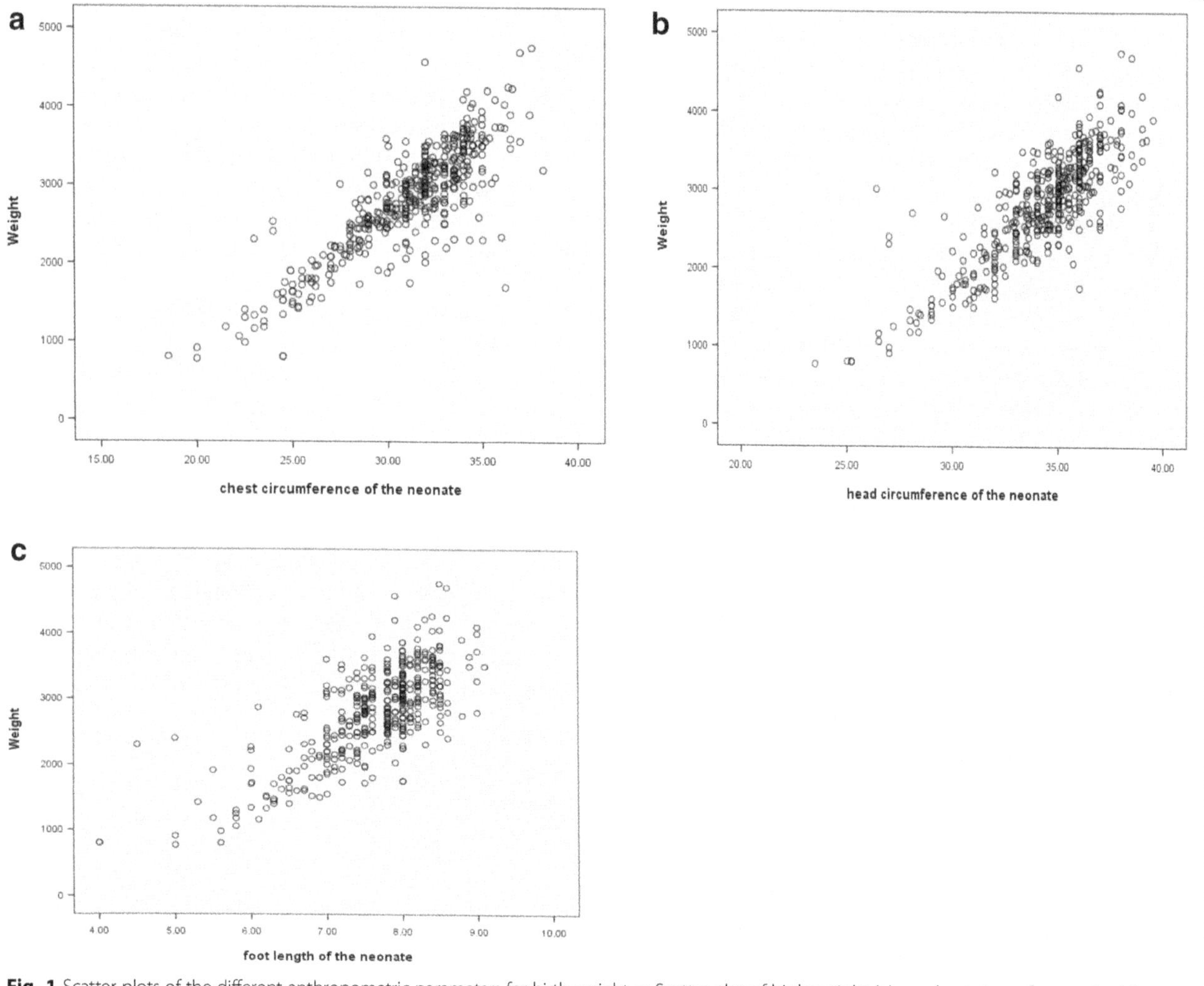

Fig. 1 Scatter plots of the different anthropometric parameters for birth weight. **a**: Scatter plot of birth weight (g) on chest circumference (cm) for neonates. **b**: Scatter plot of birth weight (g) on head circumference for neonates. **c**: Scatter plot of birth weight (g) on foot length for neonates

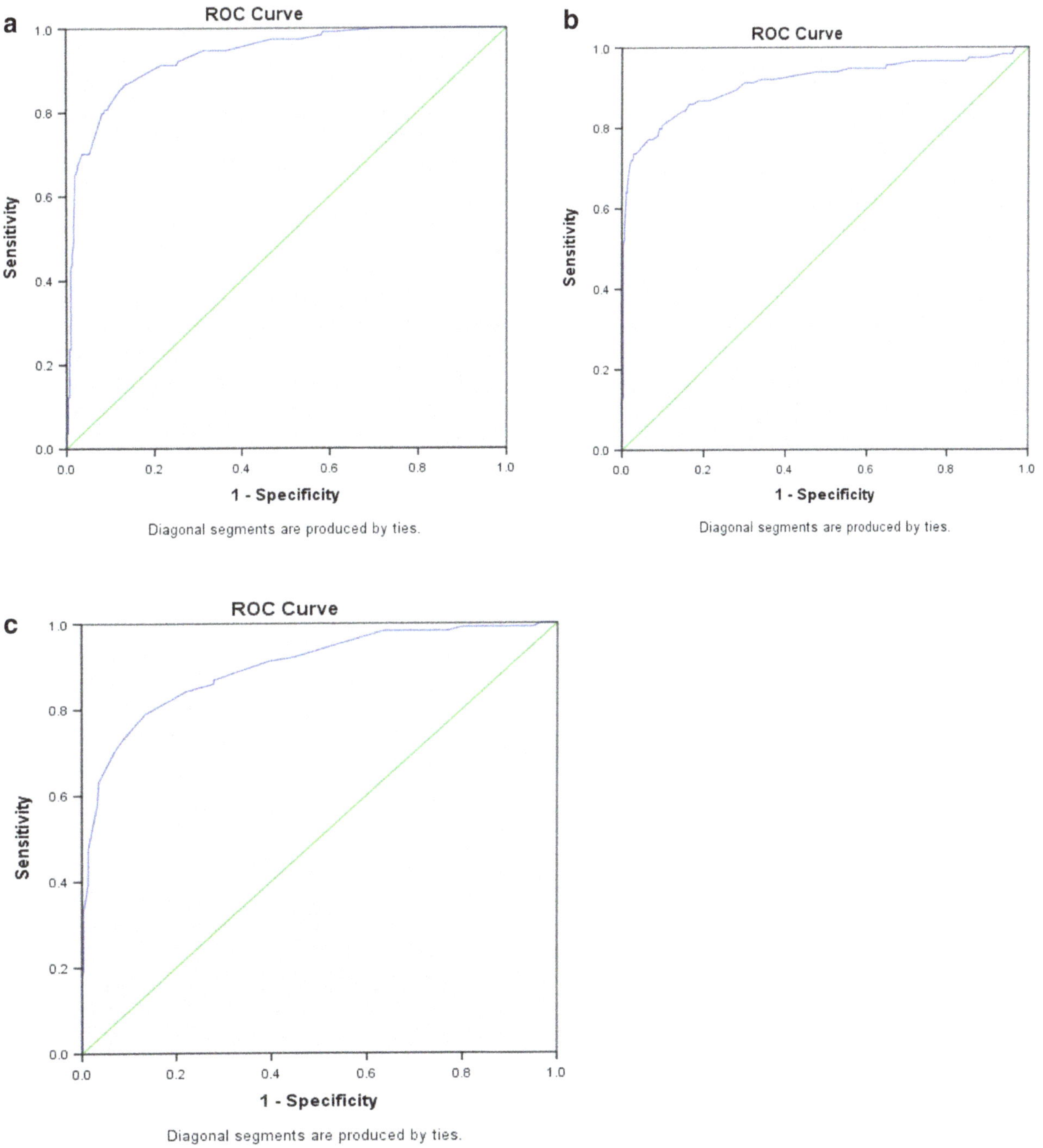

Fig. 2 ROC curve for surrogate anthropometies. **a**. CC as a surrogate for birth weigth <2500gm, **b**. HC as a surrogate for birth weigth <2500gm, **c**. FL as a surrogate for birth weigth <2500gm

measures, sensitivity and specificity at every value were calculated then the possible operational cut-off points were determined by taking the highest average of sensitivity and specificity. Then the predictive performance of each of the cut off points was calculated as outlined on Table 6.

For CC, the identified cut-off point was 30.15 cm with a sensitivity of 84.2% and 85.4% specificity. The optimal cutoff point for HC was 33.25 cm with a sensitivity of 80.7% and 90% specificity. With respect to FL the optimal cutoff point was 7.35 cm with 72.8% sensitivity and 91.6% specificity. With this CC is the most sensitive

Table 5 AUC analysis for discrimination of birth weights below 2500 g

Parameter	AUC	95% CI
Head circumference	0.933	0.908 – 0.960
Chest circumference	0.912	0.873 – 0.950
Foot length	0.897	0.861 – 0.934

measurement followed by HC which has the highest positive predictive value (Table 6).

Discussion

In this study, the prevalence of LBW was 27%; of this proportion of LBW among females were 57.9%. The mean birth weight was 2807 ± 691.82 g. Prematurity accounted for 74(17.5%) of the enrolled neonates. The LBW prevalence is a lot higher than the estimated national average which is 14% [7]. But studies show that the incidence is on an increasing trend among health institution deliveries for example in Gondar, Ethiopia the prevalence is 17.4% [15] and in the south western part of the country, Jimma it is 22.5% [7]. The higher prevalence of LBW can be attributed to the fact that the study was carried out in a referral hospital where high risk pregnancies that may result in preterm delivery are managed and where sick newborns are admitted.

Birth weight has been and is still an important screening tool for detecting newborns with LBW. Because of unavailability or inaccurate weighing scales and higher incidence of home deliveries measuring weight and detecting LBW neonates in developing countries is difficult [16]. This has led to the need for alternative measurements to assess newborns. A measuring tape is easily portable and can be used by community based health workers when they are notified of a delivery in a community under their catchment.

In the current study involving babies admitted to NICU and those born in Ayder Referral Hospital, birth weight correlated very strongly with the anthropometric variables of CC and HC. CC and HC demonstrated the best correlation with birth weight ($r = 0.85$ and AUC = 0.91) and ($r = 0.82$ and AUC = 0.93) respectively. Other analyses (sensitivity, specificity, PPV and NPV) also indicate that they are the two most appropriate measurements for identifying LBW in the study area. Though HC is not found to be the best surrogate anthropometric tool in most of the studies reviewed, the current finding is similar with a study done in Pokhara among Nepalese newborns. The study found the optimal cut-points for head circumference and chest circumference to identify LBW newborns to be 33.5 cm and 30.8 cm respectively [9]. This is comparable with the cut off points found in this study (33.25 for HC and 30.15 for CC). This is also true in a study done in newborns in Pelotas, Brazil which shows HC with cutoff point of 33 cm and CC with 31 cm to be good surrogates [6].

Table 6 Predictive performance of selected median cut-off points of CC, OFC and FL indices for birth weight <2500 g

Cutoff points	Sensitivity (%)	Specificity (%)	PPV (%)	NPV (%)
CC(30.15 cm)	84.2	85.4	67	93.5
HC(33.25 cm)	80.7	90	77	92.7
FL(7.45 cm)	78.9	86.7	72	91

PPV positive predictive value, *NPV* negative predictive value

Foot length had the least correlation among all the parameters analyzed in the current study ($r = 0.74$) and was found to be less sensitive as well (72.8%). But in a study done in Uganda it correlated strongly with birth weight ($r = 0.76$ and AUC = 0.97) and had 94% sensitivity and 83% specificity in detecting LBW [10]. The study also implied that the measurement of foot length exposes the baby less which decreases the risk of hypothermia and is technically easier which are both important points that mandates further look into this anthropometric measurement for it is the least studied as compared to the others. Other studies also found less studied surrogates to be best in detecting LBW neonates; a study done in south eastern Nigeria comparing length, head circumference, mid arm circumference and maximum thigh circumference found that maximum thigh circumference to be the best surrogate for the detection of LBW neonates [17].

CC is the best surrogate anthropometric measurement in this study. This is similar to findings in Bangladesh [14]. This is also true with findings from studies done in Pokhara [9] which have reported good correlation between CC and birth weight. The high coefficient of correlation in the current study further reinforces the recommendation of the WHO collaborative study to use CC as an alternative measurement for detection of low birth weight [16].

The cut-off point for LBW in the current study was similar to value obtained In India [12], which was 30 cm. The cutoffs in studies done in Nepal and Bangladesh were 30.3 cm and 30.5 cm respectively [14, 18] but the value is lower than Egypt and Brazil which in both cases is 31 cm [6, 8]. The findings of the current study and other studies from both Africa [8, 10, 11] and Asia [12, 14] fall between a range of 30 cm and 31.0 cm.

Though both CC and HC have good correlation with birth weight, we recommend the use of chest rather than head circumference as a surrogate for birth weight for different reasons. CC is simpler to measure because the identification of the nipple line is easier; this makes measurement more operationally feasible than that of head circumference. Unlike on the head there are no significant soft tissue changes that can happen by the delivery process on the chest. The variations in the degree of molding and edema may make HC less accurate. Moreover, the use of head circumference alone can potentially miss a number of LBW infants who have normal head circumference measures but are LBW such as in the cases of asymmetric intrauterine growth restriction or the reverse with normal birth weight but reduced head circumference as in the case of chromosomal abnormalities and prenatal infections that may result in microcephly.

Therefore a tool which is easy to use with low cost and risk to identify small babies could be an effective intervention to save the lives of neonates. This can be implemented by the development of color coded tapes which can be used by trained community based health workers (like in Ethiopia health extension workers) working at remote areas where weighing scales might not be readily available.

Study limitations

The fact that more than one data collectors were used may have an effect on the quality of data collected due to inter observer difference. But this was minimized by training the data collectors. In this study the measurements were done by health professionals but the tool will be used by health extension workers and their skill is likely to be different.

Conclusion

Chest circumference and head circumference with cut off points 30.15 cm and 33.25 cm respectively are better surrogates for detecting LBW neonates. Of the two tools this study suggests that chest circumference is the most appropriate predictor given its high correlation and sensitivity in detecting LBW babies.

Neonates who fall below the stated cut off point should be considered as high risk and referred to health institutions where they can get better service and chance of survival.

Abbreviations

ARH: Ayder referral hospital; AUC: Area under the curve; CC: Chest circumference; CI: Confidence interval; FL: Foot length; HC: Head circumference; MUAC: Mid upper arm circumference; NICU: Neonatal intensive care unit; NPV: Negative predictive value; PPV: Positive predictive value; ROC: Receiver operating characteristics; WHO: World Health Organization

Acknowledgements

We are thankful to all data collectors and study participants for taking part in the study. We would also like to thank Mekelle University, college of health science for the support that provided us in undertaking the study.

Funding

The study was conducted by the research fund obtained from Mekelle University, college of health science.

Authors' contributions

MYH was responsible for the design, statistical analysis and interpretation of the study and drafting the manuscript. AAM and AHB contributed to the design, statistical analysis and interpretation of the study and reviewing and revising the manuscript. All authors read and approved the final manuscript.

Authors' information

Marta Yemane, MD is an assistant professor of pediatrics and child health.
Araya Abrha, PhD is an assistant professor of public health.
Amanuel Hadgu, MD is assistant professor of pediatrics and child health.

Competing interests

The authors declare that they have no competing interests.

Author details

[1]School of Medicine, Mekelle Univesity, College of Health Sciences, Mekelle, Ethiopia. [2]School of Public Health, Mekelle University, College of Health Sciences, Mekelle, Ethiopia.

References

1. WHO. Handbook for guideline development. Geneva: WHO; 2008–2011.
2. UNICEF. Levels and trends in child mortality Report 2013. New York: UNICEF; 2013. 2015.
3. Negar S, Hamideh S, Farnoosh R, Ramin J, Michael G. Barakat. Anthropometric measurements at birth as predictor of low birth weight. Health. 2011;3(12):752–756.
4. Berihun MZ, Meseret Z, Nuru M. Incidence and correlates of low birth weight at a referral hospital in Northwest Ethiopia. Pan Afr Med J. 2012;12:4.
5. Louangpradith V, Yoshitoku MD, Harun-or-Rashid, Junichi S. Factors affecting Low birth weight at four central hospitals in Vientiane. Nagoya J Med Sci. 2010;72:51–8.
6. Judith P, Laura K, ACC/SCN. Low birth weight: report of a meeting in Dhaka, Bangladesh on 14–17 June 1999. 2000.
7. Negassi T, et al. Prevalence and factors associated with low birth weight in Axum and lealay maichew districts, North Ethiopia a comparative cross sectional study. Int J Nutr Food Sci. 2014;3(6):560–6.
8. Manal A, Mai M, Safaa T. Mid- upper arm, chest and head circumference cut-off points and equations for identifying low birth weight in Egypt. Int J Food Nutr Public Health. 2011;4(1)
9. Sreeramareddy CT, Neena C, Rajkumar P, Dela S, Brishna S. Anthropometric surrogates to identify low birth weight Nepalese newborns: a hospital-based study. BMC Pediatr. 2008;8:16. doi:10.1186/1471-2431-8-16.
10. Nabiwemba L, Orach Garimoi C, Kolsteren P. Determining an anthropometric surrogate measure for identifying low birth weight babies in Uganda: a hospital-based cross sectional study. BMC Pediatr. 2013;13:54.
11. Raymond EG, Tafari N, Troendle JF, Clemens J. Development of a practical screening tool to identify preterm, low birthweight neonates in Ethiopia. Lancet. 1994;344:524–7.
12. Bhargava SK, Ramji S, Lumar A, Mohan M, Marwah J, Sachdev HP. Mid-arm and chest circumference at birth as predictors of low birth weight and neonatal mortality in the community. Br Med J. 1985;1985(291):1617–9.
13. Ikenna K, Stella N, Egbuna O, Gilbert N, Benedict O, Josephat M, Isaac N, Nwachinemere D. Chest and occipito-frontal circumference measurements in the detection of low birth weight among Nigerian newborns of Igbo ethnicity. Ital J Pediatr. 2014;40:81.
14. Bishnupada D, Golam M, Shamsun N, Nazrul I. Birth-weight status of newborns and its relationship with other anthropometric parameters in a public maternity hospital in Dhaka, Bangladesh. J Health Populnutr. 2002;20(1):36–41.
15. Kahsay Z, Tadese A, Nigusie B. Low birth weight & associated factors among newborns in gondar town, North West Ethiopia: institutional based cross-sectional study. Indo Global Journal of Pharmaceutical Sciences. 2014;4(2):74–80.
16. WHO. Use of a simple anthropometric measurement to predict birth weight. WHO Collaborative Study of Birth Weight Surrogates. Bull World Health Organ. 1993;71:157–63.
17 Achebe C, Ugochukwu EF, Adogu P, Ubajaka C. Prediction of low birth weight from other anthropometric parameters in Nnewi, south eastern Nigeria. Niger J Paed. 2014;41(1):59–63.
18 Mullany LC, Darmstadt GL, Khatry SK, LeClerq SC, Tielsch JM. Relationship between the surrogate anthropometric measures, foot length and chest circumference and birth weight among newborns of Sarlahi, Nepal. Eur J ClinNutr. 2007;61(1):40–6.

2

Bacterial etiologic agents causing neonatal sepsis and associated risk factors in Gondar, Northwest Ethiopia

Tsehaynesh G/eyesus[1], Feleke Moges[2], Setegn Eshetie[2*], Biruk Yeshitela[3] and Ebba Abate[2]

Abstract

Background: Neonatal sepsis is a blood stream infection which is seen in the first month of life of the neonate. Bacterial profile of neonatal septicemia is constantly changing thus, current knowledge on the patterns of bacterial isolates, its antibiotic resistance profile, and associated factors, are essential to design and implement appropriate interventions. Therefore, the aim of this study was to identify bacterial etiologic agents, their antimicrobial susceptibility pattern and associated risk factors of neonatal sepsis among neonates.

Methods: A cross- sectional study was conducted among neonates suspected to sepsis attending University of Gondar Hospital from September/2015 to May/2016. A total of 251 consecutive neonates with clinical sign and symptoms of sepsis were included in the study. Blood sample was collected and directly inoculated into Trypton soya broth bottle and incubated at 37 °C. After 24 h of incubation it was sub- cultured in to blood agar plate, chocolate agar plate, manitol salt agar and Macconkey. The bacterial pathogens and antimicrobial susceptibility tests were identified using standard microbiological methods. Bivariate and multivariate logistic regressions were used to identify possible associated risk factors. Prior to the study ethical clearance was obtained from the School of Biomedical and Laboratory Sciences, University of Gondar.

Results: Of the 251 study participants suspected of neonatal sepsis, 117 (46.6%) showed bacterial growths, of them 120 bacteria were isolated. Gram positive bacteria were commonly isolated 81 (67.5%).The commonly isolated bacterial species were *S. aureus* 49 (40.8%) followed by coagulase negative *Staphylococci* 26 (21.6%) and *K. pneumoniae*19 (15.8%). The overall rate of multidrug resistance isolates was 78 (65%: CI 95%: 56.7–72.5%). Multidrug resistant (MDR) among Gram positive and negative bacteria were 56 (69.1%) and 22 (56.4%), respectively. Independent risk factors for the occurrence of neonatal sepsis were; Apgar score < 7/5 min (Adjusted odds ratio [AOR] =0.5), birth weight < 1.5 kg (AOR = 12.37), birth weight, 1.5–2.5 kg (AOR = 2.6), gestational week <37 weeks (AOR = 9) and caesarian section delivery (AOR = 5.2).

Conclusion: The isolation rate of bacterial pathogens in neonatal sepsis was considerably high. In addition, nearly 70% of isolates were MDR strains. Low birth weight, low Apgar score, preterm delivery and caesarian section modes of delivery were associated risk factors. Therefore, appropriate antenatal care follow up, and health education should be encouraged, especially on the importance of natural way of delivery.

Keywords: Neonate, Sepsis, Antimicrobial susceptibility, Gondar, Ethiopia

* Correspondence: wolet03.2004@gmail.com
[2]Department of Medical Microbiology, School of Biomedical and Laboratory Sciences, College of Medicine and Health Sciences, University of Gondar, Gondar, P. O. Box: 196, Ethiopia
Full list of author information is available at the end of the article

Background

Neonatal sepsis is a systemic infections of the newborn such as septicemia, meningitis, pneumonia, arthritis, osteomyelitis, and urinary tract infections [1]. The clinical syndrome of the disease can be influenced by the virulence of the pathogen, the portal of entry, the susceptibility and response of the host, and the temporal evolution of the condition [2]. Fever, temperature instability, vomiting, diarrhea, irritability, lethargy, breathing problem, low blood sugar, jaundice, reduced sucking and seizures are the most common symptoms of neonatal sepsis [3]. Neonatal sepsis may be classified according to the time of onset of the disease: early onset and late onset. Early-onset of neonatal sepsis refers to the presence of a confirmed infection in the blood or cerebrospinal fluid (CSF) of patients younger than 3 days of life, and late-onset of neonatal sepsis refers to the onset of such infection between 3 and 28 days [4, 5].

The distinction has clinical relevance, as early onset of neonatal sepsis disease is mainly occurred before and during delivery, whereas late onset of neonatal sepsis is possible due to bacteria acquired after delivery through hospital or community acquired source of infections [6, 7]. Organisms causing early onset of neonatal sepsis are typically colonizers of the maternal genitourinary tract, leading to contamination of the amniotic fluid, placenta, cervix, or vaginal canal. The pathogen may ascend when the amniotic membranes rupture or prior to the onset of labor, causing an intra-amniotic infection [8].

Bacteria, such as *Streptococcus, L. monocytogenes, E. faecalis,E. faecium*, group D *Streptococci*, α-hemolytic *Streptococci* and *Staphylococci,S. pneumoniae,H. influenzae* type B, are recognized as the principal cause of early neonatal sepsis. Less commonly, *N. meningitidis* and *N. gonorrhoeae* have been also reported as a cause of neonatal septicemia and Gram-negative enteric organisms predominantly *E. coli, Klebsiella* species are included [9, 10]. On the other hand, late-onset sepsis is predominantly caused by *Staphylococci* species and *E. coli* and most frequently related with low birth weight of infants and use of intravascular catheters, endo-tracheal intubation, assisted ventilation, surgery, contact with hand of colonized personnel and contact with contaminated equipment as the main risk factors for late onset of neonatal sepsis. Sometimes *E. cloacae* or *Citrobactor* from blood or CSF may be due to contaminated feedings. Contaminated respiratory equipment is suspected in outbreaks of hospital-acquired *P. aeroginosa* pneumonia or sepsis [11, 12].

Neonatal sepsis remains public health threat and contributing a significant challenge to the management of care groups for neonates and infants. It has been explained that neonates are at the highest risk for bacterial sepsis, with the prevalence at 1 to 10 per 1000 live births worldwide [13]. Globally each year over 4 million neonates died within 28 days of birth [14]. Neonatal mortality is still the highest mortality in human life. It has a close relation to infant mortality rate, which is used as the indicator to assess health development in countries [15]. Besides, a recent global report has also claimed that the infant mortality rate was 29 per 1000 live births [16]. The most common causes of death in the neonatal period are infections, including septicemia, meningitis, respiratory infections, diarrhea, and neonatal tetanus (32%), followed by birth asphyxia and injuries (29%), and prematurity (24%) [17].

Aside from the burden, continuous evolution of drug resistance of pathogens causing neonatal sepsis becomes a potential disastrous problem. The situation is worse in developing countries because of lack of legislation, over-the-counter sale of antibiotics and poor sanitary conditions. Notably, methicillin resistance *S.aureus* (MRSA), extended spectrum beta lactamase (ESBL) producing bacteria and MDR Gram negative organisms represent the principal setbacks to fight against infections. Most Gram negative bacteria are now resistant to ampicillin and cloxacillin and many are becoming resistant to gentamicin [18, 19].

The pattern of bacterial organisms causing neonatal sepsis constantly changes and the emergence of resistant bacteria has complicated the problem further. Therefore, this study aimed to assess bacterial etiologic agents, their antimicrobial susceptibility pattern and possible associated risk factors among neonatal patients with sepsis.

Methods

Study area, study design and study population

A prospective cross-sectional study was conducted among all admitted neonates for sepsis at the University of Gondar Hospital from September/2015 to May/2016. Diagnosis of neonatal sepsis remains challenging in this hospital, and mainly depends on clinical decision.

Inclusion criteria

Neonates with clinical sign and symptoms of sepsis at the time of admission or who develop sepsis during their stay in hospital were included in this study.

Exclusion criteria

Neonates with sepsis, who started antibiotic therapy, were excluded from the study.

Study variables

Presence of bacterial infection was dependent variable, whereas independent variable were age, sex, occupation, weight at birth, gestational week, mode of delivery, maternal health condition (fever, urinary tract infection), bottle feeding, Apgar score at 5 min, and skin or local infection.

Definition of terms

Bacteremia means the presence of bacteria in the blood stream, which may or may not be caused by infectious agents. Septicemia, on the other hand, it is serious disease characterized by systemic signs, and the presence of bacteria and their toxins in the blood stream.

Data collection and laboratory methods

Socio demographic data

Socio- demographic data of the study participants and associated risk factors for neonatal sepsis were collected using structured questionnaire. Questionnaire was checked for its completeness and validity prior to the collection of data. The pre test of the questionnaire was conducted among neonates with suspicion of sepsis in Bahirdar hospital (Additional file 1: Questionnaire).

Sample collection and processing

After getting written consent from guardian two bottle of blood samples (1 ml for each bottle) from two different sites of peripheral vein were collected aseptically (disinfecting with 70% alcohol and 2% tincture of iodine) by experienced nurses prior to any antibiotic use. The collected blood sample was inoculated directly into Trypton soya broth blood culture medium bottles (Oxoid LTD) and sent to the medical microbiology laboratory for culture and drug susceptibility testing. The blood cultures were incubated aerobically at 37 °C and observed daily for the first 3 days for the presence of visible microbial growth by one of the following: haemolysis, air bubbles (gas production), and coagulation of broth. At the same time, subcultures were made during successive days on enriched and selective media including blood agar plate (Oxoid LTD), chocolate agar plat (incubated at 5% CO_2 atmosphere), MacConkey (Oxoid Ltd. Basingstoke, Hampshire, UK), and manitol salt agar plates and examined for growth after 24–48 h of incubation.

The same protocol was repeated until the 7th day before blood cultures were considered to be free of microorganisms. Isolates obtained were identified by standard microbiological techniques namely, Gram staining, colony characteristics, and biochemical properties including catalase, coagulase (free and bound), growth on manitol salt agar, and hemolytic activity on blood agar plate for Gram positive isolates, and triple sugar iron, motility, indole, citrate utilization, urease, oxidase and H2S production for Gram negative isolates [20]. As described above two aerobic blood culture bottles were used for each patient, and growth in both bottles was considered as positive. Thus, growth of bacteria only from one bottle did not regard as pathogen and considered as contamination.

The antimicrobial susceptibility tests

Antimicrobial susceptibility test was carried out for each identified bacteria based on Clinical and Laboratory Standard Institute guideline by using disc diffusion method on Muller Hinton agar for non-fastidious organisms and Muller Hinton agar with 5% defibrinated sterile sheep blood for fastidious organisms [21].

Three to five pure colony of the test organism was taken by using a sterile wire loop and emulsify in 2 ml of nutrient broth. The bacterial suspensions turbidity was matched and checked with 0.5 McFarland standards. Then a sterile cotton swab was dipped in to the suspension and squeeze free from excess fluid against the side of test tube. The test organisms were uniformly seed on the surface of Muller-Hinton agar for non fastidious group and Muller Hinton agar with 5% defibrinated sterile sheep blood for fastidious group and expose to a concentration gradient of antibiotic diffusing from antibiotic impregnated paper disc into the agar medium and the medium was incubated at 35 °C for 18–24 h [22].

The following antimicrobial disks were used (Oxoid UK), Amoxicillin-clavulanate (AMC:20/10 μg), penicillin (P:10 unit), trimethoprim-sulfamethoxazole (SXT:1.25/23.75 μg), erythromycin (E:15 μg), tetracycline (TE: 30 μg), clindamycin (DA:2 μg), chloramphenicol (CAF:30 μg), ampicillin (AMP:10 μg), gentamicin (CN:10 μg), amikacin (AK:30 μg), ciprofloxacin (CIP: 5 μg), ceftazidime (CAZ: 30 μg),ceftriaxone (CRO:30 μg) and cefoxitin (CXT:30 μg). Grades of susceptibility pattern were interpreted by comparison of the zone of inhibition according to Clinical and Laboratory Standard Institute 2014 guideline [21].

Quality control

All materials, equipment and procedures were adequately controlled. Pre-analytical, analytical and post-analytical stages of quality assurance that are incorporated in standard operating procedures of the medical microbiology laboratory were strictly followed. The sterility of culture media was ensured by incubating 5% of each batch of the prepared media at 37°c for 24 h. Performance of all prepared media was also checked by inoculating international standard-strains such as *E.coli* (ATCC 25922) Gram negative bacteria, *S. aureus* (ATCC 25923) for Gram positive bacteria and *N. gonorrhoeae* (ATCC49226) for fastidious bacteria. To standardize the inoculums density of bacterial suspension for the susceptibility test, 0.5 McFarland standards was used [20]. To ensure the accuracy of data, double data entry method was used.

Data analysis and interpretation

Data were collected and analyzed for the presence and frequency of different bacterial isolates, antibiotic susceptibility pattern and associated risk factors. The findings were entered and analyzed using SPSS version 20. Frequencies and cross tabulations were used to summarize descriptive statistics. Univariate and multivariate logistic regression analyses were used to assess the possible risk factors of neonatal sepsis infection. Descriptive statistics was also used to explain antimicrobial susceptibility patterns. Odds ratio and 95% confidence interval was computed to assess the presence and degree of association between dependent and independent variables. *P*-value <0.05 was considered statistically significant for all cases.

Results

Characteristics of study participants

Of the total study participants (n = 251), 149 (59.4%) were male, 184 (73.3%) of the neonates were age ≤ 3 days (early onset) and146 (58.2%) were from urban residence. Of the total neonates 46 (18.3%) had very low birth weight (< 1.5 kg), 92 (36.6%) were preterm (<37 week gestation), 160 (63.7%) were delivered by spontaneous vaginal delivery. It was observed that 55 (21.9%) of the neonates mothers had history of urinary tract infection (UTI) during gestational period (Table 1).

Magnitude and bacterial profiles among neonatal septicemia

Of the study participants with neonatal septicemia, 117 (46.62%) showed bacterial growth and of these 120 different kinds of bacterial pathogens were identified. Three of blood cultures (2.5%) showed mixed growth (poly microbial), while the 114 (97.5%) showed non duplicate growth. The rest 134 (53.4%) had no bacterial growth. Gram positive bacterial species were commonly isolated 81 (67.5%) than the Gram negative bacterial species 39 (32.5%). The commonly isolated bacteria were *S. aureus* 49 (40.9%) followed by CoNS 26 (21.7%) and *K. pneumoniae* 19 (15.8%) (Table 2).

The predominant organisms during the first 3 days of life were Gram positive, accounting for 57 (65.5%) of the 87 (72.5%) isolates. Between 3 and 28 days of life, Gram negative and Gram positive isolates accounted for 9 (27.28%) and 24 (72.72%) of the 33 isolated organisms, respectively. The single predominant Gram positive organism in both age groups was *S. aureus* 49 (40.83%). Among Gram negatives, *K. pneumonia* 19 (15.83%) was the predominant causative agent in both age groups (Table 2).

Antimicrobial susceptibility pattern of bacterial isolates from neonatal septicemia

From the total isolates only 11 (9.2%, 95% CI, 4.4–15%) isolates were susceptible to all tested antibiotics. Over all in Gram positive isolates high resistance rate were observed to penicillin 42 (51.8%), ampicillin 30 (37%) and trimethoprim- sulfamethoxazole 34 (42%). On the other hand, Gram positive bacteria showed least resistance rate to clindamycin 7 (8.6%) andciprofloxacin 16 (19.7%). As indicated Table 3, species specific antibiotic resistance rates showed that more than 35% of *S. aureus* isolates were resistant to penicillin, ampicillin, Trimethoprim- sulfamethoxazole, gentamicin anderythromycin.

Susceptibility pattern in Gram negative isolates indicates that high susceptibility rate seen in amikacin 37 (94.9%), ciprofloxacin, ceftazidamide and gentamicin each 34 (87.2%) and highly resistance seen in ampicillin 33 (84.6%), ceftriaxone 22 (56.4%) and trimethoprim/sulfamethoxazole 17 (43.58%). Species specific antibiotic resistance in Gram negative has also indicated, *E.coli* were resistant to ampicillin 8 (66.7%) but relatively no resistance rates were noted to ciprofloxacin and amikacin. *K. pneumonia* was highly resistance to ampicillin 18 (94.75%), ceftriaxone 15 (78.9%) and trimethoprim/sulfamethoxazole 8 (42.1%). It was highly sensitive to ciprofloxacin and gentamicin 16 (84.2%) each (Table 4).

Multi drug resistance pattern of bacterial isolates from neonatal septicemia

Among the total isolates, 78 (65%, 95% CI: 56.7–72.5%) were resistance to three or more different class of antibiotics. Among MDR strains, 21 (17.5%) isolate were resistant to three classes of antibiotics, the rest 57 (47.5%) were resistant to greater than three classes of antibiotics. Result of drug resistance patterns compared within species specific showed that, 33 (67.3%) of *S. aureus*, 8 (66.7%) of *E. coli* and 16 (84.2%) of *K. pnuemonae* were MDR isolates. Among the total isolates of *S. aureus*, 13 (26.5%) of them were found to be MRSA (Table 5).

Associated risk factors related to neonatal septicemia

Risk factors associated with neonatal septicemia were analyzed. Univariate and multivariate analysis showed that very low birth weight with adjusted odds ratio (AOR) 12.37 (95% CI: 4.135–37.04), low birth weight with AOR 2.63 (95% CI: 1.149–6.09),caesarean section mode of delivery with AOR 5.2(95% CI: 2.36–11.37), Apgar score < 7 with AOR 0.438 (95% CI: 0.215–0.892) and preterm gestational week with AOR 8.99 (95% CI: 4.175–19.38) were associated with neonatal septicemia (Table 6).

Multivariate analysis result indicates that gestational week has significant association which means that neonates born in gestation < 37 weeks had almost nine

Table 1 Distributions of bacterial isolates per characteristics of study participants with neonatal septicemia attending the University of Gondar Hospital, North west Ethiopia, September/2015 to May/2016, (N = 251)

Characteristic		Organism isolated		
		Yes n (%)	No n (%)	Total n (%)
Age in (day)	0–3	84 (71.8)	100 (74.6)	184 (73.3)
	>3–28	33 (28.2)	34 (25.4)	67 (26.7)
Sex	Male	68 (58.1)	81 (60.4)	149 (59.4)
	Female	49 (41.9)	53 (39.6)	102 (40.6)
Residence	Urban	70 (59.8)	76 (56.7)	146 (58.2)
	Rural	47 (40.2)	58 (43.3)	105 (41.8)
Prolonged labor	No	103 (88)	114 (85.1)	217 (86.5)
	Yes	14 (12)	20 (14.9)	34 (13.5)
Prolonged rupture of membrane	No	94 (80.3)	104 (77.6)	198 (78.9)
	Yes	23 (19.7)	30 (22.4)	53 (21.1)
Fever during per partum period	No	102 (87.2)	117 (87.3)	219 (87.3)
	Yes	15 (12.8)	17 (12.7)	32 (12.7)
Mode of delivery	CS	52 (44.4)	29 (21.6)	81 (32.3)
	SVD	60 (51.3)	100 (74.6)	160 (63.7)
	Instrumental	5 (4.3)	5 (3.7)	10 (4)
History of UTI during gestational period	No	92 (78.6)	104 (77.6)	196 (78.1)
	Yes	25 (21.4)	30 (22.4)	55 (21.9)
Getting treatment for UTI	No	12 (10.3)	15 (11.2)	27 (10.8)
	Yes	13 (11.1)	15 (11.2)	28 (11.2)
Gestational week	Preterm <37 wks	75 (64.1)	17 (12.7)	92 (36.7)
	Term 37–42 wks	42 (35.9)	101 (75.4)	143 (57)
	Post term >42 wks	0 (0)	16 (11.9)	16 (6.4)
Birth Weight	Very low <1.5 kg	40 (34.2)	6 (4.5)	46 (18.3)
	Low 1.5–2.5 kg	37 (31.6)	24 (17.9)	61 (24.3)
	Normal >2.5 kg	40 (34.2)	104 (77.6)	144 (57.4)
Apgar score	Low <7/ 5 min	49 (41.9)	69 (51.5)	118 (47)
	Normal >7 /5 min	68 (58.1)	65 (48.5)	133 (53)
Previous history of neonatal admission	No	109 (93.2)	125 (93.3)	234 (93.2)
	Yes	8 (6.8)	9 (6.7)	17 (6.8)
Bottle feeding	No	112 (95.7)	127 (94.8)	239 (95.2)
	Yes	5 (4.3)	7 (5.2)	12 (4.8)
Skin/Local infection	No	108 (92.3)	126 (94)	234 (93.2)
	Yes	9 (7.7)	8 (6)	17 (6.8)

Key: *CS* Cesarean Section, *SVD* Spontaneous Vaginal Delivery

times more likely to develop sepsis compared to those neonates born in gestation ≥37 weeks. Neonates born with very low birth weight < 1.5 kg had 12 times more likely to develop neonatal sepsis as compared to normal birth weight > 2.5 kg. Neonates born with birth weight < 2500 Gram had 3 times more likely to develop sepsis than neonates with normal birth weight. Apgar score < 7 pre five minute had 0.5 times more likely to develop sepsis than neonates with normal Apgar score. Caesarian section mode of delivery had 5 time risk to develop neonatal sepsis than spontaneous vaginal delivery.

Discussion

The overall culture positivity rate of bacterial isolates identified from patients with symptoms of neonatal septicemia were 46.6%, comparable with the results reported from Addis Ababa (44.7%) and Egypt

Table 2 Distribution of bacterial isolates from neonates based on their age of admission at University of Gondar Hospital, Northwest Ethiopia, September/2015 to May/2016

Isolated organism	Age at time of admission		Total isolates N (%)
	0–3 day n (%)	>3–28 day n (%)	
S. aureus	34 (69.38)	15 (30.62)	49 (40.8)
Cons	18 (69.2)	8 (30.8)	26 (21.7)
S. pyogenes	5 (83.33)	1 (16.67)	6 (5)
E. coli	9 (75)	3 (25)	12 (10)
K. pneumoniae	13 (68.43)	6 (31.57)	19 (15.8)
Others	08 (100)	0 (0)	08 (6.7)
Total	87 (72.5)	33 (27.5)	120 (100)

Key: Others: *Serratia* ($n = 1$), *E. cloacae* ($n = 4$) and *K. rhinose* ($n = 3$), CoNs: Coagulase Negative *Staphylococcus*

(40.7%) [23, 24]. But, it is lower than study done in Sudan (61.3%) and Yemen (57%) [25, 26]. On the other hand, the present study is higher than from study done in Nepal (20.3%), Tanzania (19.2%) and Gondar (32.1%) [27–29]. This could be due to fact methodological variation, and difference in study setting might affect culture positivity rate. Besides, in previous study in Gondar, antibioti was seen that could minimize culture positivity rate.

In our finding, the predominant isolates from Gram positive and negative bacteria were *S. aureus*, 49 (40.8%) and *K. pneumoniae*, 19 (15.8%), respectively. Similarly, previous studies claimed that those isolates were also the major pathogens of neonatal septicemia [24–31]. In fact *S. aureus* is ubiquitous in nature, which is frequently found on the skin, and main cause of various type of infection in human beings, therefore, newborns can easily contaminated by this bacteria from their mothers during or after delivery [32, 33]. Likewise, *K. pneumoiae* is a normal member of gastro-intestinal flora and recently, has emerged as a significant cause of hospital acquired infections (urinary tract infection, pneumonia and septicemia). Particularly pre-mature populations are easily colonized by the bacteria, due to the fact that, infection of neonates by this bacterium is inevitable [34, 35].

Moreover, the overall MDR prevalence was 78 (65%). Among MDR Gram positive and negative bacteria, *S. aureus*, 30 (61.2%) and *K. pneumoniae*, 14 (74%) were the principal MDR strains. It is understood that *S. auerus* has remarkable feature to adapt antimicrobial pressures. Largely, it has genetic competence to acquire antibiotic resistance genes from other strains. *K. pneumonia* has also intrinsic resistance mechanisms, most importantly, it has chromosomal and plasmid encoded beta-lactam hydrolyzing enzymes (e.g. ESBLs) [36, 37]. Similarly, the issue of antibiotic resistance in the above mentioned bacteria have also documented in previous reports [28, 31, 38–40].

Specific antibiotic resistance has also indicated in the present study. Hence, ampicillin was the most ineffective antibiotics for both Gram positive and negative bacteria. It is well understood; the consequence of ampicillin resistance is mainly due to selective pressure excreted by overuse of the antibiotics. Apart from that, it is also known that bacteria showed resistance genes for beta-lactam agents including ampicllin. Similarly, consistent finding were also claimed in Addis Ababa, Gondar and Egypt with high degree of resistance to ampicillin in both Gram positive and negative bacteria [23, 28, 38, 39].

In our study, the incidence of sepsis was higher in neonates, who were born by caesarian section, thus the odds of developing sepsis among neonates born with caesarian section was five times more likely to develop sepsis to their counterparts. This finding is similar to other previous studies from Iran and Egypt [23, 38]. Reasonably, bleeding is common during surgical procedures, thus, it could be the possible factor that results to blood contamination, subsequently leads bacterial sepsis in neonates. Particularly, Neonates are vulnerable to nosocomial infections because of their reduced immunological profiles as well as the invasive procedures to which they are subjected. This is highly appreciated for those born prematurely or of low birth weight [41]. Likewise, different studies came up with the conclusion that low birth weight infants

Table 3 Antimicrobial susceptibility patterns of Gram positive bacteria from blood cultures in neonatal sepsis, University of Gondar Hospital, Northwest Ethiopia, September/2015 to May/2016

Bacterial isolates	Resistance rate N (%)											
	P	AMP	OXA	CXT	SXT	CIP	CRO	TE	CAF	E	CN	DA
S. aureus($n = 49$)	25 (51)	20 (41)	13 (27)	13 (27)	18 (37)	10 (20)	12 (24.5)	16 (33)	15 (30.6)	18 (37)	19 (38.8)	04 (8.1)
CoNs ($n = 26$)	17 (65)	10 (38)	10 (38)	10 (38)	12 (46)	05 (19)	08 (30.8)	11 (42)	10 (38)	11 (42)	14 (53.8)	02 (7.7)
S.pyogenes($n = 6$)	0 (0)	0 (0)	1 (17)	1 (17)	4 (67)	1 (17)	2 (33.3)	1 (17)	1 (17)	1 (17)	2 (33.3)	1 (17)
Total = 81	42 (52)	30 (37)	24 (30)	24 (30)	34 (42)	16 (20)	22 (27.2)	28 (34)	22 (27)	30 (37)	28 (35)	07 (8.6)

Keys: *CoNS* Coagulase negative *Staphylococcus DA* Clindamycin, *CXT* Cefoxitin, *E* Erythromycin, *OXA* Oxacillin, *P* penicillin, *SXT* Trimethoprim-sulfamethoxazole, *TE* Tetracycline, *Amp* Ampicillin, *CRO* Ceftriaxon, *CAF* Chloramphenicol, *CN* Gentamicin, *CIP* Ciprofloxacin

Table 4 Antimicrobial susceptibility patterns of Gram negative bacteria from blood cultures in neonatal sepsis, University of Gondar Hospital, Northwest Ethiopia, September/2015 to May/2016

Bacterial isolates	Number of resistance to antimicrobial agents (%)									
	SXT	AMC	TE	CIP	CN	CRO	AK	AMP	CAZ	CAF
E.coli (*n* = 12)	04 (33.3)	3 (25)	2 (16.7)	0 (0)	1 (8.3)	3 (25)	0 (0)	8 (66.7)	1 (8.3)	2 (16.7)
K.pneumoniae (*n* = 19)	8 (42.1)	6 (31.6)	7 (36.8)	3 (15. 8)	3 (15.8)	15 (78.9)	2 (10.52)	18 (94.7)	2 (10.5)	6 (31.6)
Others (*n* = 08)	05 (62.5)	02 (25)	01 (12.5)	02 (25)	01 (12.5)	04 (50)	0 (0)	07 (87.5)	02 (25)	02 (25)
Total = 39	17 (43.58)	11 (28.2)	10 (25.6)	5 (12.8)	5 (12.8)	22 (56.4)	2 (5.1)	33 (84.6%)	5 (12.8)	10 (25.6)

Key: *SXT* Trimethoprim- sulfamethoxazole, *AMC* Amoxicillin-clavulanate, *TE* Tetracycline, *Amp* Ampicillin, *CIP* Ciprofloxacin, *CN* Gentamicin, *AK* Amikacin, *CRO* Ceftriaxon, *CAZ*: Ceftazidamide, *CAF* Chloramphenicol, Others:*Seratia*species (01), *Enterobactor* species (04) and *K. rhinose* (03)

are at high risk of developing sepsis compared to normal birth weight [42].

It is largely understood that prolonged rupture of membrane and prolonged labor are the commonly associated risk factors for the occurrence of neonatal sepsis because of the danger of ascending infection. However, the present study indicated that no significant associations with the above mentioned variables. This study showed that low Apgar score at 5th minute had a significant effect on the development of neonatal sepsis; this result is consistence with study conducted in Mekelle, Indonesia and Nepal [43–45]. In general Apgar score at the first minute associated with the Hydrogen Potential (pH) cord blood and intra partum depression and not associates with the outcomes, whereas the Apgar score/5 min then reflects the infants' changes condition on the resuscitation performed [44].

In the present study, gestational week <37 was also the risk factor with nine times higher risk to develop sepsis than gestational week >37. Similarly, studies conducted in Addis Ababa, Nepal, Mexico and Indonesia, have also documented that gestation <37 weeks had significant association with neonatal sepsis [39, 43, 44, 46]. Evidently, preterm baby may have a limited capacity to increase neutrophil production in accordance to demand to overcome the problem. Neutropenia and depleted neutrophil storage pools have been found to be associated with neonatal bacterial sepsis and are predictive of a poor prognosis [47].

In this study very low birth weight and low birth weight had significant association with the occurrence of sepsis; this is consistent with studies conducted in Nepal and Indonesia [43, 44]. Immunological barriers began to mature around 32–34 weeks of gestation and accelerated after birth. That's why the level mucosal antibody is low in underweight neonates [48]. the deficiency of molecular reactants phase such as C- reactive proteins, inhibitor protein and several of the coagulation proteins have been also demonstrated in immature neonates. Moreover, pre-term baby had a lot of neutrophil in circulatory pool but it reserves in the bone marrow is only about 20% compared to the term baby and adults so that the state of sepsis occur severe neutropenia [48–50].

Limitation of the study

A specific characterization MDR bacterium (MRSA, ESBL) has not been done due to lack of well-established methodological techniques. Moreover, molecular based specification for some bacterial groups (CoNS) was not done.

Table 5 Multi drug resistance pattern of bacterial isolates in neonatal septicemia, University of Gondar Hospital North West Ethiopia, from September/2015 to May/2016

Organism isolated	Degree of resistance								Total MDR isolates ≥R3
	R0 (%)	R1 (%)	R2 (%)	R3 (%)	R4 (%)	R5 (%)	R6 (%)	R7 (%)	
S. aureus (*n* = 49)	08 (16.3)	02 (4)	09 (18.3)	09 (18.3)	06 (12.2)	06 (12.2)	06 (12.2)	03 (6.1)	30 (61.2)
CoNS (n = 26)	02 (7.7)	02 (7.7)	01 (3.8)	00 (0)	07 (26.9)	09 (34.6)	03 (11.5)	02 (7.7)	21 (81.0)
S. pyogenes (n = 6)	-	-	01 (16.7)	03 (50)	02 (33.3)	_	_	_	05 (83.3)
E. coli (n = 12)	-	04 (33.3)	05 (41.7)	02 (16.7)	_	_	01 (8.3)	_	03 (25.0)
K.pnuemoniae(n = 19)	01 (5.2)	02 (10.5)	02 (10.5)	05 (26.3)	04 (21)	01 (5.2)	02 (10.5)	02 (10.5)	14 (74.0)
Others (*n* = 8)	_	01 (12.5)	02 (25)	02 (25)	_	01 (12.5)	02 [25]	_	05 (62.5)
Total *n* = 120	11 (9.2)	11 (9.2)	20 (16.7)	21 (17.5)	19 (15.8)	17 (14.2)	14 (11.6)	07 (5.8)	78 (65.0)

Key:*CoNS Coagulase Negative Staphylococcus*, others: *Seratia*species, *E. cloaca*, *K. rehinose*, R0: susceptible to all antibiotics, R1–7: resistance to 1,2, 3, 4, 5, 6 & 7 antibiotics, ≥ R3: resistance to 3 or more antibiotic

Table 6 Univariate and multivariate analysis on risk factors associated with positivity rate of neonatal Septicemia at University of Gondar Hospital, Northwest Ethiopia September/2015 to May/2016

Variable	Bacterial isolates		Univariate analysis		Multi variate analysis	
	Yes = 117	No = 134	COR(95% CI)	*P*- value	AOR(95% CI)	*P*-value
Mode of delivery						
CS	52	29	2.989 (1.714,5.21)	<0.001	5.191 (2.36,11.37)	<0.001
I	5	5	1.667 (0.463,599)	0.434	5.26 (0.875,31.7)	0.070
SVD	60	100	1		1	
Gestational week						
Pre term	75	17	10.7 (5.607,20.074)	<0.001	8.99 (4.175,19.38)	<0.001
Term	42	101	1		1	
Birth weight						
Very low	40	6	17.3 (6.823,44.03)	<0.001	12.37 (4.135,37.04)	<0.001
Low	37	24	4.0 (2.135,7.526)	<0.001	2.63 (1.149,6.09)	0.022
Normal	40	104	1		1	
Apgar score						
Low	49	69	0.679 (0.412,1.12)	0.129	0.438 (0.215,0.892)	0.023
Normal	68	65	1		1	

Key: *COR* crude odds ratio, *AOR* Adjusted odds ratio, *CI* Confidence interval, *APGAR score* Appearance, pulse, grimace, activity and respiration, *CS* caesarean section, *SVD* Spontaneous Vaginal Delivery, *I* Instrumental

Conclusion

High prevalence of bacterial isolates was observed in this study. *S. aureus* was the predominant pathogen from Gram positive and *K. pneumonia* was from Gram negative. The overall prevalence of MDR was high. Comparably high level of resistance to ampicillin was observed among Gram positive and Gram negative bacteria.The most common risk factors for neonatal sepsis infection observed in this study were caesarian section mode of delivery, Apgar score < 7, birth weight < 2.5 kg and gestational week <37 weeks. Substantially, strengthening of antenatal screening of mothers, prenatal care of newborns and interventions of babies born with complications are the key elements to control the problem. Moreover, Empirical regimens for neonatal sepsis using ampicillin and gentamicin must be taken into consideration due to the risk of resistance, misdiagnosis and mismanagement.

Abbreviations

CoNS: Coagulase negative *Staphylococcus* species; CSF: Cerebrospinal fluid; ESBL: Extended spectrum beta lactamase; MDR: Multi Drug resistant; MRSA: Methicilin resistant *staphylococcus aureus*; UTI: Urinary tract infection

Acknowledgements

We would like to thank study participants and University of Gondar for allowing us to use the laboratory facilities.

Ethical approval and consent to participate

Ethical clearance was obtained from the research and ethics committee of the School of Biomedical and Laboratory Sciences, University of Gondar prior the initiation of the study. There is no additional sample to be taken from the study participants for the sake of this study. The blood sample collected in the study was part of the routine patient investigation and management at the neonatology ward. A written informed consent was obtained from mothers/caretakers of neonates after explaining the purpose and objective of the study. The blood sample was collected by experienced pediatric nurses as part of the routine sample collection at neonatology ward. The result was communicated to the treating physician for immediate and appropriate treatment. Confidentiality was kept through using codes instead of names in all the study process.

Funding

The study was supported by the mega project of the University of Gondar in Reference number of VP/RCS/05/192/2015 and by Armauer Hansen Research Institute.

Authors' contributions

TG and FM conception of research idea, study design, data collection, analysis and interpretation. SE conception of research idea, study design data collection, analysis, interpretation and the drafting of manuscript. FY and EA data collection, analysis and interpretation and supervision. All authors read and approved the final manuscript.

Competing interests

The authors declare that they have no competing interests.

Author details

[1]Amhara Regional Health Bureau, South Gondar Zonal Health Bureau, Debre Tabor, , Ethiopia. [2]Department of Medical Microbiology, School of Biomedical and Laboratory Sciences, College of Medicine and Health Sciences, University of Gondar, Gondar, P. O. Box: 196, Ethiopia. [3]Armauer Hansen Research Institute (AHRI), Addis Ababa, , Ethiopia.

References

1. Sankar MJ, Agarwal R, Deorari AK, Paul VK. Sepsis in the newborn. Indian J Pediatr. 2008;75(3):261-6.
2. Lever A, Mackenzie I. Sepsis: definition, epidemiology, and diagnosis. Br med J. 2007;3(7):879.
3. Shaha C, Dey S, Shabuj H, Chisti J, Mannan M, Jashimuddin M, et al. Neonatal sepsis review. Bangladesh J Child Health. 2012;36(2):82–9.
4. Puopolo K. Epidemiology of neonatal early-onset sepsis. Neo Reviews. 2008; 9(12):571–9.
5. Zakariya B, Bhat V, Harish N, Babu T, Joseph M. Neonatal sepsis in a tertiary care hospital in South India: bacteriological profile and antibiotic sensitivity pattern. Indian J Pediatr. 2011;78(4):413–7.
6. Tallur S, Kasturi A, Nadgir S, Krishna B. Clinico-bacteriological study of neonatal septicemia in Hubli. Indian J Pediatr. 2000;67(3):169–74.
7. Karunasekera K, Pathirana D. A preliminary study on neonatal septicaemia in a tertiary referral hospital paediatric unit. Ceylon Med J. 1999;44(2):81–6.
8. Shah BA, Padbury JF. Neonatal sepsis: An old problem with new insights. Virulence. 2014;5(1):170-78. doi:10.4161/viru.26906.
9. Simonsen KA, Anderson-Berry AL, Delair SF, Davies HD. Early-onset neonatal sepsis. Clin Microbiol rev. 2014;27(1):21–47.
10. Stoll BJ, Hansen N, Fanaroff AA, Wright LL, Carlo WA, Ehrenkranz RA, et al. Late-onset sepsis in very low birth weight neonates: the experience of the NICHD neonatal research network. Pediatrics. 2002;110(2):285–91.
11. Mohammad S, Aletayeb H, Khosravi AD, Dehdashtian M, Kompani F, Mortazavi M, et al. Identification of bacterial agents and antimicrobial susceptibility of neonatal sepsis: a 54-month study in a tertiary hospital. Afr J Microbiol res. 2011;5:528–31.
12. Shaw G, Sim K, Randell P, Cox J, McClure Z, Li M-S, et al. Late-Onset Bloodstream Infection and Perturbed Maturation of the Gastrointestinal Microbiota in Premature Infants. PloS one. 2015;10(7):e0132923.
13. Afsharpaiman S, Torkaman M, Saburi A, Farzaampur A, Amirsalari S, Kavehmanesh Z. Trends in incidence of neonatal sepsis and antibiotic susceptibility of causative agents in two neonatal intensive care units in tehran, Iran. J Clin Neonatol. 2012;1(3):124–30.
14. Knippenberg R, Lawn J, Darmstadt L, Begkoyian G, Fogstad H, Walelign N, et al. Systematic scaling up of neonatal care in countries. Lancet. 2005;36(9): 1087–98.
15. Shah GS, Budhathoki S, Das BK, Mandal RN. Risk factors in early neonatal sepsis. Kathmandu Univ med J. 2006;4(2):187–91.
16. World Health Organization. Countdown to 2015, maternal, newborn & child survival-fulfilling the health agenda for women and children: the 2014 report. Geneva: WHO press; 2014.
17. Costello A, Francis V, Byrne A, Puddephatt C. State of the World's Newborns: A Report from Saving Newborn Lives: 2001. Available at http://files.eric.ed.gov/fulltext/ED458972.pdf.
18. Jyothi P, Basavaraj C, Basavaraj P. Bacteriological profile of neonatal septicemia and antibiotic susceptibility pattern of the isolates. J Nat sc Biol med. 2013;4(2):306.
19. Paolucci M, Landini P, Sambri V. How can the microbiologist help in diagnosing neonatal sepsis? Int J Pediatr. 2012;120139(10):26.
20. Cheesbrough M. District laboratory practice in tropical countries: Cambridge university press; 2006. Available at http://fac.ksu.edu.sa/sites/default/files/Book-District_Laboratory_Practice_in_Tropical_Countries_Part-2_Monica_Cheesbrough.pdf
21. Clinical and laboratory standard inustitut. Performance standards for antimicrobial susceptibility testing:twenty-forth informational supplement CLSI document M100-S24CLS. 2014;34(1).
22. Clinical and Laboratory Standards Institute (CLSI). Methods for dilution antimicrobial susceptibility tests for bacteria that grow aerobically: approved standard-Tenth Edition. CLSI document M07-A10. Wayne: CLSI; 2015.
23. Shehab E, El-Sokkary A, Bassiouny R, Hassan R. Epidemiology of neonatal sepsis and implicated pathogens: a study from Egypt. Biomed res Int. 2015; 509484(10):4.
24. Shitaye D, Asrat D, Woldeamanuel Y, Worku B. Risk factors and etiology of neonatal sepsis in Tikur Anbessa university hospital, Ethiopia. Ethiop Med J. 2010;48(1):11–21.
25. Al-Shamahy H, Sabrah A, Al-Robasi B, Naser M. Types of bacteria associated with neonatal sepsis in al-Thawra university hospital, Sana'a, Yemen, and their antimicrobial profile. Sultan Qaboos Univ med J. 2012;12(1):48.
26. Kheir A, Khair R. Neonatal sepsis; prevalence and outcome in a tertiary neonatal unit in Sudan. Time J Med Sci. 2014;2:21–5.
27. Khanal R, Manandhar S, Acharya G. Bacteriological profile of neonatal sepsis in a tertiary level Hospital of Nepal. J Nepal Paediatr soc. 2015;34(3):175–80.
28. Gebrehiwot A, Lakew W, Moges F, Anagaw B, Yismaw G, Unakal C. Bacterial profile and drug susceptibility pattern of neonatal sepsis in Gondar University hospital, Gondar Northwest Ethiopia. Der Pharmacia Lettre. 2012; 4(6):1811–6.
29. Mkony F, Mizinduko M, Massawe A, Matee M. Management of neonatal sepsis at Muhimbili National Hospital in Dar es salaam: diagnostic accuracy of C–reactive protein and newborn scale of sepsis and antimicrobial resistance pattern of etiological bacteria. BMC Pediatr. 2014;14(1):1.
30. Khan M, Khan A, Shah F, Munir A. Neonatal sepsis: a study of causative pathogens and their antimicrobial sensitivity pattern at tertiary hospital. Gomal J Med Sci. 2012;10(2):244–7.
31. Onyedibe KI, Bode-Thomas F, Nwadike V, Afolaranmi T, Okolo M, Uket O. High rates of bacteria isolates of neonatal sepsis with multidrug resistance patterns in Jos Nigeria. Ann Tropl Pediatr Int Child Health. 2015;3:1052.
32. Naber C. *Staphylococcus aureus* Bacteremia: epidemiology, pathophysiology, and management strategies. Clin Infect Dis. 2009;48(4):231–7.
33. Jimenez N, Tedeschi S, Saye EJ, McKenna BD, Langdon W, Wright JP, et al. Relationship between maternal and neonatal *Staphylococcus aureus* colonization. Pediatrics. 2012;129(5):1252–9.
34. Zaidi K, Thaver D, Ali S, Khan T. Pathogens associated with sepsis in newborns and young infants in developing countries. Pediatr Infect Dis J. 2009;28(1):10–8.
35. Ghotaslou R, Ghorashi Z, Nahaei M. *Klebsiella pneumoniae* In neonatal sepsis: a 3-year-study in the pediatric hospital of Tabriz Iran. Jpn J Infect Dis. 2007; 60(2/3):126.
36. Thenmozhi S, Moorthy M, Sureshkumar B, Suresh M. Antibiotic resistance mechanism of ESBL producing Enterobacteriaceae in clinical field: a review. In J Pure Appl Biosci. 2014;2:207–26.
37. Östholm Balkhed Å. Extended-Spectrum ß-Lactamase-Producing Enterobacteriaceae: Antibiotic consumption, Detection and Resistance Epidemiology. Linköping: Linköping University Electronic Press; 2014.
38. Aamir M, Ali E, Hamouda M, Mourad F. Prevalence of multi drug resistant bacteria causing late-onset neonatal sepsis. Int J Curr Microbiol app Sci. 2015;4(5):172–90.
39. Yusuf A, Worku B. Descriptive cross–sectional study on neonatal sepsis in the neonatal intensive care unit of Tekur Anbessa hospital, Addis Ababa, Ethiopia. Ethiop J Pediatr Child Health. 2010;6(6):50–4.
40. Kayange N, Kamugisha E, Mwizamholya DL, Jeremiah S, Mshana SE. Predictors of positive blood culture and deaths among neonates with suspected neonatal sepsis in a tertiary hospital, Mwanza-Tanzania. BMC pediatrics. 2010;10(1):1.
41. Vergnano S, Sharland M, Kazembe P, Mwansambo C, Heath P. Neonatal sepsis: an international perspective. Arch Dis Child Fetal Neonatal Ed. 2005; 90(3):220–4.
42. Dhumal P, Ujagare M, Gandham N, Nagdawane R, Sardar M, Sharma M, et al. Incidence and antimicrobial susceptibility pattern of neonatal septicaemia from tertiary care hospital of India. Int J Med Clin Res. 2012;3(7):207.
43. Shah G, Budhathoki S, Das B, Mandal R. Risk factors in early neonatal sepsis. Kathmandu Univer Med J (KUMJ). 2005;4(2):187–91.
44. Muhammad Hayun, Ema Alasiry, Dasril Daud, Dwi Bahagia Febriani, Djauhariah Madjid, The Risk Factors of Early Onset Neonatal Sepsis, American Journal of Clinical and Experimental Medicine. 2015;3(3): 78-82. doi:10.11648/j.ajcem.20150303.11.
45. Gebremedhin D, Berhe H, Gebrekirstos K. Risk Factors for Neonatal Sepsis in Public Hospitals of Mekelle City, North Ethiopia, Unmatched Case Control Study. PloS one. 2016;11(5):e0154798.
46. Leal Y, Álvarez VJ, Rosado U, Diego N, Paz E, et al. Risk factors and prognosis for neonatal sepsis in southeastern Mexico: analysis of a four-year historic cohort follow-up. BMC Pregnancy Childbirth. 2012;12(1):1.
47. Petrova A, Mehta R. Dysfunction of innate immunity and associated pathology in neonates. Indian J Pediatr. 2007;74(2):185–91.
48. Benitz W, Gould B, Druzin L. Risk factors for early-onset group B *Streptococcal* sepsis: estimation of odds ratios by critical literature review. Pediatrics. 1999; 103(6):77.

3

Screening for glucose-6-phosphate dehydrogenase deficiency in neonates: a comparison between cord and peripheral blood samples

Saif AlSaif[1], Ma. Bella Ponferrada[1], Khalid AlKhairy[4], Khalil AlTawil[2], Adel Sallam[3], Ibrahim Ahmed[1], Mohammed Khawaji[1], Khalid AlHathlol[1], Beverly Baylon[1], Ahmed AlSuhaibani[4,6] and Mohammed AlBalwi[4,5,6*]

Abstract

Background: The use of cord blood in the neonatal screening for glucose-6-phosphate dehydrogenase (G6PD) deficiency is being done with increasing frequency but has yet to be adequately evaluated against the use of peripheral blood sample which is usually employed for confirmation. We sought to determine the incidence and gender distribution of G6PD deficiency, and compare the results of cord against peripheral blood in identifying G6PD DEFICIENCY neonates using quantitative enzyme activity assay.

Methods: We carried out a retrospective and cross-sectional study employing review of primary hospital data of neonates born in a tertiary care center from January to December 2008.

Results: Among the 8139 neonates with cord blood G6PD assays, an overall incidence of 2% for G6PD deficiency was computed. 79% of these were males and 21% were females with significantly more deficient males ($p < .001$). Gender-specific incidence was 3.06% for males and 0.85% for females. A subgroup analysis comparing cord and peripheral blood samples ($n = 1253$) showed a significantly higher mean G6PD value for peripheral than cord blood (15.12 ± 4.52 U/g and 14.52 ± 4.43 U/g, respectively, $p = 0.0008$). However, the proportion of G6PD deficient neonates did not significantly differ in the two groups ($p = 0.79$). Sensitivity of cord blood in screening for G6PD deficiency, using peripheral G6PD assay as a gold standard was 98.6% with a NPV of 99.5%.

Conclusion: There was no difference between cord and peripheral blood samples in discriminating between G6PD deficient and non-deficient neonates. A significantly higher mean peripheral G6PD assay reinforces the use of cord blood for neonatal screening since it has substantially low false negative results.

Keywords: Glucose-6-phosphate dehydrogenase deficiency, Screening, Neonates, Cord blood

* Correspondence: balwim@ngha.med.sa
[4]Department of Pathology and Laboratory Medicine, King Abdulaziz Medical City, Ministry of National Guard Health Affairs, P.O. Box 22490, Riyadh 11426, Kingdom of Saudi Arabia
[5]Medical Genomics Research Department, King Abdullah International Medical Research Center, Ministry of National Guard Health Affairs, P.O. Box 22490, Riyadh 11426, Kingdom of Saudi Arabia
Full list of author information is available at the end of the article

Background

Despite the wide variability in the assessment methods for glucose-6-phosphate dehydrogenase deficiency, it remains the most prevalent enzyme deficiency in the world. It is estimated that nearly 330 million people may be affected by G6PD deficiency worldwide with a global prevalence of 4.9% [1]. G6PD deficiency in neonates is particularly important because it may have fatal consequences. It could cause severe neonatal jaundice, and if not recognized and managed early, it could lead to kernicterus with permanent neurologic sequelae, if not death [2, 3] In the Middle East, the prevalence estimates of G6PD deficiency is the second highest in the world at 6% (95% CI: 5.7–6.4, $p < 0.001$), the first being Sub Saharan Africa [1, 4]. For males alone, it is estimated to be 7.2% (95% CI: 6.6–7.7, $p < 0.001$). Local studies in Saudi Arabia have shown a wide variability in the region-specific prevalence. Riyadh has a prevalence of 2.0% to 3.8%, Qatif with 30.6%, and AlHasa with 14.7% [3, 5–7]. Most of these studies made use of the cord blood for screening in the neonates. The use of cord blood in the neonatal screening for metabolic diseases including G6PD deficiency is being done with increasing frequency in some centers [6, 8–12]. This method of specimen collection is convenient, easy, and more importantly it spares the neonate of unnecessary pain and stress. The premise is that; coming from the same individual, cord blood should reflect the same glucose-6-phosphate dehydrogenase (G6PD) levels as in the peripheral sample. This may not be entirely accurate; however, considering the tremendous physiologic changes in the newborn period that could affect G6PD activity. In this study, we sought to determine the incidence and gender distribution of G6PD deficiency among neonates using cord blood, and compared cord against peripheral blood in identifying G6PD deficiency in neonates using a quantitative enzyme activity assay.

Methods

We carried out a retrospective, cross-sectional study employing review of primary hospital data of term and near term neonates born (>35 weeks of completed gestation) in a tertiary care center from January to December 2008. King Abdullah International Medical Research Center (KAIMRC), Ministry of National Guard Health Affairs (MNGHA), International Review Board (IRB) has approved this study protocol (RC09/106), and all patients were provided with written informed consent through their guardian/parent.

Cord blood is defined as a specimen collected from the umbilical artery at the time of delivery and peripheral blood is the blood obtained from any other site of the body within one week of age. Unless otherwise specified, we define G6PD deficiency as a G6PD quantitative assay by spectrophotometric analysis of ≤5.7 U/g Hb (unit of enzyme activity/g hemoglobin), as per laboratory recommendation.

Cord and venous blood samples were collected from each patient using conventional techniques into Vacutainer (BD Plymouth, PL6 7BP, U.K.) or Microtainer (Becton, Dickinson and Co., Franklin Lakes, NJ 07417, USA) tubes with K2EDTA as anticoagulant at a concentration of 1.8 mg/ml. Samples were accessioned into the Laboratory Information System (LIS), then their hemoglobin (Hb) levels were determined on same time and day as the G6PD analyses using Cell-Dyn Sapphire blood analyzers (Abbot Diagnostics Division, Abbot Park, IL 60064, USA). All samples were stored at 2-8C, batched and analyzed for G6PD enzymatic activity within 4–6 h of collection. Sadly, three infants died before the peripheral blood sample could be obtained for measurement of the G6PD.

One hundred microliters of well-mixed whole blood was pipetted in a test-tube containing 400 μl of a proprietary lysing reagent, mixed well and let stand for 5 min. An aliquot of this was poured into a sample cup using the only G6PD assay kit designed for both newborn and adults, which then was placed in the Udilipse Random Access Analyzer (United Diagnostics Industry, P.O. Box 9466, Dammam 31,413, Kingdom of Saudi Arabia). Once hemolysates were made, analysis was carried out immediately and strictly within an hour.

The principle of the test involves the catalysis of glucose-6-phosphate to 6-phosphogluconate by G6PD and reduction of NADP to NADPH in the following reaction [10] (**Glucose-6-phosphate + NADP → 6-Phosphogluconate + NADPH + H^+**).

The activity of G6PD was proportional to the rate of production of NADPH which possesses a peak Ultraviolet (UV) light absorption at 340 nm. Results from the Analyzer were automatically transmitted to LIS permitting access to patient's previously estimated blood hemoglobin level, computed and reported results in units/g (of hemoglobin).

In carrying out the study, we collected the names and medical record numbers (MRN) of all newborns with G6PD quantitative assays (cord or peripheral) for the specified time interval (January to December 2008). This was the year that our institution began implementing universal G6PD deficiency neonatal screening. We then selected the neonates with cord G6PD assays and from this pool, the overall incidence and the gender distribution of G6PD deficiency was computed. However, due to the unavailability of G6PD molecular genotyping in our institute DNA analysis was not possible. There is a future plan to include DNA genotyping in a forthcoming study.

From among the newborns with cord blood G6PD assays, we picked out those who also had peripheral samples taken (presumably within one week of age). A subgroup analysis was carried out on this particular subset of patients (n = 1, 253) comparing the cord and peripheral G6PD values.

Statistical analysis

Statistical analysis was performed using SPSS v.20 (IBM Corp., Armonk, NY, USA). The data were statistically tested by descriptive statistics. Kolmogrov-Smirnov test was used for normality and found that it was normally distributed. The Quantitative G6PD analysis and correlation between deficient and non-deficient groups for both cord and peripheral blood samples were performed using Student T-test and Pearson chi-square. P-value of <0.05 was considered statistically significant. Data was expressed as mean ± SD unless indicated otherwise (see Tables 1, 2 and 3).

Results

There were a total of 8396 neonates admitted to the hospital between January and December 2008 whose G6PD assays were obtained. Cord blood samples for G6PD activity were actually available from 8139 patients. The remainder either had non-optimal cord specimens (clotted or insufficient) or were born outside our Hospital from whom cord bloods could not be taken.

Among the 8139 with cord blood samples successfully taken, the mean result for G6PD assay was 14.6 with a minimum value of 0.2 and a maximum value of 45.4. As we had a standard deviation of 3.28, 2 standard deviations from the mean (~2.5 percentile) give us a cut-off value of 8.05 (at 95% CI) below which defined a G6PD deficient neonate. It was well known that G6PD deficient variants were grouped into different classes corresponding with disease severity [1, 2].

Using a cut-off value of 8.05 Units/g Hemoglobin (U/g Hb), the overall incidence of G6PD deficiency was 3.13% of which 60% were males and only 40% were females. There was a significantly higher proportion of deficient males ($p < 0.001$) with significantly lower values as well ($p < 0.001$).

Presently however, when we applied using normal adult cut-off value of 5.7 U/g Hb, the overall incidence of G6PD deficiency was 2% of which 79% were males and only 21% were females (Fig. 1). There was a significantly higher proportion of deficient males ($p < 0.001$) with significantly lower values as well ($p < 0.001$).

We ran the analysis looking at gender differences in G6PD levels in both cut-off value of 5.7 and 8.05 U/g Hb for cord and peripheral blood samples and we found that there were equally highly significant differences ($p < 0.001$) in the levels between males and females in both samples (Table 2). Pearson chi-square test revealed a significantly higher proportion between gender groups of affected males ($p = 0.001$) consistent with an X-linked pattern of inheritance (M:F ratio) equal to 1.5–3.7:1 respectively. Among males alone, the computed incidence of the disease was 3.06% while female patients had an incidence of only 0.85% female neonates) with a male to female ratio of 3.7:1. The gender-specific incidence for males reinforces the universal screening practice also applied in our institution since it is within the WHO recommendation; that is, to screen for all neonates in populations with prevalence of ≥3% in males [2].

To make a comparison between results obtained using cord blood and peripheral blood samples, we used the subset of patients from whom both samples were taken (Fig. 2, Table 1). A total of 1253 observations were analyzed. The mean result of G6PD activity assay was 14.52

Table 1 Subgroup analysis of G6PD Quantitative Assay for Neonates with both Cord and Peripheral blood samples

Description		Cord	Peripheral blood	p-value
G6PD Quantitative Assay (U/g)				0.0008*
Overall		14.52	15.12	
Mean		4.43	4.52	
Incidence of G6PD % at two cut-off values	5.7 U/g	5.83	5.59	0.796[a]
	8.05 U/g	7.98	7.18	0.450
Mean G6PD Quantitative Assay (U/g Hgb), at 5.7 U/g cut-off	Deficient	1.45 ± 1.16 (n = 73)	1.64 ± 1.27 (n = 70)	0.3711
	Non - Deficient	15.33 ± 3.09 (n = 1180)	15.92 ± 3.18 (n = 1183)	<0.001*
Mean G6PD Quantitative Assay (U/g Hgb), at 8.05 U/g cut-off	Deficient	2.95 ± 2.68 (n = 100)	2.85 ± 2.56 (n = 90)	0.8001
	Non - Deficient	15.52 ± 2.85 (n = 1153)	16.07 ± 3.01 (n = 1163)	<0.001*

*Level of significance: p = < 0.05

The cord results are statistically lower than the peripheral results (*p = 0.0008*). This also holds true among the non-deficient subgroup of patients (*p < 0.001*) but NOT among the deficient neonates (*p = 0.3711 and p = 0.8001 using cut-off of 5.7 and 8.05 U/g Hb respectively*)

[a]Pearson chi^2 test did not reveal any significant difference in the proportion of G6PD deficient neonates between cord and peripheral blood samples

Table 2 Gender distributed Differences in G6PD levels

Gender	Cut-off value	Cord		PB		P.value
		Mean	Range	Mean	Range	
Male	5.7 U/g	15.29 ± 3.28	(6–27)	15.78 ± 3.35	(5.8–30.5)	
Female		15.36 ± 2.90	(6–29)	16.02 ± 2.87	(5.7–27.7)	P < 0.001*
Male	8.5 U/g	15.45 ± 2.77	(8–27)	16.05 ± 2.7	(8.10–30.5)	
Female		15.57 ± 2.95	(8.10–29)	16.08 ± 3.12	(8.10–27.7)	P < 0.001*

*Level of significance: $p = < 0.05$, *Cord* Cord Blood, *PB* Peripheral Blood. Normal G6PD level distributed among different gender between the cord blood and peripheral blood samples

(U/g Hb) for cord and 15.12 (U/g Hb) for peripheral blood samples. There was a significant difference between the mean results of the two samples ($p = 0.0008$). The G6PD activity assay was statistically lower in the cord than in the peripheral blood. This was consistent with the result of the concordance correlation coefficient of Lin with Rho c = 0.774 ($p < 0.001$, 95% CI: 0.752, 0.796) which only fell under the poor category (Pearson's $p = 0.78$). However, when we dichotomized our patients into deficient and non-deficient, chi-square analysis revealed statistically comparable proportions of G6PD deficiency between the two samples using both cut-off points ($p = 0.796$ and $p = 0.45$ for cut-off 5.7 and 8.05, respectively). It was interesting to note that if we compared the mean G6PD values of the cord and peripheral blood samples in the deficient patients alone, no statistically relevant results were obtained using t-test ($p = 0.3711$) as opposed to the results obtained for the non-deficient group ($p < 0.001$, Table 1). Validity indices of cord blood G6PD assay, with peripheral blood as the gold standard, was confirmed as shown in Table 3.

Discussion

The prevalence of G6PD deficiency is high in the Saudi Arabian population we think because of high consanguinity and the prevalence of endemic malaria. This justifies our thinking that neonatal screening is important for early diagnosis and identification of G6PD deficiency in infants before hospital discharge.

Table 3 Screening Indices for Cord Blood G6PD Assay at two cut-off values

	Cut-off values	
	5.7 U/g Hb	8.05 U/g Hb
Sensitivity	98.6%[a]	90%
	(CI:91.2, 99.9)	(CI:81.4, 95)
Specificity	99.7%	98.4%
	(CI:99.1%, 99.9%)	(CI:97.4%, 99%)
Positive Predictive Value	94.5%	81%
	(CI:85.8%, 98.2%)	(CI:71.7%, 87.9%)
Negative Predictive Value	99.5%	99.2%
	(CI:99.5%, 100%)	(CI:98.5%, 99.6%)
Accuracy	99.6%	97.77%

CI Confidence intervals
[a]98.6% of all the patients with truly deficient peripheral G6PD assays had deficient cord blood results with cut-off 5.7 U/g Hb once compared to 8.05 U/g Hb

There are important observations that we have arrived at in this study. First, we note the preponderance of the disease in males which is congruent with an X-linked pattern of inheritance of G6PD deficiency. Moreover, the enzyme assays in the affected males are significantly lower than in the affected females which could explain the more severe nature of the disease in the male population.

Second, G6PD activity in the peripheral blood samples appears to be higher than in cord blood especially among non-deficient patients. This could reflect an up-regulation of G6PD activity as a response to oxidative stress in the newborn period by way of enhanced G6PD gene expression (i.e. transcription) [12–16]. Other possibilities are increased erythropoiesis resulting in normoblastemia, reticulocytosis, or possible other characteristics peculiar to fetal and neonatal erythrocyte metabolism [15, 17]. Cappellini and colleagues cite this as a diagnostic issue among neonates which could lead to false negative results [17]. This even raises doubts as to whether the peripheral neonatal blood is reflective of the true value or it could be a falsely elevated estimate. Therefore, we have used the 5.7 cut-off value as it is much more stringent and is based on the adult values. Using a much higher cut-off value would indeed show more number of G6PD deficient infants some of which could be false positive. Cut-off values used as described in the literature of <2.0 U/g Hb for profound and between 2 U/g to 7 U/g Hb for partial deficiency in the neonate may Indeed be too low.

Among the deficient group of neonates, regardless of the sample, they would have consistently low enzyme assays. We could only speculate that among this group of neonates, the same physiologic changes do not result in increased G6PD activity since the enzyme function is not optimal from the start. These observations reinforce the use of cord blood sample for G6PD deficiency screening among neonates since having a generally lower value than the peripheral blood samples, false negative results are minimized (i.e. negative predictive value of 99.5%, CI: 99.5%, 100%).

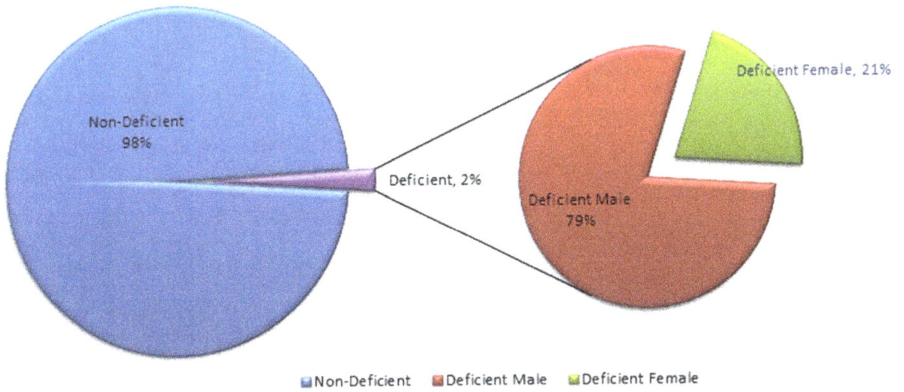

Fig. 1 Incidence and Distribution of G6PD DEFICIENCY among neonates admitted in KAMC, during 2008 ($N = 8139$)

While we observed a statistically substantial discrepancy in the mean of G6PD assay between cord and peripheral blood samples using t-test, a chi-square analysis of the proportion of G6PD deficiency failed to show any meaningful difference. We also noticed that there were different normal G6PD level distributed among gender between cord blood and the peripheral blood samples.

This suggests that in so far as discriminating between deficient and non-deficient patients is concerned; there is no significant difference between the two groups. Again, this underscores the usefulness of cord blood in the universal neonatal G6PD deficiency screening.

Conclusion

In this study, we found no difference between the cord and peripheral blood samples in discriminating between G6PD deficient and non-deficient neonates using quantitative enzyme activity assay. However, peripheral blood appears to have a higher G6PD quantitative assay than the cord blood. This reinforces the practice of using cord blood for neonatal screening since, having a generally lower value, the chances of missing a G6PD deficient neonate will be less (i.e. substantially low false negative results).

Recommendation

The results of this study are best understood in the light of the following limitations. No randomization was carried out so the recommendations would not be as robust. The subset of patients for whom we analyzed correlation between the cord and peripheral blood for G6PD assay were mostly those for whom jaundice work-up was carried out, or those with borderline G6PD values in the cord blood, so that both cord and peripheral G6PD values had to be drawn. This may have imparted a sampling bias in this study.

An important question raised in this study which could be worth looking into in the future is establishing the relationship between cord and peripheral neonatal blood with that of older children. Should we be able to prove that the neonatal peripheral blood G6PD assay is indeed an overestimate of the true mature value? It might be plausible to set a higher cut-off point for labeling a newborn as G6PD deficient using a peripheral blood sample?

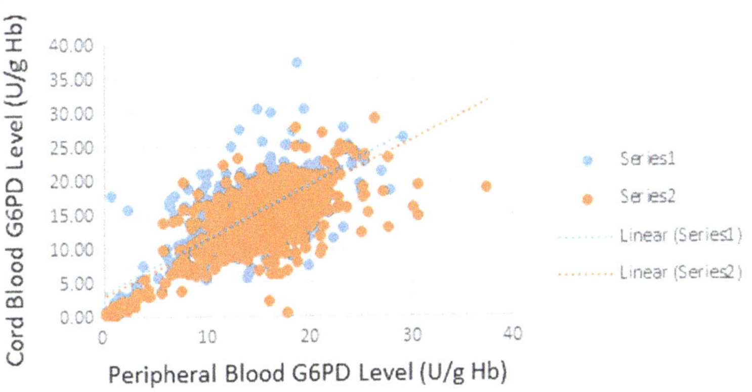

Fig. 2 Concordance of G6PD Quantitative assay between Cord and Peripheral Blood Samples of KAMC neonates

Abbreviations

G6PD DEFICIENCY: glucose-6-phosphate dehydrogenase deficiency; G6PD: glucose-6-phosphate dehydrogenase; IRB: International Review Board; KAIMRC: King Abdullah International Medical Research Center; KAMC: King Abdulaziz Medical City; LIS: Laboratory Information System; MNGHA: Ministry of National Guard Health Affairs; MRN: medical record numbers

Acknowledgments

The authors gratefully acknowledge Ms. Zoe P. Camarig for her secretarial assistance in reviewing and editing the manuscript.

Funding

This study is funded by King Abdullah International Medical Research Center (KAIMRC) protocol # RC09/106.

Authors' contributions

SS, BP and KK: drafted the manuscript, and contributed in the preparation of manuscript figures and tables; KT and IA contributed to the gathering and interpretation of data; AS and BB: contributed to the project design; MK, KH and AS conducted the analysis and carried out the interpretation of results; MB: aided in the project design and the overall review, editing and submission of manuscript. All authors read and approved the final manuscript.

Competing Interest

The authors declare that they have no competing interests.

Author details

[1]Division of Neonatology, Department of Pediatrics, King Abdulaziz Medical City, Ministry of National Guard Health Affairs, P.O. Box 22490, Riyadh 11426, Kingdom of Saudi Arabia. [2]Division of Neonatology, Department of Pediatrics, Prince Mohammad bin Abdulaziz Hospital, Ministry of National Guard Health Affairs, P.O. Box 40740, Al Madinah, Al Medina 41511, Kingdom of Saudi Arabia. [3]Division of Neonatology, Department of Pediatrics, King Abdulaziz Medical City, Ministry of National Guard Health Affairs, P.O. Box 9515, Jeddah 21423, Kingdom of Saudi Arabia. [4]Department of Pathology and Laboratory Medicine, King Abdulaziz Medical City, Ministry of National Guard Health Affairs, P.O. Box 22490, Riyadh 11426, Kingdom of Saudi Arabia. [5]Medical Genomics Research Department, King Abdullah International Medical Research Center, Ministry of National Guard Health Affairs, P.O. Box 22490, Riyadh 11426, Kingdom of Saudi Arabia. [6]College of Medicine, King Saud bin Abdulaziz University for Health Sciences, P.O. Box 3660, Riyadh 11481, Kingdom of Saudi Arabia.

References

1. Nkhoma E, Poole C, Vannappagari V, Hall SA, Beutler E. The global prevalence of glucose-6-phosphate dehydrogenase deficiency: a systematic review and meta-analysis. Blood Cells Mol Dis. 2009;42:267–78.
2. Glucose-6-phosphate dehydrogenase deficiency. WHO Working Group. Bull World Health Organ. 1989;6796:601–11.
3. Kaplan M, Hammerman C. Glucose-6-phosphate dehydrogenase deficiency and severe neonatal hyperbilirubinemia: a complexity of interactions between genes and environment. Semin Fetal Neonatal Med. 2010;15:148–56.
4. Kosaryan M, Mahdavi MR, Jalali H, Roshan P. Why does the Iranian national program of screening newborns for G6PD enzyme deficiency miss a large number of affected infants? Pediatr Hematol Oncol. 2014 Feb;31(1):95–100.
5. As W, El-Hazmi MA. G6PD deficiency, distribution and variants in Saudi Arabia: an overview. Ann Saudi Med. 2001;21:174–7.
6. Muzaffer MA. Neonatal screening of glucose-6-phosphate dehydrogenase deficiency in Yanbu. Saudi Arabia J Med Screen. 2005;12:170–1.
7. Alharbi KK. Genetic polymorphisms in paraoxonase 1 and G protein-coupled receptor 77, and the risk of glucose-6-phosphate dehydrogenase deficiency in a Saudi population. Saudi Med J. 2015 May;36(5):544–8.
8. Gari MA, Chaudhary AG, Al-Qahtani MH, Abuzenadah AM, Waseem A, Banni H, et al. Frequency of Mediterranean mutation among a group of Saudi G6PD patients in western region-Jeddah. Int J Lab Hematol. 2010;32:17–21.
9. Niazi GA, Adeyokunnu A, Westwood B, Beutler E. Neonatal jaundice in Saudi newborns with G6PD Aures. Ann Trop Paediatr. 1996;16:33–7.
10. Kaddari F, Sawadogo M, Sancho J, Lelong M, Jaby D, Paulin C. Etal. Neonatal screening of glucose-6-phosphate dehydrogenase deficiency in umbilical cord blood. Ann Biol Clin. 2004;62:446–50.
11. Sanpavat S, Nuchprayoon I, Kittikalayawong A, Ungbumnet W. The value of methemoglobin reduction test as a screening test for neonatal glucose 6-phosphate dehydrogenase deficiency. J Med Assoc Thail. 2001;84:S91–8.
12. Lohr GW, Waller HD. Glucose-6-phosphate Dehydrogenase. In: Bergmeyer HU, editor. Methods of Enzymatic Analysis. 2nd English ed. New York: We ran the analysis looking at gender differences in G6PD , Weinheim, and Academic Press; 1974. p. 636–43.
13. Lin LI. A note on the concordance correlation coefficient. Biometrics. 2000; 56:324–5.
14. Preville X, Salvemini F, Giraud S, Chaufour S, Paul C, Stepien G, et al. Mammalian small stress proteins protect against oxidative stress through their ability to increase glucose-6-phosphate dehydrogenase activity and maintaining optimal cellular detoxifying machinery. Exp Cell Res. 1999;247:61–78.
15. Ko CH, Wong RP, Ng PC, Li K, Chui KM, Yuen PM, et al. Oxidative challenge and glucose-6-phosphate dehydrogenase activity of preterm and term neonatal red blood cells. Neonatology. 2009;96:96–101.
16. Miyazono Y, Hirono A, Miyamoto Y, Miya S. Erythrocyte enzyme activities in cord blood of extremely low-birth-weight infants. Am J Hematol. 1999;62:88–92.
17. Cappellini MD, Fiorelli G. Glucose-6-phosphate dehydrogenase deficiency. Lancet. 2008;371:64–74.

4

Knowledge and practice of immediate newborn care among health care providers in eastern zone public health facilities, Tigray, Ethiopia, 2016

Abadi Kidanemariam Berhe[1*], Fitiwi Tinsae[2] and Gebremedhin Gebreegziabher[3]

Abstract

Background: According to WHO (2013) report the number of under five-year mortality in Ethiopia was 195,504, out of this 84,437 was from neonatal death and this mortality is related to immediate obstetric and newborn care of babies provided by health care providers; But little was known about the level of knowledge and practice related to immediate newborn care and their associated factors among health care providers generally in Tigray region and specifically in the Eastern Zone so the aim of this study was to assess knowledge and practice of immediate newborn care and associated factors among health care providers in the Eastern zone public health facilities, Tigray, Ethiopia.

Methods: A cross-sectional study was conducted from December 2015 to February 2016. A total of 16 health care facilities were selected for study using simple random sampling techniques and all health care providers in the selected health care facilities who participated in immediate newborn care were involved in the study. Data were entered, cleaned and analyzed using SPSS version 20.0. Ethical clearance was obtained from Adigrat University institutional ethical review board and Tigray regional health bureau. Consent was obtained from participants to conduct the study.

Result: In this study 215 participants were contacted, with a response rate of 99.1%. Generally, from the health care providers who participated in this study, 74.65% had adequate knowledge on newborn care and overall 72.77% of the participants were having good newborn care practice. Among the health care providers participated in the study, 151 (70.9%) were getting access to newborn care national guideline and only 99 (46%) of the health care providers get training in newborn care within the past two years before the study. Availability of national guideline, having adequate materials, the period of taking training and type of health facility were significant predictors for the health care providers newborn care practice.

Conclusion: Even though some improvement observed in the knowledge and practice of health care providers on newborn care, but still this study identified knowledge and practice gap. Regional health bureau and district health offices should provide refreshment training on immediate newborn care regularly, equipping all health facilities with necessary materials and national guideline of newborn care and there should be sharing experience between hospital and health center staffs working on newborn care through mentoring.

Keywords: Knowledge, Practice, Immediate newborn care, Tigray, Ethiopia

* Correspondence: abadik021@gmail.com
[1]Adigrat University, College of Medicine and Health Sciences , Adigrat, Ethiopia
Full list of author information is available at the end of the article

Background

According to WHO 2015 report globally every year, 2.7 million neonates die during the neonatal period which constitutes 45% of under-5 mortality and approximately 58% of infant mortality and 75% of the deaths occur during the first week in the neonatal period [1, 2]. Most neonatal deaths were in low and middle-income countries, which account for a growing proportion of all under-five mortality [3]. If the trend continues like this the share of neonatal deaths to under-five death is projected to increase from 45% in 2015 to 52% in 2030 [4]. Similarly, according to WHO (2013) report, the number of under five-year mortality in Ethiopia was 195,504, out of this 84,437 was from neonatal death [5]. According to the 2011 Ethiopia Demographic and Health Surveys (EDHS), the neonatal mortality rate was 37 per 1000 live births and the perinatal mortality rate was 46 per 1000 this is high compared to the African region average neonatal mortality rate which was 35.9 per 1000 live births [6].

A study conducted in Ethiopia on trend and determinants of neonatal mortality identified sepsis, asphyxia, birth injury, tetanus, preterm birth, congenital malformations as a cause of early neonatal mortality [7]. Immediate newborn care interventions are part of essential newborn care used to protect against newborn morbidity and mortality by using clean cord care, thermal care including drying and wrapping of the newborn immediately after delivery and delaying the newborn's first bath for at least 24 h or several days to reduce hypothermia risk), and initiation of breastfeeding within the first one hour of birth, management of immediate asphyxia, management of early sepsis [8]. Immediate newborn care aims at addressing poor care practices immediately following delivery [9],

Approximately 50 million were dying each year in the late 1980s, but two-thirds of this has been saved through the application of immediate newborn care [10].

Wide acknowledgments were showed that the MDG 4 target for child survival cannot be achieved without a particular focus on newborn health, especially during the first seven days of life [11]. Newborn complications resulting from hypothermia, infection, birth asphyxia and low birth weight that occurs within the first seven days following birth contribute to the highest burden of morbidity and mortality [12, 13].

A study conducted in Uganda among health workers practice with immediate newborn care showed that appropriate implementation is dependent upon levels of knowledge [14]. A similar study conducted in India showed a high level of knowledge among community health workers was considered as very important for improving coverage and adherence to recommended newborn care practices [15]. Other studies conducted in eastern Uganda also showed that neonatal mortality autopsies indicated the low levels of knowledge among health workers regarding prenatal and newborn care as a major determinant of death [16]. A similar study in Uganda showed that 52% of deliveries take place at the health facility, and neonatal mortality remains relatively high at 29 per 1000 live births this might be related to the immediate newborn care and obstetric care [17]. Critically ill newborn babies often present for care at the formal health facilities where general nurses and midwives are routinely deployed [18]. Studies showed that in the neonatal period more than 70% of the current deaths could be prevented through evidence-based procedures (e.g. exclusive breastfeeding and hypothermia management) [19].

Generally, Ethiopia like other countries in the sub-Saharan region has a high perinatal mortality and specifically the study area Tigray regional state is among the top three regional states with a high burden of perinatal mortality and second highest stillbirth from all regional states of Ethiopia according to EDHS 2011.Perinatal deaths have multi-factorial etiology, therefore, to address the high perinatal mortality there is a need for careful analysis of contributing factors in order to design appropriate interventions. Identifying the level of knowledge and practice was important for deciding the implementation strategy and for effective and sustainable implementation of knowledge into practice but only a few studies has evaluated strategies for knowledge translation in low-income countries [1]. Similarly, little is known about the level of knowledge and practice related to immediate newborn care and associated factors among health care worker providing service in intrapartum and postnatal care generally in Tigray region and specifically in Eastern Zone.

Moreover, this study will be used as a baseline data for district health office, human resource of regional health bureau to provide capacity building to health care providers based on the identified gap and used as a baseline for researchers of the further study. So, the aim of this study was to assess knowledge and practice of immediate newborn care and associated factors among health care providers in Eastern zone public health facilities, Tigray, North Ethiopia 2016.

Methods

A cross-sectional study design was conducted from December 2015 to February 2016 in Eastern zone of Tigray Region; to assess knowledge and practice of immediate newborn care and associated factors among health care providers.

According to the 2014 report of Tigray region health bureau, health service coverage in the eastern zone is approximately 80%, with two general hospitals, 4 primary hospital, 26 health centers and 116 health posts. Midwives, Nurses, and public health officers are responsible for providing basic delivery and postnatal service both in hospitals and health centers in the study area. A total of 16 health care facilities providing delivery service (1 general hospital, 2 primary hospitals, and 13 health centers) were selected for study using simple random sampling techniques from 32 health facilities in the eastern zone, health posts were not included in the study since they did not provide delivery service. All health care providers in the selected health care facilities who participated in immediate newborn care were involved in the study.

Observational questionnaire to assess the practice of immediate newborn care and interviewer guided structured and pre-tested questionnaire to assess knowledge of newborn care on Breastfeeding, immediate postnatal care, newborn infection management, care of low birth weight baby.

Ten-degree Midwives and Nurses were recruited for data collection and two BSc degree Nurse and four masters in midwifery as a supervisor. The overall data collection process was coordinated and supervised by supervisors, co-investigators and the principal investigator.

The validity of the questionnaire was maintained by adapting the questionnaire from different relevant kinds of literature that were used by other researchers and modified in the local context. 5% of the calculated sample size was pre-tested in another health facility which is not included in the study before the actual application for data collection. Data completeness and accuracy was checked on a daily basis by supervisors.

After the fieldwork completed and coded, then the data were entered and cleaned using SPSS version 20.0.

The data analysis methods used were descriptive analysis for frequencies, percentage, mean, standard deviation and percentage, Bivariate logistic regression analysis to see the relationship of each independent variable with practice of immediate newborn care and finally variables which are found significant at $p < 0.05$ in bivariate analysis was taken to multivariate logistic regression analysis to determine the final predictors with practice of immediate newborn care.

Model assumption fulfillment and multicollinearity test were done prior to multivariate logistic regression. The final logistic model goodness of fit was assessed using the Hosmer-Lemeshow goodness of fit test, an omnibus test of model coefficients and the result shows the model is fit.

Compute score was done to assess the result of knowledge and practice of health care providers involved in the study.

There were ten procedures to assess the immediate newborn care practice on observation (see Table 2) and operationally defined as.

Good practice: if the health care providers perform more than or equal to 70% the practice procedures.

Poor practice: if the health care providers performs less than 70% of the practice procedures.

There were 12 questions to assess knowledge of health care providers' on immediate newborn care assessed using interview and operationally defined as.

Adequate knowledge: if the health care provider answers the knowledge question above or equal to mean.

Inadequate knowledge: – if the health care provider answers the knowledge questions below mean.

Finally, the result of the study was presented using tables and text.

Result

Socio-demographic characteristics

In this study 221 participants were eligible, but at the time of data collection six of the eligible study participants were not available due to office work and annual leave. Overall, among the eligible study participants, 215 were contacted, 2 interrupted between the interviews. A total of 213 participants has completed the survey, with a response rate of 99.1%, out of those 150 (70%) were females. The median age of the participants was 30.00 [IQR: 22–38] years. Approximately half of the participants were working in health center 116 (54.5%) and 44 (20.7%) of participants were trained in newborn care within the past two years. Moreover, the the majority of the participants 194 (91.1%) were Orthodox in religion and concerning the educational status of respondents 148 (69.5%) were diploma and 69 (29.1%) was degree. Working experience of the participants ranges from 1 to 39 years; median 5 years [IQR 3–12 years]. Other details are shown in Table 1.

Practice of health care providers on immediate newborn care

The result of this survey showed that 155 (72.8%) of respondents generally have good newborn care practice; specifically 180 (84.5%) of the participants have properly practice putting a baby on to mother's abdomen immediately after delivery, 184 (86.4%) of the participants place the baby in skin-to-skin contact and on the breast to initiate breastfeeding, 156 (73.2%) of participants apply Tetracycline eye ointment and 141 (66.2%) give Vitamin K IM on anterior mid-thigh but only 18 (8.5%) of participants apply chlorhexidine to cord after cord cutting (Table 2).

Knowledge of health care providers on immediate newborn care

Regarding knowledge of health care providers on option of breastfeeding of newborn 91.5% of the participants stated breastfeeding should start within one hour after delivery, 93% choice exclusive breastfeeding for six months option, 55.9% of participants stated breastfeeding should stop completely at two years from the

Table 1 Socio-demographic characteristics of healthcare providers in public health facilities at Eastern zone, Tigray regional state, Ethiopia, 2016

Variable		Frequency (N)	Percent (%)
Age (in year)	20–30	116	54.5
	31–40	71	33.3
	41–50	23	10.8
	≥51	3	1.4
Sex	Male	63	29.6
	Female	150	70.4
Religion	Orthodox	194	91.1
	Muslim	6	2.8
	Catholic	13	6.1
Educational status	Diploma	148	69.5
	Degree	62	29.1
	MSc	3	1.4
Monthly salary(USD)	75–108	79	37.1
	108.10–174	65	30.5
	174.10–207	41	19.2
	207.10–240	22	10.3
	≥240.10	6	2.8
Type health facility	General Hospital	56	26.3
	Primary Hospital	41	19.2
	Health Center	116	54.5
Working experience (in year)	1–5	111	52.1
	6–10	43	20.2
	11–15	17	8.0
	16–20	16	7.5
	21–30	25	11.7
	≥31	1	.5

duration of breastfeeding options and 78.4% of the participants choice breastfeed more frequently as option to the care of mother with inadequate breast milk during the first few days after delivery (See Table 3).

Regarding knowledge of health care providers in the immediate postnatal care of newborn babies, 38.97% of the participants have knowledge about prevention of newborn bleeding and 41.8% have knowledge about the correct dose of Vitamin K to be given to a term newborn and preterm baby. In addition, the Knowledge of health care providers about infection management of newborn baby shows 35.2% of the participants know how to apply eye drops (silver nitrate) after cleaning eyes to prevent eye infections after delivery and 87.3% of the participants have knowledge about the the care of umbilical cord after delivery. Other details are shown in Table 4.

Health care providers' knowledge about the care of a low birth weight baby, 75.6% of the study participants

Table 2 Practice of health care providers on Immediate Newborn Care in public health facilities at Eastern zone, Tigray regional state, Ethiopia, 2016

Variable		Frequency (N)	Percent (%)
Deliver baby on to mother's abdomen	Yes	180	84.5
	No	33	15.5
Dry baby's with dry towel, Wipe eyes, Wrap with dry one and cover head	Yes	184	86.4
	No	13	13.6
Assess breathing and color	Yes	187	87.8
	No	26	12.2
If the baby breath normally delay cord cutting 1–3 min	Yes	148	69.5
	No	65	30.5
Tie the cord two fingers from abdomen and another tie two fingers from the 1st one cut the cord between the 1st & 2nd tie	Yes	161	75.6
	No	52	24.4
Place the baby in skin-to-skin contact and on the breast to initiate B/feeding	Yes	184	86.4
	No	29	13.6
Apply chlorhexidine to cord after cord cutting	Yes	18	8.5
	No	195	91.5
Apply Tetracycline eye ointment once	Yes	156	73.2
	No	57	26.8
Give Vitamin K IM on anterior mid- thigh	Yes	141	66.2
	No	72	33.8
Weigh the baby	Yes	195	91.5
	No	18	8.5

have knowledge on ways to stabilizing the temperature of a newborn baby, 81.2% of participants have knowledge of the definition of low birth weight of newborn child and 68.5% participants stated bath more frequently as not important when taking care of a low birth weight baby. Other details are shown in Table 5.

The overall knowledge of health care providers of Immediate Newborn Care in public health facilities of Eastern zone was 74.65%.

Factors that affect the practice of immediate newborn care among health care providers

In bivariate logistic regression analysis age, sex, educational status, type of health facility, working experience, availability of national guideline, shortage of materials and the period of taking training were significant predictors but after controlling for the effects of potentially confounding variables using multivariate logistic regression only availability of national guideline, shortage of materials, the period of taking training and type of health facility were found to be significant predictors for practice of immediate newborn care. Those health facilities having adequate materials for newborn care were 4.69 times more likely practicing good newborn care

Table 3 Knowledge of health care providers about Breastfeeding of newborn baby in public health facilities at Eastern zone, Tigray regional state, Ethiopia, 2016

Variable		Freq. (N)	Percent (%)
Initiation of breastfeeding after birth	Within the first hour	195	91.5
	1–6 h after birth	12	5.6
	6–12 h	3	1.4
	More than 12 h after birth,	0.00	0.00
	Other	3	1.4
Mother inadequate breast milk during the first few days after delivery	Give formula while waiting for breast milk	19	8.9
	Breastfeed more frequently	167	78.4
	Give rice water, herbal fluids or honey water	8	3.8
	Advise the mother to ask someone else to breastfeed her baby	19	8.9
	Other	0.00	0.00
Period of exclusively breastfeed	2 months	4	1.9
	4 month	6	2.8
	6 months	200	93.9
	More than 6 months	2	0.9
	Other	1	0.5
After how long should a mother stop breastfeeding her child completely	24 months	119	55.9
	More than 2 years	78	36.6
	18 months	12	5.6
	6 months	3	1.4
	12 months	0.00	0.00
	I have no opinion	1	0.5

compared to health facilities having a shortage of materials for newborn care [AOR; 4.69 95% CI: (1.5, 14.6)]. Similarly, facilities having a national guideline about newborn care were 28.4 times more likely practicing good newborn care than those did not have national guideline [AOR = 28.495% CI: (5.10,15.22)].

But those health care providers taking newborn care training before two years were 76% lower odds of newborn care practice compared to those taking training within two years [AOR = 0.2495% CI: (0.09,0.66)]. In addition, those health care providers working in health centers were lower odds of newborn care practice compared to health care providers working in General hospitals [AOR = 0.089, 5% CI: (0.01,0.65)]. For detail see (Table 6).

Discussion

The first few hours since birth is the most crucial period in the life of an infant for further growth and development, which is largely determined by the quality of care that the newborn receives [20].

Table 4 Knowledge of health care providers about immediate postnatal care and Infection management of newborn baby in public health facilities at Eastern zone, Tigray regional state, Ethiopia, 2016

Variable		Freq. (N)	Percent (%)
Prevent newborn children from bleeding	Breastfeeding the child,	130	61.03
	Not necessary to give any drugs,	0.0	0.00
	Give Vitamin K	83	38.97
	I have no opinion,	0.0	0.00
Dose of Vitamin K to give to a term newborn baby	0.5 mg	102	47.90
	1 mg	89	41.80
	2 mg	4	1.90
	5 mg	0.0	0.00
	10 mg	1	0.50
	I have no opinion,	8	3.80
	Other	9	4.20
Prevention of eye infections after delivery	Do not apply anything	36	16.90
	Apply breast milk in the babies' eyes	4	1.88
	Clean eyes with sterile gauze only	83	38.97
	Apply eye drops (silver nitrate) or TTC after cleaning eyes	75	35.20
	I have no opinion	4	1.88
	Other	10	4.7
Which care of the umbilical cord of newborn after delivery is important	Cut the cord with a clean instrument (for example, a razor, blade)	186	87.3 0
	Use any sharp instrument for cutting the cord	7	3.30
	After cutting the cord, apply for traditional herbs/medicines	1	0.50
	Always put a bandage on the cord,	8	3.80
	I have no opinion,	1	0.50
	Other	10	4.70

In this study an effort has been made to assess knowledge, the practice of newborn care and associated factors among health care providers in public health facilities of eastern zone, Tigray, Ethiopia.

Overall, 74.65% of the health care providers participated in the study was having adequate knowledge on newborn care. This result is more or less similar to the study conducted in Addis Ababa 2013 which was 68% [21] but it is higher than the study conducted in Egypt (52.2%), Uganda (46.5%), and Khartoum (50.6%) [22]. This difference might be due to the difference in the

Table 5 Knowledge of health care providers about Care of a low birth weight baby in public health facilities at Eastern zone, Tigray regional state, Ethiopia, 2016

Variable		Freq. (N)	Percent (%)
Way to stabilizing the temperature of a newborn baby	Bathing the baby in water of appropriate temperature	6	2.80
	By putting on clothes and cover head,	0.0	0.00
	Having the baby skin-to-skin with her/his mother,	161	75.60
	Keep the baby in a room with a temperature of 28–30 °C,	15	7.00
	Have the baby close to heat (radiator, fire, etc.),	31	14.60
	Other	0.0	0.00
Definition of low birth weight for newborn child	Weight is less than 3000 g,	5	2.30
	Weight is less than 2500 g,	173	81.20
	Weight is less than 1500 g,	20	9.40
	Weight is less than 1000 g,	3	1.40
	I have no opinion,	7	3.30
	Other	5	2.30
Not important when taking care of a low birth weight baby	Start breastfeeding early and frequently	36	16.9
	Bath the baby often	146	68.5
	Keep the child warm	13	6.1
	Apply skin to skin contact	6	2.8
	Prevent infection from developing	4	1.9
	None	8	3.8

period of study and a slight difference in the data collection tools we used.

Knowledge of breastfeeding initiation was 91.5%, this finding is in line with a study conducted in Uganda which was 86.4% [13]. The findings of this study reveal that the knowledge of Exclusive breastfeeding and age of a child to stop breastfeeding are 11.2% and 9.9% respectively. This result is lower than the study conducted in Uganda (2011) which was 64%, 19.1% respectively [13]. This difference might be due to the difference in access to short-term training provided to health care providers on breastfeeding.

Our study showed that 71.2% of the health care providers were having knowledge on the immediate postnatal care of a newborn; compare to study conducted in Uganda which was reported 72.5% knowledge of health care provides its more or less similar finding [13]. But it is lower than the study conducted in Sudan 98% [9], this difference might be due to the gap capacity building like in-service training on a newborn. Similarly, in this study the health care providers' knowledge of vitamin K was 41.8% this was more or less similar to study conducted in Uganda which was 49.7% [13]. But it is lower than the study conducted in Haryana India 76% [23]. These variations could be largely due to the difference in the educational level of the participants and access to newborn care training provided to health care providers.

Knowledge about low birth weight management (75.6%) among health care providers reported from this study was more or less similar to study conducted in Uganda 71% [13].

In this study practice of newborn care among health care providers was 72.77%: this result is more or less similar to the study conducted in Vietnam (64%) [1], Egypt (69.2%) [20] But this finding was much higher than the study conducted in Haryana, India, Khartoum Sudan, Addis Ababa which was 55%, 41.1%, and 30% respectively [13, 21, 24]. Differently, this finding was much lower than the study conducted in Tanzania which was 88.2%. This difference might be due to a difference in materials, type of health facility and variation in the study period.

From the multivariate logistic regression analysis availability of national guideline was found a significant predictor of newborn care practice [AOR = 28.495% CI: (5.10, 15.22)]. This result is different from Vietnam, which shows the availability of national guideline was not significantly associated with newborn care practice [1].

In addition, those health care providers working in health centers were lower odds of newborn care practice compared to health care providers working in General hospitals. This finding is different from the study conducted in Uganda, which shows the type of health facility has no significant association with newborn care practice [21].

Those health facilities having adequate materials for newborn care were 4.69 times more likely practicing good newborn care compared to health facilities having

Table 6 Multivariate analysis to identify factors associated with Practice of health care providers on Immediate Newborn Care in public health facilities at Eastern zone, Tigray regional state, Ethiopia

Variable	Practice of newborn care		Cured OR (95% CI)	Adjusted OR (95% CI)
	No N (%)	Yes N (%)		
Work experience				
1–5	35 (60.3%)	76 (49.0%)	1.00	1.00
6–10	8 (13.8%)	35 (22.6%)	2.01 (0.84,4.79)	1.85 (0.28,11.95)
11–15	4 (6.9%)	13 (8.4%)	1.49 (0.45,4.92)	4.87 (0.24,97.20)
16–20	8 (13.8%)	8 (5.2%)	0.46 (0.16,1.32)	0.40 (0.02,6.63)
21–30	3 (5.2%)	22 (14.2%)	3.37 (1.23,12.03)*	9.6 (0.78,12.24)
≥ 31	0 (0.0%)	1 (0.6%)	2.17 (0.71,10.40)	24.4 (0.001,14.3)
Age				
20–30	24 (41.4%)	92 (59.4%)	1.00	1.00
31–40	28 (48.3%)	43 (27.7%)	0.40 (0.20.0.77)*	0.23(0.04,1.32)
41–50	6 (10.3%)	17 (11.0%)	0.73 (0.26,2.07)	0.21 (0.01,2.71)
≥ 51	0 (0.0%)	3 (1.9%)	3.80 (0.63,7.23)	7.29 (0.001, 15.1)
Shortage of material				
No	48 (82.8%)	46 (29.7%)	1.00	1.00
Yes	10 (17.2%)	109 (70.3%)	11.3 (5.3,24.4)*	4.69 (1.5,14.6)*
Guideline				
No	46 (79.3%)	15 (9.7%)	1.00	1.00
Yes	12 (20.7%)	139 (90.3%)	35.5 (15.5,81.3)*	28.4 (5.10,39.22)*
When do you take training				
Within two years	11(28.2%)	86 (79.6%)	1.00	1.00
Before two years	28(71.8%)	22 (20.4%)	0.10 (0.04,0.23)*	0.24 (0.09,0.66)*
Education				
Diploma	51(87.9%)	97 (62.6%)	1.00	1.00
Degree	7(12.1%)	55 (35.5%)	4.13 (1.75,9.72)*	1.74 (0.27, 10.89)
MSc	0 (0.0%)	3 (1.9%)	1.9 (0.67,5.24)	1.04 (0.04, 8.23)
Sex				
Male	10(17.2%)	53 (34.2%)	1.00	1.00
Female	48(82.8%	102(65.8%)	0.40 (0.18,0.85)*	0.39 (0.06,2.57)
Type of health				
General hospital	1 (1.7%)	63 (40.6%)	1.00	1.00
Primary hospital	2 (3.4%)	57 (36.8%)	0.45 (0.04,5.12)	0.32 (0.28.3.78)
Health center	55 (84.8%)	35(22.6%)	0.01 (0.001,0.76)*	0.08 (0.01,0.65)*

* = $P \leq 0.05$ (* indicate level of significance), 1 = Ref.cat

a shortage of materials for newborn care. This finding is consistent with the study done in Addis Ababa [21].

The odds of newborn care practice were less by 76% for those health care providers taking training before two years compared to those taking training within two years.

Conclusion

Majority health care providers in the public health facilities eastern zone of Tigray have adequate knowledge on initiation of breastfeeding, cord care, but they have a knowledge gap on prevention of eye infection and prevention and management of early bleeding. Generally, among the health care providers who participated in this study, 74.65% had adequate knowledge of newborn care.

Even though 72.77% of the participants have adequate newborn care practice, but specifically the study participants showed a gap in the practice of vitamin K administration and application of chlorhexidine to cord after delivery.

The health care providers practice of immediate newborn care were affected by the availability of the national guidelines, shortage of materials for newborn care, the time of taking training on newborn care and type of health facility.

Based on findings of the study, we recommend to Tigray regional health bureau and district health offices in collaboration with other stakeholders: to strengthen providing refreshment in-service training on immediate newborn care regularly and follow up, equipping all health facilities with national guideline of newborn care and necessary materials to provide immediate newborn care and there should be sharing experience between Hospital staffs and health centre staffs working on newborn care through mentoring.

Abbreviations

AOR: Adjusted odd ratio; EDHS: Ethiopia demographic and health surveys; ENC: Essential newborn care; IM: Intramuscular injection; IQR: Inter quartile range; MDG: Millennium development goal; SPSS: Statistical package for social science; TTC: Tetracycline; WHO: World Health Organization

Acknowledgments

We would like to thank Adigrat University for their financial support to carry out our research.

We would like also to extend our gratitude to eastern zone administration and respective weredas/district/health office for providing us the necessary information and cooperative support for the accomplishment of our research work.

Our gratitude also goes to data collectors and supervisors for their hard work patience in obtaining necessary information. Our special thanks also go to participants who generously shared their thoughts and feelings despite other commitments.

Funding

The source of funding to carry out for this research was Adigrat University. The funding organization has no role in the design of the study and collection, analysis, and interpretation of data and in writing the manuscript this was the role of authors.

Authors' contributions

AK was the principal investigator who contributed to the conception and design of the study, collected, entered, analyzed, interpreted the data, prepared the manuscript and acted as the corresponding author. FT & GG contributed to data analysis, interpretation and drafted the manuscript. All authors read and approved the final manuscript.

Ethics approval and consent to participate

Ethical approval and clearance for the study were obtained from Adigrat University institutional ethical review board and Tigray regional health bureau. An official letter of cooperation was obtained from regional health bureau to hospital and each woreda/district/health office. Verbal consent from the Medical Directors of each health centers and CEO of the hospital was obtained too.

The study participants were approached individually and given information regarding the purpose of the study, confidentiality of study, their right to participate or withdraw from the study and then finally written consent was obtained for the study.

Competing interests

The authors declare that they have no competing interests.

Author details

[1]Adigrat University, College of Medicine and Health Sciences , Adigrat, Ethiopia. [2]Department of Nursing, College of Medicine and Health Sciences, Adigrat University, Adigrat, Ethiopia. [3]Department of Midwifery, College of Medicine and Health Sciences, Adigrat University, Adigrat, Ethiopia.

References

1. Leif Eriksson et al. Evidence-based practice in neonatal health: knowledge among primary health care staff in northern Viet Nam Human Resources for Health 2009, 7:36 doi:10.1186/1478-4491-7-36.
2. Level and trends of child mortality, UNICEF, WHO, UN and World bank report 2015 accessed on http://www.childmortality.org/files_v20/download/IGME%20report%202015%20child%20mortality%20final.pdf.
3. Kim et al. Assessing the capacity for newborn resuscitation and factors associated with providers' knowledge and skills: a cross-sectional study in Afghanistan BMC Pediatrics 2013, 13:140.
4. UNICEF, WHO, World Bank Group and UN. Levels and trends in Child mortality, 2015 report. Available at http://www.childmortality.org/files_v20/download/igme%20report%202015_9_3%20lr%20web.pdf..
5. World health organization report on under five mortality 2013 accessed by http://apps.who.int/maternal_child_adolescent/epidemiology/profiles/neonatal_child/eth.pdf.
6. Oestergaard MZ, Inoue M, Yoshida S, Mahanani WR, Gore FM, Cousens S, Lawn JE, Mathers CD. Neonatal mortality levels for 193 countries in 2009 with trends since 1990: a systematic analysis of progress, projections, and priorities. PLoS Med. 2011;8(8):e1001080.
7. Mekonnen et al. Neonatal mortality in Ethiopia: trends and determinants BMC Public Health 2013, 13:483.
8. WHO recommendations on ways to improve quality of newborn care in health facilities, 2016 accessd at http://www.who.int/features/2017/quality-care-facilities/en/.
9. MahamaSaaka and Mariam Iddrisu, Patterns and Determinants of Essential Newborn Care Practices in Rural Areas of Northern Ghana International Journal of Population Research Volume 2014, Article ID 404387, 10.
10. Grant J. Opening session, world summit on medical education, Edinburgh 8–12 August, 1993. Medical Education. 1994;28(11).
11. Ganatra HA, Zaidi AK. Neonatal infections in the developing world. SeminPerinatol. 2010;34(6):416–25.
12. Shiffman J. Issue attention in global health: the case of newborn survival. Lancet. 2010;375:2045–9.
13. Ayiasi et al. Primary healthcare worker knowledge related to prenatal and immediate newborn care: a cross sectional study in Masindi, Uganda BMC Health Services Research 2014, 14:65.
14. Lutwama GW, Roos JH, Dolamo BL. A descriptive study on health workforce performance after decentralisation of health services inUganda. Hum Resour Health. 2012;10(1):41.
15. Agrawal PK, Agrawal S, Ahmed S, Darmstadt GL, Williams EK, Rosen HE, Kumar V, Kiran U, Ahuja RC, Srivastava VK, et al. Effect of knowledge of community health workers on essential newborn health care: a study from rural India. Health Policy Plan. 2012;27(2):115–26.
16. Waiswa P, Kallander K, Peterson S, Tomson G, Pariyo GW. Using the three delays model to understand why newborn babies die in eastern Uganda. Tropical Med Int Health. 2010;15(8):964–72.
17. MoH: Health Sector Strategic and Investment Plan III: Promoting People's Health to Enahnce Socio-Economic Transformation (2010/2011–2014/2015). Kampala: The Ministry of Health; 2010.
18. Rutebemberwa E, Pariyo G, Peterson S, Tomson G, Kallander K. Utilization of public or private health care providers by febrile children after user fee removal in Uganda. Malar J. 2009;8:45.
19. Darmstadt GL, Bhutta ZA, Cousens S, Adam T, Walker N, de Bernis L. Evidence-based, cost-effective interventions: how manynewborn babies can we save? Lancet. 2005;365:977–88.

20. Neamaabd El Fattah1 and Nagwa A. Zein El Dein. Assessment of Quality of Nursing Care Provided Immediately after Birth at University Hospital in El kom-Minoufiya, Egypt. Life Science Journal. 2012; 9(4).
21. Mirkuzie et al. Current evidence on emergency obstetric and new born care services in Addis Ababa Ethiopia BMC Pregnancy and Childbirth 2014, 14:354.
22. Taha FAN. Assessment of knowledge, attitude and practices of nurse midwives towards immediate Care of the Newborn in Khartoum state teaching hospitals. 2016.
23. Louis D, Kumar P, Gupta A. Knowledge and practices of healthcare providers about essential newborn care and resuscitation in a district of Haryana. J Indian Med Assoc. 2013;111(2):114–7.
24. Deepak Louis, Praveen Kumar and Ashish Gupta. Practitioners' Series Knowledge and practices of health care providers about essential newborn care and resuscitation in a district of Haryana. J Indian Med Assoc. February 2013.vol 111(2).

5

Transition to parenthood in the neonatal care unit: a qualitative study and conceptual model designed to illuminate parent and professional views of the impact of webcam technology

Susan Kerr[1*], Caroline King[1], Rhona Hogg[2], Kerri McPherson[1], Janet Hanley[3], Maggie Brierton[4] and Sean Ainsworth[4]

Abstract

Background: Complications during pregnancy, childbirth and/or the postnatal period may result in the admission of a baby to a neonatal unit (NNU). While the survival and long-term prospects of high-risk infants are enhanced by admission, the enforced separation of the parent and child may have psychological consequences for both. There is a need to develop and evaluate interventions to help parents 'feel closer' to their infants in circumstances where they are physically separated from them. In this paper we present findings from an in-depth, theoretically-driven, evaluation of a technological innovation designed to address this need. The study sought to explore parent and professional views of the impact of the technology, which transmits real-time images of the baby via a webcam from the NNU to the mother's bedside in the post-natal care environment.

Methods: A qualitative approach was adopted, guided by a critical realist perspective. Participants were recruited purposively from a NNU located in East-central Scotland. Thirty-three parents and 18 professionals were recruited. Data were collected during individual, paired and small group interviews and were analysed thematically. Following the initial analysis process, abductive inference was used to consider contextual factors and mechanisms of action appearing to account for reported outcomes.

Results: Views on the technology were overwhelmingly positive. It was perceived as a much needed and important advancement in care delivery. Benefits centred on: enhanced feelings of closeness and responsiveness; emotional wellbeing; physical recovery; and the involvement of family/friends. These benefits appeared to function as important mechanisms in supporting the early bonding process and wider transition to parenthood. However, for a small number of the parents, use of the technology had not enhanced their experience and it is important, as with any intervention, that professionals monitor the parents' response and act accordingly.

Conclusions: With a current global increase in premature births, the technology appears to offer an important solution to periods of enforced parent-infant separation in the early post-natal period. The current study is one of a few world-wide to have sought to evaluate this form of technology in the neonatal care environment.

Keywords: Neonatal unit, Technology, Perceptions, Parents, Professionals, Qualitative

* Correspondence: s.m.kerr@gcu.ac.uk
[1]School of Health & Life Sciences, Glasgow Caledonian University, Cowcaddens Road, Glasgow G4 OBA, Scotland
Full list of author information is available at the end of the article

Background

Complications during pregnancy, childbirth and/or in the postnatal period may result in the admission of a baby to a neonatal care unit (NNU). Recent estimates suggest that 8–12% of babies in the developed world receive some form of care in a NNU, with the most common reason for admission being premature birth [1, 2]. While the survival and long-term prospects of high-risk infants are enhanced by admission to the NNU, the separation of the mother and child, enforced by different care environments, can have psychological consequences for both [3].

"Transition to motherhood" has been described as a process of change that occurs as a woman begins to care for her child, to problem solve and to appraise herself as a mother [4, 5]. Mothers with infants admitted to a NNU are known to experience greater difficulties in transitioning to the maternal role than mothers with healthy babies [6, 7]. Reasons include periods of separation and reduced opportunities for early bonding that may lead to decreased levels of maternal responsiveness and sensitivity [8, 9]. Also, concern for the immediate and long-term health and development of their baby has been shown to result in higher levels of stress, anxiety and depression in mothers, which may persist after the baby has been discharged [9, 10]. Importantly, the psychological well-being of mothers is known to influence early parent-child interactions and can impact the social, emotional, behavioural and cognitive development of children in the short and longer term [9].

In Western societies, there have been significant changes in family structures and compositions in the past 30–40 years and this includes shifting expectations of the roles of fathers in the post-natal period [11]. As a consequence, the "transition" of fathers, as they seek to establish a relationship with the new baby and support their partner, has increasingly been explored [11]. While research on the psychological adjustment of fathers of children admitted to NNU is limited, elevated rates of depression and anxiety have been identified [12]. Also, similar to their partner, periods of enforced separation from their new-born baby can function as a barrier to the establishment of the early parent-child relationship [8].

A range of interventions designed to promote physical and emotional closeness between parents and their babies has been developed for use in NNUs. These interventions include: kangaroo care, which facilitates skin to skin contact; infant massage, designed to promote parent-child interaction; and, diaries written by staff on behalf of babies, which parents can access online [13–15]. While these interventions have been shown to be useful, further research is required to develop and evaluate interventions to help parents 'feel closer' to their infants when they are physically separated from them [9]. In recent years, interest has grown in the use of webcam technology to address this need, with this form of technology being used in the United States of America (USA), Australia, Singapore, the Netherlands [16–18] and most recently in Ireland [19] and the United Kingdom (UK) [20].

In this paper findings are presented from an in-depth evaluation of the impact of webcam technology used in a UK setting. The intervention, named *mylittleone*, involves an Internet Protocol (IP) camera being placed over a cot/incubator in the NNU, which transmits real-time images of the baby, wirelessly and securely, to a dedicated network hub, coupled to a tablet device kept by the mother in the post-natal care environment. To ensure confidentiality, the camera is fixed so that the images transmitted are of the individual cot/incubator and no sound is transmitted. The camera is switched off when nursing and/or medical procedures are undertaken, otherwise it is in constant operation and therefore allows a mother to view her baby whenever she wishes. The *mylittleone* technology was developed with the intention of promoting increased feelings of closeness, and, in turn, facilitating the parent-infant bonding process.

While technological innovations in the health field are generally introduced with laudable intentions, a critique of the literature suggests that the expected advantages are not a given and indeed there may be uncertainties or anxieties associated with their use [21]. Reactions appear to be influenced by a complex and inter-related array of social, psychological and technical factors, situated within the healthcare environment into which the new technology has been introduced [22]. For example, the introduction of new technologies may influence care expectations, re-define interpersonal relationships and/or impact feelings of agency [23]. It is therefore important that new technologies are evaluated to determine whether their anticipated benefits are realised and to identify any unanticipated consequences of their use. The views of those classified as 'end users' of the new product are particularly relevant in this regard. When considering the use of webcams in NNUs, while some important evaluative work exists, this has focused on implementation issues, including parental 'satisfaction' with the technology [16, 18], the impact on the workload of nurses [14, 15], and views of parents, nurses and doctors prior to the introduction of the technology [19]. To the best of our knowledge, there has, to date, been no theoretically driven, in-depth exploration of the impact of this form of technology on the parental role in the early postpartum period.

In light of the above, the aim of the current study was to explore parent and professional views of the impact of the *mylittleone* technology on the transition to parenthood and to uncover likely mechanisms of action. The study also sought to identify contextual factors that appeared to have influenced views of the technology.

Methods

Design

A qualitative approach, informed by a critical realist ontological perspective, was adopted [24]. In a critical realist study reality is considered to be largely, but not wholly, social constructed with the conditions and social relations involved in the production of knowledge (e.g. during a research interview) acknowledged as influencing its content [25, 26].

Sample, setting and recruitment

Participants were recruited from a NNU located in east-central Scotland. At the time of recruitment this was the only NNU in the UK using the *mylittleone* technology.

Parents were recruited purposively [27] based on age, family size, socio-economic status, the medical condition of the baby and the length of stay/anticipated length of stay in the neonatal unit. Purposive sampling was used to ensure the views expressed were from a heterogeneous group of parents and thereby to enhance the potential transferability of the findings [27]. The only inclusion criterion was experience of using the *mylittleone* technology; there were no exclusion criteria. Staff working in the NNU distributed Study Information Sheets to mothers of the babies they were caring for; this included mothers who had been discharged (prior to their baby) and those who had not yet been discharged. Mothers who were interested in taking part, or who wished to receive further information before making up their minds, were asked to complete a form that gave permission for their contact details to be passed to the study researcher (CK). Participation was on a voluntary basis; parents were informed that if they did not wish to take part it would not affect their own or their baby's care in any way. Those who agreed to participate were asked to invite their partner to take part in the study, if they wished. The aim was to recruit 30 parents, including fathers. All participants provided written consent.

Purposive sampling was also used to recruit members of the multi-disciplinary team of professionals caring for babies in the neonatal unit and parents in the postnatal care environment (e.g. neonatal nurses, midwives, doctors). The professionals were provided with an Information Sheet (distributed in the NNU and post-natal care environment by the study researcher) and were informed that participation was on a voluntary basis. The aim was to recruit c.20 professionals. Again, all participants provided written consent.

Data collection

Data were collected from the parents during individual or paired semi-structured, face-to-face interviews (n = 25). Paired interviews were undertaken when both the mother and father had been recruited. The majority of the interviews (n = 17) were conducted in a private setting in the NNU, with eight conducted in the family home, as this was the parents' preference. The professionals participated in individual, paired or small group face-to-face, semi-structured face-to-face interviews (n = 8), depending on their availability and/or preference. The decision to interview the professionals in this manner was largely pragmatic. The interviews with the professionals were conducted in a private location in the neonatal/postnatal care environment. Interview guides were used to facilitate the interview process and to ensure similar issues were addressed across the participant groups (see Table 1). The data were collected by the project researcher CK, between January and July 2015; the technology had been fully functional in the neonatal unit from November 2014. The researcher was unknown to the participants prior to the study commencing.

Data analysis

The audio-recorded interviews were transcribed verbatim and checked for accuracy. Names and any identifying information were removed prior to the analysis. The data were analysed thematically, in NVivo version 10, using the process described by Braun & Clarke [28]. Familiarisation with the data was followed by a coding process that drew on a priori reasoning and was linked, deductively, to questions in the interview guide. The data were then indexed thematically (and inductively) based on what was discussed by the study participants. In the final stage, and in line with the critical realist approach underpinning the study [24], 'abductive' inference was used to consider the contextual factors and mechanisms of action that appeared to account for the reported outcomes [29]. This final stage in the analysis process was viewed through a theoretical lens informed by literature on the transition to parenthood [6, 7], parent-child bonding [30–32] and the experience of

Table 1 Interview Guides (outline of content)

Parents	Professionals
Health during pregnancy	Own views and experience of *mylittleone* - expectations before introduced - reality of its use
Admission to NNU (anticipated/unanticipated)	Observations of parents' experiences - general views/experience - any aspects of care made easier - any aspects of care made more difficult - partners/extended family
Experience of baby being cared for in NNU	- Impact on own caring role
Views and experience of *mylittleone* - general views/experience - any aspects of care made easier - any aspects of care made more difficult - views/experience of extended family	Other issues professionals wished to discuss
Other issues parents wished to discuss	

'new technologies' in the health field [22, 33], with a conceptual model developed to explain the relationships.

The analysis was undertaken by the project researcher (CK). Other members of the research team (SK, RH, KMcP) provided peer-review and assisted with the interpretation of the data, to ensure rigour in the process.

Ethical approval

The study was considered to be a service evaluation by the East of Scotland Ethics Committee (Ref: CYA/AG/13/GA/127) and so did not require NHS ethical approval. Ethical approval was therefore sought and granted from the School of Health & Life Sciences Ethics Committee at Glasgow Caledonian University.

Results

Participant characteristics

Thirty-three parents were recruited (25 mothers and 8 fathers). A profile of the participants is presented in Table 2. As noted, the age of the parents ranged from 19 to 44 years, with the majority being married or living with a partner. Eighteen of the babies (including one set of twins) were born before 37 weeks' gestation. Those born after 37 weeks were most commonly admitted to the neonatal unit because they were jaundiced, had a suspected infection, breathing difficulties, low blood sugar, and/or because they were of low birth weight.

Eighteen professionals were recruited. A profile of the professional participants can be found in Table 3. The professionals were neonatal nurses, midwives, nursery nurses and doctors.

The themes that emerged from the analysis of the data are presented under three broad categories: Benefits of *mylittleone*; Potential disadvantages of *mylittleone*; and, Extending *mylittleone's* reach to the home environment. When presenting the findings, the accounts from the parents and professionals have been integrated, where appropriate, to allow similarities and differences in the views and experiences of the participant groups to be highlighted. The conceptual model is presented in the Discussion, with the findings considered, in light of extant empirical and theoretical literature.

Table 2 Parent participants and their babies (*n* = 33)

Mother's age (*n* = 25)	Frequency
19 years and younger	1
20–29 years	13
30–39 years	10
40 years and older	1
Range 18–44 years	
Father's age (*n* = 8)	
19 years and younger	1
20–29 years	5
30–39 years	2
Range 19–39 years	
Marital Status	
Married/living with partner	22
Single	3
Baby's gestation at birth in completed weeks	
< 28 weeks	2
28 < 32 weeks	6
32 < 37 weeks	9
37 + weeks	8
Range 26 weeks–41 weeks	
Baby's sex	
Female	16
Male (includes 1 set of twins)	10
Other children	
Yes	14
No	11
Scottish Index of Multiple Deprivation (SIMD)[a]	
1–2	10
3	9
4–5	6

[a][49] Participants' postcodes were used to calculate scores. Areas scoring 1 are the most deprived; areas scoring 5 are the least deprived

Benefits of *mylittleone*

The majority of the participants believed the development and deployment of *mylittleone* was an important advancement in the provision of neonatal care. The manner in which the technology had enhanced the parents' experience was central in the accounts of both the parents and professionals. Themes that emerged from the data included: Being present when you're not; Keeping mums (and dads) on an even keel; Helping mums to take care of themselves; and, "Showing off" the new baby.

Being present when you're not

Mothers in the post-natal care environment most commonly have their babies with them immediately following the birth and throughout their hospital stay. However, when a baby is admitted to a neonatal care unit, periods of separation result and, depending on the mother's physical health, these periods can be lengthy. The impact of separation from their child was discussed at length in the interviews, by both the mothers and fathers and, as exemplified in the following quotes, *mylittleone* was reported as helping them 'feel closer' to their babies when they could not be with them:

[Mother 1; baby 6 weeks premature] Oh, it was brilliant, absolutely brilliant ... I was so tired, that I couldn't sit for longer than half an hour [in neonatal care] ... I

Table 3 Professional participants (n = 18)

Place of work	Frequency
Neonatal Unit	10
Postnatal Ward	8
Professional Background	
Neonatal Nursing	8
Midwifery	3
Nursery Nursing[a]	5
Medicine	2
Gender	
Female	17
Male	1

[a]In the UK, neonatal nursery nurses (who have undertaken certified training) are responsible for the care and daily living needs of babies from admission to discharge, under the guidance of the nurse manager. Tasks include bathing, nappy changing, observations and providing parents with advice and support

didn't feel well, I was sick and I was dizzy, so when I got up the stairs [to post-natal ward], I put [mylittleone] right next to the bed, and even though I fell asleep pretty quick, it was like ... it was like she was near me, because I could see her. Instead of being completely cut off from her, she was still there.

[Mother 12; baby 4 weeks premature] [It's hard] when you've not got your baby with you, when everybody else does.

[Father 12] [But] you actually feel like you're with them basically because you're getting a live feed.

[Mother 12] Yes, so you're present even when...

[Father 12] Even when you're not.

In addition to the increased feeling of proximity, there was a belief that *mylittleone* helped the mothers, in particular, to be more responsive to their baby's needs and this included responding physically through the production of breast milk. As indicated below, mothers who had had previous experience of the neonatal environment were able to make useful comparisons.

[Mother 2; baby 8+ weeks premature] It's so different this time. With my little boy [also admitted to a neonatal unit] I couldn't see him straightaway ... whereas this time having the mylittleone camera ... I can see her constantly, she's right beside my bed, really. [Also], I've found with things like expressing milk, I've found that a lot easier.

[Professional interview 5, post-natal ward] I think it's excellent ... it's like [the mothers] are really close to their babies ... A lot of the mums...when the baby's upset will go down the nursery. You know, they'll say, the baby's really upset I'm away down to see if it's needing fed or what's wrong with it. So, they'll toddle away down and see.

The feelings of 'closeness' and 'responsiveness' that *mylittleone* engendered appeared to be important in facilitating the process of 'transitioning to parenthood,' and relatedly, to encourage the early bonding process between the parents (both mothers and fathers), and their babies, which, from what was described, would have been more challenging had the physical separation not been bridged by the technology.

Keeping mums (and dads) on an even keel

There was much discussion of the positive emotions associated with parents seeing their baby for the first time using the *mylittleone* technology.

[Mother 24; baby 15+ weeks premature] You couldn't wipe the smile off [husband's] face when the doctor brought the tablet round.

[Father 24] It was like an overwhelming thing. I was just so happy and proud that I could see her, if that makes sense.

[Mother 2; baby 8+ weeks premature] As soon as the doctor [gave me the tablet] ... I couldn't speak, I just kept crying ... it was amazing just to see this tiny little baby that you knew was yours, but there she was.

The parents also discussed how the technology had enabled them to keep more stable emotionally in the days following the delivery. A key benefit appeared to be the reassurance connected with being able to see their baby was 'okay,' that is, there had been no worsening of their condition. The comfort associated with this is clear in the narratives below.

[Mother 1; baby 6 weeks premature] I'm not just saying this, but if I didn't have the camera ... I think I would have cracked up, because it's been...I've been waking up during the night and kind of looking and being able to see that she was there and that she was sleeping, and I would be able to fall back asleep again.

[Father 19; baby full-term] It provides reassurance. You can see her snoozing and, as long as you can see the quilt going up and down, you know she's breathing okay. We don't fret when we are away from her because we can see her.

Discussions of emotions extended to the low emotional state, commonly referred to as the 'baby blues,' that mothers may experience a few days after the birth of their baby.

[Mother 16, baby 5 weeks premature, also low birth weight] Everyone was kind of saying I would have a 'baby blue day' and I think I didn't get that because I knew she was okay and I was able to see her ... So I was waiting on that and I think that having [mylittleone] and watching her probably helped quite a bit, I didn't ever have down days ... I don't quite know what I would've done without it.

Also, seeing their baby on the tablet device allowed parents to prepare themselves emotionally for visiting the neonatal unit for the first time.

[Mother 23; baby 9+ weeks premature] He was born at 11 min past four and my boyfriend went to see him about five and then brought [mylittleone] straight down,

and I got to come up at about 11 to see him, so it was really good because I got to prepare myself by looking on the screen of what I was coming up to see, like the tubes and stuff, so it was quite nice.

The continuous ability to monitor their baby's progress was also reported by some as giving them 'hope' in terms of the immediate and longer-term health and development of their child. The baby referred to in the quote below had had a serious respiratory problem at birth and this had required intensive and prolonged medical interventions.

[Father 21; baby full-term] Just little things isn't it [to mother]? Because where we are it's little steps, really little steps at a time, just like her hand moving and she's trying to grab things and you can see.

[Mother 21] Or she's trying to touch her face or things like that ... It's just these things that's giving us that wee bit of hope.

Finally, staff in the neonatal care unit stressed the almost 'gift like' quality of *mylittleone*, something which again appeared to enhance the emotional well-being of the parents.

[Professional interview 8; neonatal unit] You get such a great reaction the minute the baby's stable ... if I've had to take the [tablet] round, the mum's just so happy, you know, she knows she wasn't going to see her baby for [maybe] another 12 h and you have appeared and said, here she is here and you can watch her.

From what was described, the positive impact on the parents' emotional well-being appeared to be an important outcome associated with their use of *mylittleone*. Use of the technology allowed them to feel more connected to their baby, monitoring their welfare and progress, and thus to function in a parenting role, despite periods of separation imposed by the location of the baby in the NNU. Also, the ability to view their baby on the tablet device, in what they commonly perceived as the 'alien' environment of the neonatal unit, was considered important as it allowed parents to prepare themselves for an unanticipated transition, that of being the parent of a sick and/or premature baby.

Helping mums to take care of themselves

Another benefit related to the scope *mylittleone* provided in assisting the physical recovery of the mothers following the birth of their baby. The main issues discussed were sleep, rest, nourishment and the reduction of pain/discomfort.

[Mother 25; baby 8+ weeks premature] After having a C-section, and being on a lot of medication ... I was in a wheelchair, and I had my lovely catheter bag, and everything ... I managed to sit with her for five minutes, but it's more comfortable sitting in your own room ... You're very sore, and things.

[Mother 19; baby full-term] I would definitely have got less sleep if I couldn't see her on the tablet.

[Father 19] And that's not good because you need to rest, as part of the recovery process.

Mothers who had had a baby in neonatal care previously were able to compare their experiences.

[Mother 24; baby 15+ weeks premature] This time [with mylittleone] it felt much better, like going back up to the ward, you know like you weren't so...I wasn't so reluctant to leave her ... So, if you had to go for painkillers or...lunch or food or anything like that it was easier to do that than you would have found it previously.

The professionals also emphasised the importance of *mylittleone* in assisting the mothers' recovery, and similar to the mother above, commented on the situation prior to the technology being available.

[Professional interview 5, post-natal ward] Before [mylittleone], they would go down to the unit and they would sit there for hours and hours and they would have to really pull themselves away to come back, but now they're coming back and having a rest in the afternoon or coming back for lunch. Before, we used to have to really chase ladies to say, you need to come back for your lunch, you know? But now, because they've got the [tablet], they're quite happy to come back because their baby is almost in the room with them, really. ... So, that's helping.

The ability of the mothers to address their own physical needs was perceived as important in aiding their early postnatal recovery, thus enabling them to better care for their babies. Use of the *mylittleone* technology was reported as being important in easing/facilitating the early process of transition to motherhood by giving the mothers time and space to take care of themselves. The ability to care of themselves whilst also monitoring their baby appeared to be important in supporting the early bonding process.

"Showing off" the new baby

Finally, the parents discussed the benefits that *mylittleone* afforded in allowing them to share 'real-time' pictures of the baby with their wider family and friends. This was important as restrictions on visiting, linked to infection control measures, meant that siblings, members of the extended family, such as grandparents, and/or friends of the family, were not permitted entry to the neonatal care unit to see the baby.

[Mother 4; baby 5+ weeks premature] [My partner] loves [mylittleone] ... just being able to see her all the time ... and my mum and dad, they were up visiting yesterday and they thought it was a fantastic idea as well ... because she's in neonatal and they can't [go in] and they can't touch her or anything like that but it meant they didn't have to wait to see her sort of thing.

[Mother 21; baby full-term] Our son was able to have a look at her on the tablet when he visited.

[Father 21] He was upset, because he's only four, and he wasn't allowed in to the neonatal unit.

[Mother 21] So seeing her on the tablet helped.

Being able to introduce/show the baby off (via *mylittleone*) to their wider family and friends appeared to be important in 'normalising' the situation for parents. The ability to view and discuss moving images of the baby helped create a shared experience that was valued.

In sum, most parents and professionals talked about the *mylittleone* technology as a positive development in the neonatal care environment. From what was discussed, the relationship with their new baby and the parents' emotional wellbeing appeared to have been enhanced by addressing feelings of 'closeness', the ability to identify and respond to the baby's needs and by engendering a shared experience among the parents and their wider family and friends, including siblings.

Potential disadvantages of using *mylittleone*

Importantly, while most parents believed that *mylittleone* was a positive development, for a small minority, its use had not enhanced their experience of parenting in the neonatal care environment. While they could see some benefits in its use, a few parents had decided not to use it for the duration of their hospital stay and/or would not use it again if they found themselves in a similar circumstance. The central issue was that for some, rather than providing reassurance, the ability to see the baby whenever they wanted appeared to increase anxiety levels. The themes that emerged from the parents' and professionals' narratives focused on: Dealing with dilemmas; Interpreting what was being seen on screen; Wondering if there was something to be concerned about; and, Parents seeing something they would rather have not.

Dealing with dilemmas

The following account, which is necessarily long, demonstrates some of the tensions associated with seeking to be responsive to a baby's needs, particularly when these needs were highlighted by use of the *mylittleone* technology and might otherwise have gone unnoticed.

[Mother 17; baby full-term] I remember at one point that I got quite upset and the reason was it was night time and I'd just been down to breastfeed him, and .... and by the time I got back up the stairs I could see that he was crying on the screen and it really upset me ... and ... the staff member that was on that night, she ... sort of kept putting his dummy back in and, you know, and sort of trying to shoogle the cot as it were, but you ... could tell he wasn't settling. ... And it just, yeah, it really upset me because I was kind of in two minds ... can I go back down again, can I not, you know, even though they've said that I can come and go whenever I please ... would it be a case that, you know, would she not think, "Oh you've just been here why are you here again?", you know, so you were in that awkward sort of stage of will I or won't I type of thing. What I had to do was literally just put the tablet down so that I could go to sleep.

[Interviewer] And did you feel you could have turned the tablet off?

[Mother 17] Yeah but again it was almost like the sort of curiosity killed the cat, so it was like I don't want to turn it off but I just don't want to see it just now ... And ... you would almost feel like you were ... like sort of not being a mother if you turned it off. You know it was almost like you don't care enough.

The issue of not feeling it was 'appropriate' to turn off the tablet device was discussed by a small number of the mothers. Concerns seemed to be linked to feeling that they were not fulfilling expectations associated with their parenting role i.e. identifying and being responsive to their baby's needs, if they did not constantly 'observe' their baby.

Interpreting what was being seen on screen

Other concerns raised by a small number of parents, linked to their ability to make sense of what they we seeing on the tablet device.

[Father 9; baby 6 weeks premature] It's a double edged sword [using mylittleone], I would say.

[Mother 9] Yeah.

[Father 9] You can see what's happening but you don't know what's happening. ... So every time they're doing something [to the baby], it might be routine, it either gets switched off or you see a pair of hands coming in [to the incubator/cot] with the gloves and then it gets switched off and you think, is it just something routine, is it not? And then you'd wait for maybe ten, fifteen minutes and it would come back on ... and then you might see five minutes later something else happening again. As I say, you're never quite sure ... It wasn't for us, no; it wasn't for us.

The ability of parents to interpret what they were seeing was also discussed by the professionals.

[Professional interview 2; neoanatal unit; Participant A] I think for the anxious mums it [can] make them even more anxious.

[Professional interview 2; neoanatal unit; Participant B] I think a lot of the interpretation of [what they see on the tablet] and certainly where mum's anxiety comes from, comes from mum's experience, whether she's a first time mum or not, whether she's had a complicated pregnancy or not, whether there's been pre or post anxiety or complications and things. I think that alters their interpretation of what they see on the tablet.

Again, what was discussed demonstrates that for some, albeit a small number of parents, use of the technology was not perceived as beneficial, and in some instances, not desirable. Use of the technology appeared to give them access to information about the care of their baby that they were either not able to make sense of or they were struggling to deal with, having found themselves unexpectedly taking on the role of parent to a sick and/or premature.

Wondering if there is something to be concerned about

The switching off and on of the *mylittleone* camera by staff was the focus of much discussion and some debate among the parents and professionals. As noted above, when staff were undertaking a medical/nursing procedure, the policy was that the camera should be switched off. When the camera was switched off a notice appeared on the tablet device letting the parents know a procedure was underway. However, the notice was a standardised message that did not indicate what the procedure was or why it was being undertaken and there was no indication of how long the procedure would last. Procedures could vary from the changing of a nappy to resuscitation of the baby.

It was not uncommon for parents to report delays in the camera being switched back on after a procedure. For some this raised concern as they began to wonder if there was 'something wrong' with their baby.

[Mother 11] One thing I didn't like was sometimes they turned the camera off ... and they would forget to turn it on again ... and you had a sense of anxiousness when you couldn't see him ... I didn't want to make a fuss and be like a neurotic mother ... but I was like please can you turn it on [so I can see he's okay].

Parents seeing something they would rather have not

A final concern was that staff occasionally forgot to switch the camera off when undertaking a procedure. This meant that a small number of parents had seen procedures that had the potential to cause stress and anxiety. This issue was discussed by both the parents and professionals.

[Mother 9; baby 6 weeks premature] Sometimes you see stuff you don't want to see. I saw them taking blood from his heel and he was screaming the place down, he wasn't happy.

[Father 9] Then he got a blockage in his oxygen tube so they started putting another tube in to suck things out.

[Professional interview 7; post-natal ward] I know of two instances where the mum got upset because someone had taken bloods and forgotten to turn the camera off.

Linked to the above, there was discussion in all of the interviews with staff about what would happen in relation to the switching off of *mylittleone* in an emergency situation, where a baby required immediate attention. The scenario of an emergency clearly caused staff concern thinking about the possibility and (perceived/assumed negative) consequences of forgetting to turn off *mylittleone* as they sought to ensure the safety and well-being of the baby in their care.

In sum, while parents framed the 'downsides' of using *mylittleone* in different ways, there was a commonality in relation to the situations discussed. Most often the downsides related to witnessing something on screen which they otherwise would not have seen, for example, their baby crying or a medical procedure being undertaken. Importantly, some parents downplayed the significance of any negative aspects of *mylittleone* in light of their overall positive experience and other parents talked about similar events as having been more problematic for them.

Staff agreed that while for most parents, use of *mylittleone* reduced their anxiety levels, for a small number it had the opposite effect. Some had observed that it was often late at night that they would receive calls from parents about what they had seen on *mylittleone*. Similarly, they often received calls immediately the camera was switched off to undertake a procedure. The professionals felt the hyper-vigilance that could be associated with the constant ability to monitor the baby had the potential to impact negatively on the well-being of a small number of the mothers. The staff were aware that they needed to be able to identify these mothers and take appropriate action (e.g. encouraging the mothers to switch the tablet off for periods of time; asking if they wished not to use it).

The findings on the benefits and disadvantages of the *mylittleone* technology clearly demonstrate that the parents reacted differently to the same or similar events, when taking into account the health and developmental progress of their baby. Contextual factors that appears to be influential included: the health of the mother in the early post-natal period; the level of parenting experience, including experience of parenting a child in the neonatal care environment previously; and, relatedly, levels of stress and associated coping resources. For the majority, use of the technology brought with it a level of comfort and reassurance that impacted positively on their relationship with their newborn baby. However, there were two sides to the use of the new technology, for a small minority of parents *mylittleone* did not reduce and may have increased anxiety levels by providing 24/7 access to their sick and/or premature child that they did not feel they benefitted from and/or could cope with.

Extending *mylittleone's* reach to the home environment

At the time the interviews were conducted the *mylittleone* technology could only be used in the hospital setting. However, as it was anticipated that, in the future, video images of the baby could be transmitted to family homes when, for example, the mother had been discharged and her baby remained in hospital; parents and professionals were asked to share their views on this potential development. The two themes that emerged from the parent and professional accounts were: Going home without the baby; and, Mothers taking matters into their own hands.

Going home without the baby

The majority of parents felt that being able to use *mylittleone* at home would be beneficial and desirable.

[Parent 19; baby full-term] I [am] starting to get really anxious about going home without her and thinking when I've been here I've had this camera that I've been able to just use all the time. Whereas at home I'm going to have absolutely nothing and I can't imagine having like a night's sleep. I [will] be having to phone the unit, like two or three times a night just to check on her.

[Mother 19] You've had the experience of having to go home and not being able to see her [to partner], how did you find that?

[Father 19] It was really tough, especially after seeing her for like the first 48 h [stayed in the hospital with mother]. It's tough when you go home and can't see them anymore.

The majority of the parents had other children and they discussed the difficulty associated with being with the new baby whilst caring for older siblings. Again, the *mylittleone* technology was believed to be something that could assist.

[Father 24; baby 15+ weeks premature] We've not been able to be there very much for them [older children], they have been minded by somebody else. If we were able to have mylittleone at home we would be able to work things better and they would be able to see her.

[Mother 24] And I wouldn't be sat at home anxious all of the time, you could see if she was settled.

Although parents were mostly positive about such a development, the possibility of not being able to respond to their baby's needs from the distance of home was raised as an issue.

Staff in the post-natal ward were well-positioned to comment on the potential for *mylittleone* to be used at home as they frequently witnessed mothers being discharged before their baby.

[Professional interview 5; post-natal ward] Ideally, the mothers would like to know that they could take it home and then see their baby from home. None of the mothers want to go home [leaving] their baby in the hospital.

The fact that the mothers were not able to able to have regular contact via the *mylittleone* technology following their discharge was something that the professionals felt was a barrier to the continued establishment of the relationship between the parents and their baby. While parents were encouraged to visit as much as possible, the ability to connect with their baby whenever they wanted, included first thing in the morning and last thing at night, was considered to be important. The professionals also emphasised that mothers are often discharged weeks or even months in advance of their baby.

Mothers taking matters into their own hands

Interestingly, some of the mothers had used FaceTime® while in the post-natal care environment as a way of involving the baby's father in seeing what they could see on the tablet device.

[Mother 16; baby 5 weeks premature + low birth weight] [When I was in hospital] I would FaceTime® my husband [from my phone when he was at home] so he could watch her as well. So we could watch it at the same time. ... Yeah, it would basically be, like, look what she's doing now or did you see that? ... And she made good improvements all the time, you know, we'd see a difference in her and she would have a bit of equipment removed and things like that and we'd just talk about her, what will happen next and how soon until she gets out and things like that.

[Interviewer] So it was like a wee, sort of, bonding session between the three of you?

[Mother 16] Yeah, [a] three way conversation, except you couldn't talk [of course].

Hence mothers, to an extent, had already extended the use of the *mylittleone* technology to enable their partners to 'view' the baby from home.

In sum, the ability to extend use of *mylittleone* to the home environment was generally viewed positively by parents and professionals. The technology appeared to have an important potential in helping parents to feel closer to their baby following the mothers' discharge from hospital and thus to assist the ongoing transition process.

Discussion

The current study sought to explore parent and professional views of the impact of the *mylittleone* technology, to uncover mechanisms of action, and to determine factors that appeared to influence perceptions of the technology. Based on the study results, an empirically informed conceptual model of the impact of the *mylittleone* technology was developed and is presented below (Fig. 1).

Positive mechanisms and outcomes

As indicated, the majority of the parents and professionals who participated in the study spoke very positively about *mylittleone*, believing that it assisted the process of transition to motherhood. Perceived positive outcomes associated with its use included: an enhanced relationship with the baby; enhanced emotional wellbeing; enhanced physical recovery; and, a greater level involvement of the mother's partner and extended family. The mechanisms of action that resulted in these perceived benefits included feelings of closeness and responsiveness engendered by the ability to see their baby on the tablet device, the constant ability to monitor the welfare and progress of their baby, the ability of the mothers to address their own physical needs, whilst monitoring their baby, and the ability to share the images of the baby, and thus the experience of being a new parent, with their partner and extended

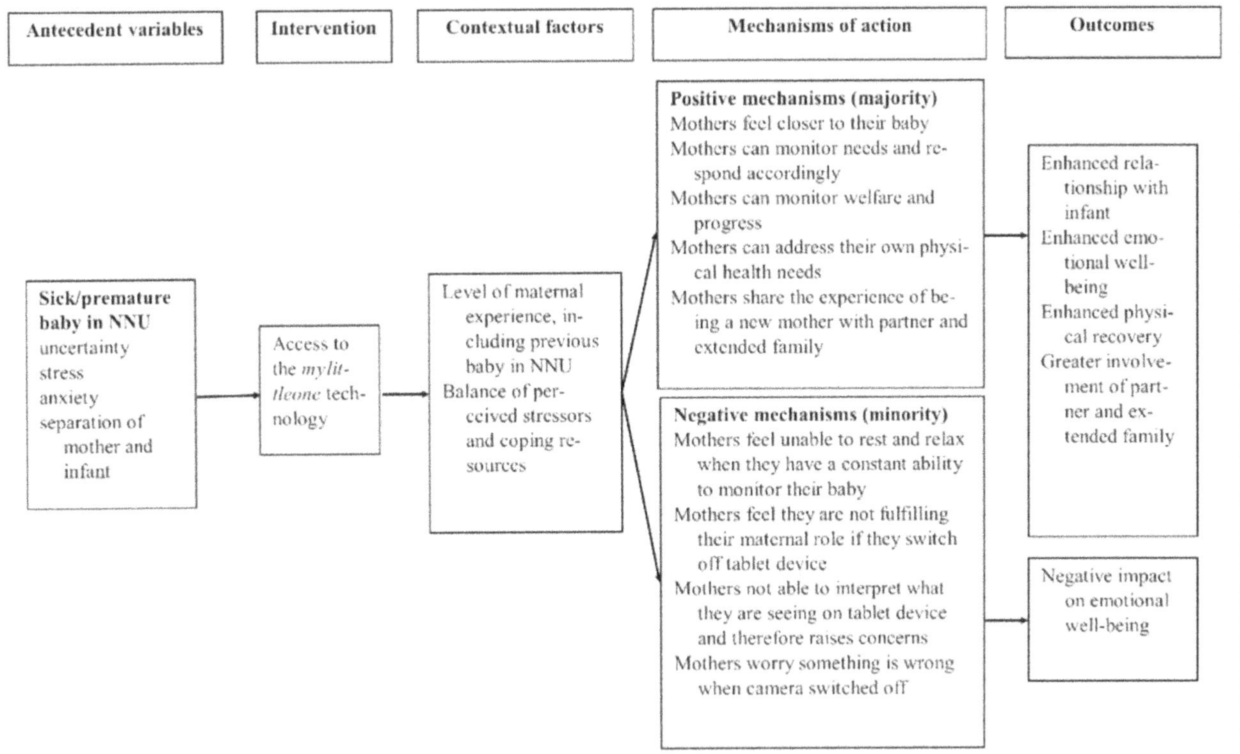

Fig. 1 Perceived impact of *mylittleone* - empirically informed conceptual model

family. The perceived benefits of the *mylittleone* technology are discussed below in light of existing literature.

The developing relationship between a parent and their new-born baby is believed to be a central and important psychological process of the puerperium; however, the early establishment of the bond between the parent and infant is known to be compromised when a child is admitted to a NNU [4, 11, 30, 34]. Bonding is the term commonly used to describe the mother (and father) coming to know, love and accept her new infant and has been defined as an enduring relationship that is positive, unique to the child and occurs through the process of attachment [35, 36]. Importantly, three attributes have been identified as central to the bonding process and these are proximity, reciprocity and maternal commitment [37]. Physical proximity is required to allow a parent to bond with her baby. From what was described by the mothers and fathers in the current study, use of the *mylittleone* technology helped them to feel closer to their baby when they could not physically be with them. Reciprocity refers to the mutual/shared behaviours of the parent and infant. Again, from what was described, use of the technology allowed the mothers, in particular, to identify and respond to their infant's needs demonstrating both reciprocity and maternal commitment. Interestingly, as noted in the Results section, engagement with the baby via the tablet device appeared to assist with milk production, encouraging the let-down reflex. While this allowed the mothers to be responsive to her babies' needs, it is important to note that the production of breast milk is linked to levels of the hormone oxytocin and that oxytocin has also been implicated in the establishment of the maternal-infant bond [32].

As bonding and attachment have been shown to influence an infant's emotional, cognitive and physical development, in the short and longer term, it is important that efforts are made to encourage the process [38, 39]. Findings from the current study suggest that the *mylittleone* technology may have an important contribution to make in helping to facilitate the early bonding process when periods of separation are imposed. It also appears to aid the wider transition by helping mothers be responsive to their baby's needs. Responding to their baby's needs is in turn likely to result in a more positive appraisal of their newly established role as mother to the infant in the NNU.

When considering maternal emotional well-being, the distress experienced by many when their child is admitted to a NNU is well-established (e.g. [8, 40]). Importantly, recent research has also demonstrated the emotional impact on fathers [12]. Parents of children who are very sick or premature often struggle with the uncertainty associated with their child's short and longer term prognosis and the highly technical and somewhat 'alien' environment of the neonatal unit [41]. From what was described, the ability to see their baby was 'stable' when they were not with them provided the majority of parents with an important level of reassurance that, in turn, impacted positively on their emotional well-being. Use of the technology also allowed parents to prepare themselves for seeing the baby for the first time in the neonatal unit, and this was reported as helping to diminish the stress which has been shown to be associated with this event [8]. The reduction in stress and anxiety appeared to be important in enhancing the emotional well-being of the mothers and fathers and, consequently, in supporting the bonding process. The *mylittleone* technology therefore appeared to be functioning as an important coping resource, assisting the transition to parenthood.

Another perceived benefit, discussed by the majority of parents and professionals related to the scope *mylittleone* provided in assisting the mothers' recovery. The ability that the technology provided in allowing mothers to relax and recover physically, whilst still 'keeping in touch' with their babies appeared to assist the bonding process. Previous research has demonstrated an association between rest and recuperate in the early post-natal period, emotional well-being, bonding and the production of breast-milk [42, 43].

Finally, parents spoke of the benefits of being able to introduce the baby (via *mylittleone*) to the wider family, including siblings and friends, who, due to issues associated with infection control, were not allowed access to the neonatal unit. This appeared to be important in normalising the situation. Previous research has shown that mothers, in particular, often feel bereft when, unlike the other mothers in the post-natal environment, they do not have a baby at their bedside to show to family members [8]. From what was discussed, the ability to see the baby may also have encouraged the number of visitors and visits. Access to existing support networks has been highlighted as important for maternal well-being in previous research and may help protect mothers who are confined to hospital from feelings of isolation [8]. In the current study, the shared experience of viewing and discussing the 'real time' images of the baby appeared to be important in this regard and was discussed by both the mothers and fathers.

Negative mechanisms and outcomes

While the majority of the parents found the *mylittleone* technology to be advantageous, for a small minority of parents, the almost constant ability to see their baby that *mylittleone* provided appeared to increase rather than decrease feelings of stress and anxiety and so did not assist the process of transition to motherhood. The parents and professionals referred to what might be described as a state of hyper-vigilance i.e. a heightened level of watchfulness and feelings of protection for the baby. This form of response in parents of babies admitted to a neonatal unit has been identified in review-level evidence and generally 'relaxes' as the parents' form trusting relationships with the professionals caring for their child/ren [41, 44]. However, the fact that a small number of parents decided that they did not wish to use the technology after trying it out, with others saying that they would not use the technology in the future, if they found themselves in similar circumstances, is obviously something that is important to note.

Contextual factors influencing the maternal response

It is important to consider the factors responsible for differences in the experience of the *mylittleone* technology. When seeking to explain the wide variation in parental reactions to the same or similar events research has increasingly drawn upon models of stress and coping, with Lazarus and Folkman's [45] theory, being one of the most commonly utilised [46]. Lazarus and Folkman [45] view stress as resulting from the transaction between an individual and the environment. The stress process is based on a number of appraisals made by the individual, in which the nature of the demands faced is compared with their perceived ability to cope. Stress is considered to be based primarily on subjective perceptions of events rather than objective circumstances. 'Coping' refers to an individual's cognitive and behavioural efforts to manage the internal and external demands of the stressful situation. Coping has two major functions, that is, to reduce stressful emotions (emotion-focused coping) and to alter the demanding situation (problem-focused coping). Examples of emotion-focused coping include: distancing; escape-avoidance; exercising self-control over the expression of feelings; seeking social support and positive reappraisal. Problem-focused coping targets the cause of stress in a practical way to remove or reduce the stress. Coping is influenced not only by an individual's appraisal of the actual demands of the situation but also by the internal and external resources s/he is able to draw upon. These resources can be categorised as material physical (e.g. maternal health in the postpartum period), psychological (e.g. beliefs, personality) and social (e.g. support from partner and family) [45].

As noted, what is described above, helps to explain why some mothers valued the use of the *mylittleone* technology and others did not. From what was described parents appraised the same or similar situations (in terms of the baby's health and prognosis) in different ways based on the access that they had to coping resources. For example, if a mother who was particularly anxious about her baby's health/prognosis wished to employ a coping strategy that involved 'distancing' herself from the situation she found herself in, the 24/7 ability that the *mylittleone* technology afforded was not perceived as beneficial. If, however, a mother who was anxious about her baby's health/prognosis was reassured by the ability to see her baby and monitor their needs and progress, *mylittleone* functioned as a useful coping resource.

When considering the contextual factors that influenced views of the technology, maternal experience of the NNU environment previously appeared to be consistent in encouraging the mothers to compare experiences and to view *mylittleone* positively. Otherwise, views of the technology (mothers and fathers) appeared to be based on the unique balance of perceived stressors and coping resources associated with their individual circumstances.

Key, of course, is the important role that professionals have in discussing the care package offered to mothers and their partners and ensuring that it is tailored to their individual needs and preferences. Ensuring, therefore, that staff are skilled in understanding the different needs and reactions of mothers and vigilant to potentially negative outcomes is an important consideration for future implementation of this form of technology. Importantly, professionals should also consider whether difficulty in observing the baby via the technology is linked in any way to an ambivalent parenting response. In some instances, avoidance of the technology may be predictive of maladaptive coping, insecure bonding, the development of post-traumatic stress, anxiety and/or depression.

Strengths and limitations of the study

A key strength of the current study is that it is one of few world-wide to have sought to evaluate technology to help parents feel closer to their babies when periods of separation are enforced [20]. To our knowledge, this is the first study to have undertaken an in-depth, theoretically driven, exploration of perceived outcomes. As discussed previously, a critique of the literature on the introduction of technological innovations suggests that there may be both positive and negative consequences and it is important, therefore, that clinicians and/or researchers seek to give voice to the views and experience of those for whom the technology was developed [27].

When considering methodological issues, the use of purposive sampling techniques helped to ensure heterogeneity in the parents and professionals recruited and thereby to enhance the potential transferability of the results [47]. That said, none of the parents who were recruited were from black and/or minority ethnic groups and this may limit transferability.

Conclusion

In conclusion, we believe that this study makes a valuable contribution to the evidence base on the use of webcam technology in NNUs. To the best of our knowledge, there has, to date, been no theoretically-driven, in-depth exploration of the perceived impact of this form of technology on the parental role in the early post-natal period.

While views of the technology varied, for most (parents and professionals) it was viewed as a much needed advancement in care delivery in NNUs, functioning as an important coping resource. With a current global increase in premature births [48], webcam technology appears to offer an important solution to periods of enforced parent-infant separation in the early post-natal period.

Further work is however required, to assess cost-effectiveness. Also, if use of the technology is extended to the family home, following the mother's discharge, and when the baby remains in hospital, it is essential that its impact in this setting is evaluated. One small scale trial undertaken, to date, found that its use in this manner was feasible and acceptable and did not reduce the number of visits made by the parents to the NNU [18].

Abbreviations

NHS: National Health Service; NNU: Neonatal Unit; Ref: Reference; SIMD: Scottish index of multiple deprivation; UK: Uniting Kingdom; USA: United States of America

Acknowledgements

The *mylittleone* technology was developed by Integrated Care 24, England, UK, a not for profit 'gold' social enterprise. The setting up, use and evaluation of the *mylittleone* technology were facilitated by the Digital Health & Care Institute, Scotland, UK. We would like to thank the parents and professionals who participated in the study. We would also like to acknowledge the important contribution made by members of the project Steering Group.

Funding

The reported study is an independent evaluation funded by the Digital Health & Care Institute, Scotland, UK. The views expressed in the paper are those of the authors and do not necessarily reflect those of the funding body.

Authors' contributions

All authors contributed to the study's conception and design. CK recruited participants, collected and analysed the data. SK, RH and KMcP contributed to the peer review and interpretation of the data. SK lead on the drafting of the manuscript, with input from CK and KMcP. RH, JH, MB, SA critically reviewed the manuscript. All authors read and approved the final version of the manuscript.

Competing interests

The authors declare they have no competing interests.

Author details

[1]School of Health & Life Sciences, Glasgow Caledonian University, Cowcaddens Road, Glasgow G4 OBA, Scotland. [2]National Health Service (NHS) Greater Glasgow & Clyde, West House, Gartnavel Royal Hospital, 1055 Greater Western Road, Glasgow G12 0YN, Scotland. [3]School of Health and Social Care, Edinburgh Napier University, Sighthill Campus, Sighthill Court, Edinburgh EH11 4BN, Scotland. [4]Victoria Hospital, NHS Fife, Hayfield Road, Kirkcaldy KY2 5AH, Scotland.

References

1. Harrison W, Goodman D. Epidemiologic trends in neonatal intensive care, 2007-2012. JAMA Pediatr. 2015;169:855–62.
2. Royal College of Paediatrics and Child Health (RCPCH) Your baby's care: measuring standards and improving neonatal care. London: RCPCH;2015.
3. Obeidat HM, Bond EA, Callister LC. The parental experience of having an infant in the newborn intensive care unit. J Perinat Educ. 2009;18:23–9.
4. Sanders LM, Buckner EB. The newborn behavioural observation system as a nursing intervention to enhance engagement in first-time mothers: feasibility and desirability. Pediatr Nurs. 2006;32:455–9.
5. Pridham KF, Chang AS. Transition to being the mother of a new infant in the first 3 months: maternal problem solving and self-appraisals. J Adv Nurs. 1992;17:204–16.
6. Nelson AM. Transition to motherhood. J Obstet Gynecol Neonatal Nurs. 2003;32:465–77.
7. Shin H, White-Taut R. The conceptual structure of transition to motherhood in the neonatal intensive care unit. J Adv Nurs. 2006;58:90–8.
8. Aagaard H, Hall EOC. Mothers' experiences of having a preterm infant in the neonatal unit: a meta-synthesis. Int J Pediatr Nurs. 2008;23:e26–36.
9. Flacking R, Lehtonen L, Thomson G, Axelin A, Ahlqvist S, Moran VH, Ewald U, Dykes F. Closeness and separation in neonatal intensive care. Acta Paediatr. 2012;101:1032–7.
10. Borghini A, Pierrehumbert B, Miljkovictch R, Muller-Nix C, Forcada-Guex M, Ansermet F. Mothers' attachment representations of their premature infants at 6 and 18 months after birth. Infant Ment Health J. 2006;27:494–508.
11. Chinn R, Hall P, Daiches A. Fathers' experiences of their transitions to fatherhood: a metasynthesis. J Reprod Infant Psychol. 2011;29:4–18.
12. Pace CC, Spittle AJ, Molesworth CM, Lee KJ, Northam EA, Cheong JLY, Davis PG, Doyle LW, Treyvaud K, Anderson PJ. Evolution of depression and anxiety symptoms in parents of very preterm infants during the newborn period. JAMA Pediatr. 2016;170:863–70.
13. Feldman R, Eidelman AL, Sirota L, Weller A. Comparison of skin-to-skin (kangaroo) and traditional care: parenting outcomes and preterm infant development. Pediatr. 2002;110:16–26.
14. Ferber SG, Feldman R, Kohelet D, Kuint J, Dollberg S, Arbel E, Weller A. Massage therapy facilitates mother-infant interaction in preterm infants. Infant Behav Dev. 2005;28:74–81.
15. Freer Y, Lyon A, Stevenson B, Russell C. BabyLink – improving communication among clinicians and with parents with babies in intensive care. British Journal of Healthcare Computing and Information Management. 2005;22:34–6.
16. Rhoads SJ, Green AL, Lewis SD, Rakes L. Challenges of implementation of a web-camera system in the neonatal intensive care unit. Neonatal Netw. 2012;31:223–8.
17. Joshi A, Chyou P, Tirmizi Z, Gross J. Web camera use in the neonatal intensive care unit: impact on nursing workflow. Clin Med Res. 2015;14:1–6.
18. Yeo CL, Ho SKY, Khong KC, Lau YY. Virtual visitation in neonatal intensive care: experience with the use of internet and telemedicine in a tertiary neonatal unit. Perm J. 2011;15:32–6.
19. Hawkes GA, Livingstone V, Ryan CA, Dempsey EM. Perceptions of webcams in the neonatal intensice care unit: Here's looking at you kid! Am J Perinatol. 2015;32:131–6.
20. Kerr S, King C, Hogg R, McPherson K, Hanley J, Brierton M, Ainsworth S. Helping parents 'keep in touch' with their babies in the neonatal unit: evaluation of the *mylittleone* digital solution. Glasgow: Glasgow Caledonian University; 2016.
21. Webster A. Innovative health technologies and the social: redefining health, medicine and the body. Curr Sociol. 2002;50:443–58.
22. Cresswell K, Sheikh A. Organizational issues in the implementation and adaption of health information technology innovations: an interpretive review. Int J Med Inform. 2013;82:e73–86.
23. Webster A. Health, technology and society: a sociological critique. Basingstoke: Palgrave Macmillan; 2007.
24. McEvoy R, Richards D, McEvoy P. Critical realism: a way forward for evaluation research in nursing. J Adv Nursing. 2003;2003(43):411–20.
25. Sayer A. Realism and social science. London: Sage; 2000.
26. Benton T, Craib I. Philosophy of social science. Hampshire: Palgrave; 2001.
27. Byrne M. Sampling for qualitative research. AORN. 2001;73:497–8.
28. Braun V, Clarke V. Using thematic analysis in psychology. Qual Res Psychol. 2006;3:77–101.
29. Timmermans S, Tavory I. Theory construction in qualitative research: from grounded theory to abductive analysis. Sociol Theory. 2012;30:167–86.
30. Klauss MH, Kennell JH. The impact of early separation or loss on family development. CV Mosby: St. Louis; 1976.
31. Crouch M, Maderson L. The social life of bonding theory. Soc Sci Med. 1995; 41:837–44.
32. Feldman R, Weller A, Leckman JF, Kuint J, Eidelman AI. The nature of the mother's tie to her infant: maternal bonding under conditions of proximity, separation and potential loss. J Child Psychol Psychiatry. 1999;40:929–39.
33. Lehoux P. The problem of health technology: policy implications for modern health care systems. London; Routledge. 2006;
34. Brockington IF, Aucamp HM, Fraser C. Severe disorders of the mother–infant relationship: definitions and frequency. Arch Women's Mental Health. 2006; 9:243–51.
35. Bowlby J. Attachment and loss. New York: Basic Books; 1969.
36. Kennell JH, Klauss MH. Bonding: recent observations that alter perinatal care. Pediatr Rev. 1998;19:4–12.
37. Goulet C, Bell L, Tribble D, Paul D, Lang A. A concept analysis of parent-infant attachment. J Adv Nurs. 1998;28:1071–81.
38. Bowlby J. Attachment and loss: separation. New York: Basic Books; 1973.
39. Bienfait M, Maury M. Haquet, Faillie JL, franc N, comes C, Daude H, Picaud JC, Rideau a, Cambonie G. Pertinence of the self-report mother-to-infant bonding scale in the neonatal unit of a maternity ward. Early Hum Dev. 2011;87:281–7.
40. Holditch-Davis D, Miles MS. Mothers' stories about their experiences in the neonatal intensive care unit. Neonatal Network. 2000;19:13–21.
41. Cleveland LM. Parenting in the neonatal intensive care unit. J Obstet Gynecol Neonatal Nurs. 2008;37:666–91.
42. Brown S, Lumley J. Physical health problems after childbirth and maternal depression at six to seven months postpartum. British J Obstet Gynaecol. 2000;107:1194–201.
43. Grassley JS, Clark M, Schlies J. An institutional ethnography of nurses' support of breastfeeding. J Obstet Gynecol Neonatal Nurs. 2015;44:567–77.
44. Higgins I, Dullow A. Parental perceptions of having a baby in the neonatal intensive care unit. Pediatr Child Health Nursing. 2003;6:15–20.
45. Lazarus R, Folkman S. Stress, appraisal and coping. New York: Springer; 1984.
46. Kerr SM. An exploration of parental coping and adaptation following the birth of a child with a congenital limb deficiency. Glasgow: Glasgow Caledonian University; 2004.
47. Polit DF, Beck CT. Generalisation in quantitative and qualitative research: myths and strategies. Int J Nurs Stud. 2010;47:1451–8.
48. World Health Organization (WHO). Born too soon. The global action report on preterm birth. Geneva: WHO; 2012.
49. Scottish Government. Scottish index of multiple deprivation. Scottish Government: Edinburgh; 2010.

6

Reduced glutathione and glutathione disulfide in the blood of glucose-6-phosphate dehydrogenase-deficient newborns

Zhen-hua Gong[1*], Guo-li Tian[2], Qi-wei Huang[3], Yan-min Wang[2] and Hong-ping Xu[2]

Abstract

Background: Glucose-6-phosphate dehydrogenase (G6PD) deficiency is commonly detected during mass screening for neonatal disease. We developed a method to measure reduced glutathione (GSH) and glutathione disulfide (GSSG) using tandem mass spectrometry (MS/MS) for detecting G6PD deficiency.

Methods: The concentration of GSH and the GSH/GSSG ratio in newborn dry-blood-spot (DBS) screening and in blood plus sodium citrate for test confirmation were examined by MS/MS using labeled glycine as an internal standard.

Results: G6PD-deficient newborns had a lower GSH content (242.9 ± 15.9 μmol/L)and GSH/GSSG ratio (14.9 ± 7.2) than neonatal controls (370.0 ± 53.2 μmol/L and 46.7 ± 19.6, respectively). Although the results showed a significance of $P < 0.001$ for DBS samples plus sodium citrate that were examined the first day after preparation, there were no significant differences in the mean GSH concentration and GSH/GSSG ratio between the G6PD deficiency-positive and negative groups when examined three days after sample preparation.

Conclusion: The concentration of GSH and the ratio of GSH/GSSG in blood measured using MS/MS on the first day of sample preparation are consistent with G6PD activity and are helpful for diagnosing G6PD deficiency.

Keywords: Glucose-6-phosphate dehydrogenase deficiency, Blood, Glutathione, Tandem mass spectrometry

Background

Glucose-6-phosphate dehydrogenase (G6PD) deficiency, an X-chromosome-linked genetic disorder, is the most prevalent mutation in humans, affecting more than 400 million people worldwide [1]. This disorder is characterized by decreased activity of the G6PD enzyme, which is the central factor of the antioxidant defense system in red blood cells (RBCs). The enzyme is responsible for maintaining high levels of reduced glutathione (GSH) and nicotine adenine dinucleotide phosphate (NADPH), which protect the cell from the oxidative damage caused by reactive oxygen species. Because G6PD-deficient RBCs are unable to generate NADPH through other pathways, these cells lack the ability to tolerate excessive amounts of oxidative stress [2, 3]. The most common clinical manifestation associated with G6PD deficiency is hemolytic anemia, which is generally triggered by the intake of oxidative drugs or foods. Occasionally, the defect can result in such complications as kidney failure, severe neonatal jaundice, or gallstones, and may require blood transfusion [4].

The diagnosis of G6PD deficiency is commonly based on the results of a fluorescent spot test for NADPH generation and a quantitative spectrophotometric assay of G6PD activity. Although these tests provide some perspective on the severity of a patient's clinical symptoms, they are based on measurements of G6PD specific activity under normal conditions, and do not reflect the status of the patient's antioxidant defense system, predominantly GSH/glutathione disulfide (GSSG). Furthermore, such tests also do not

* Correspondence: gongzh1963@163.net
[1]Department of general surgery, Shanghai Children's Hospital, Shanghai Jiao Tong University, road, West Lane 1400, number 24. Shanghai, Beijing 200040, China
Full list of author information is available at the end of the article

specifically predict the dynamic response of metabolite and enzyme activity levels in RBCs during the intake of oxidative agents. Indeed, not all G6PD-deficient patients detected via neonatal screening will develop neonatal jaundice or hemolytic anemia, even when oxidative drugs or foods are consumed [4, 5].

GSH is the major low molecular weight thiol in cells, with intracellular concentrations typically in the millimolar range. GSH acts as a recyclable antioxidant through the formation of glutathione disulfide (GSSG) and subsequent enzymatic reduction by glutathione reductase. Due to its relatively high concentration within cells and favorable reaction rates, GSH is a strong antioxidant in vivo [6]. All of the reduced GSH present in plasma (and other extracellular fluids) is of intracellular origin. However, the physiological pathways that regulate the supply of GSH to extracellular fluids are complex, as several organs may contribute to extracellular GSH to varying extents [7, 8]. RBCs can synthesize GSH from cysteine, glycine, and glutamic acid because these cells contain all of the enzymes necessary for GSH biosynthesis, and a significant percentage of RBC GSH is produced de novo daily, significantly contributing to the plasma pool of GSH [9]. Although plasma lacks reductases and coenzymes, such as NADPH, that provide reducing equivalents to reduce disulfides to thiols [10], both GSSG and glutathione conjugates (GS-X) are actively exported from RBCs when their intracellular concentration is high [11, 12]. This de novo re-synthesis may balance GSH loss due to GSSG and GS-X export and is regulated by a feedback mechanism [13].

Changes in redox state are commonly used as an index of oxidative stress within biological systems, and numerous methods have been established to quantify GSH and GSSG levels. The majority of techniques use reverse-phase chromatography for separation, with detection is based on the UV absorbance of the compound or the fluorescence of an adduct [14]; liquid chromatography coupled with mass spectrometric detection is also utilized to assay a variety of biological sources [15–17]. However, no tandem mass spectrometry (MS/MS) method that is suitable for screening or detecting G6PD deficiency is available for the quantification of these compounds in the blood. In the present study, we developed a high throughput MS/MS method for diagnosing G6PD deficiency in patients using dry-blood-spot (DBS) samples.

Materials and methods

Materials

GSH was obtained from AMRESCO (Solon, OH, USA). NeoBase non-derivatized MS/MS kits were purchased from PerkinElmer (Boston, MA, USA) and included isotopically labeled glycine (^{15}N, 2-^{13}C-glycinem, 762.2 μmol/l as the working solution) as an internal standard. The DBS extraction solution and the flow solvent were composed of methanol(1000 ml),water (2 ml), and formic acid(0.2 mmol/L).

The endogenous concentration of GSH in whole blood by this method is as low as 200 μmol/L, and as high as 500 μmol/L. The GSH recovery test samples were prepared with the extraction solution. GSH was added to vials containing 0.1 ml of extraction solution to produce GSH concentrations of 0,200,400,600,800,1000,2000,and 4000 μmol/L. All of the samples were dropped onto S&S Grade 903 filter paper using a 100-μl pipette without overlap, dried at room temperature, prepared in dry-spot, and stored at 4 °C until the MS/MS analysis.

Methods

The blood samples for newborn G6PD screening, including 12 positive and 623 negative, were collected by puncturing the heel on the third to seventh day of age. The blood was dropped directly onto S&S Grade 903 filter paper without overlapped by another drop of blood and dried at room temperature. The DBS samples were transferred to our newborn screening center and stored for 2 to 4 days at 4 °C. A quantitative spectrophotometric assay of G6PD activity was used for G6PD deficiency screening (Neonatal G6PD KIT, PerkinElmer Life and Analytical Sciences; WallacOy, Turku, Finland).

Thirty seven blood samples were collected from the veins of neonates who tested positive during the G6PD screening (These 37 samples were not all from the 12 babies above, other patients were added). Thirty seven control blood samples from their parents and from 21 neonates control without G6PD deficiency were also intravenous collected. In each case, the blood was drawn into a tube containing sodium citrate as an anticoagulant and mixed immediately. The blood samples were transferred to the laboratory within 3 h and dropped onto S&S Grade 903 filter paper using a 100-μl pipette without overlap and dried at room temperature for 6–24 h until examination by MS/MS. The G6PD activity for the confirmation test was measured immediately when the blood arrived at the laboratory using a method that measures the G6PD/6-phosphogluconate dehydrogenase (6PGD) ratio [18]. The clinical and neonatal samples were obtained from maternity hospitals and the Children's Hospital of Shanghai. This study approved by the ethics committee of the participating hospitals.

We extracted GSH and GSSG, use with one 3 mm DBS disk per analysis, using 100 μl extraction solution containing isotopically labeled glycine working solution (11:1) per sample in 96-well plate (NUNC),incubating in 45 °C, shaking at 700 rpm for 45 min. The extractions were transfer to another 96-well plate for mass spectrometry analyses.

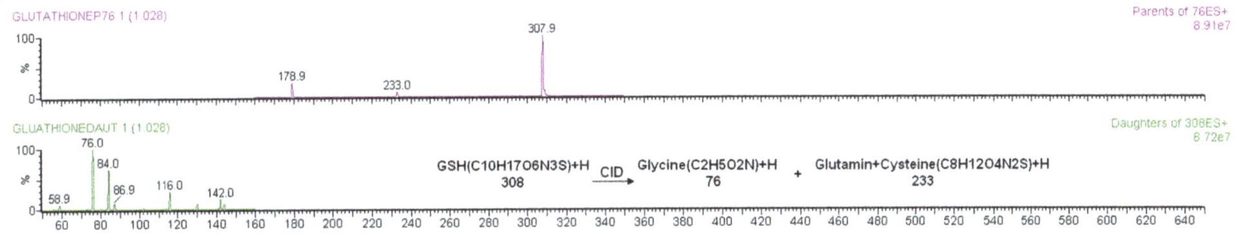

Fig. 1 The MS/MS fragment ions assumed and fragment generated by collision-induced dissociation of GSH. The MS scans of the GSH solution show a peak at m/z 307.9(GSH307+H1). The product scan of m/z 308 shows a peak at m/z 76 (glycine75+H1$^+$)

Mass spectrometry analyses were performed using a Waters MICROMASS Quattro micro™API, (Manchester, UK). The electrospray needle was maintained at +3.5 kV, and the desolvation temperature was set to 350 °C. The desolvation gas flow was 650 L/Hr, the cone potential was 30 V, the collision energy was 3.0 eV, and the dwell time was 50 ms. Nitrogen, the sheath gas, was set at 50 units. The collision gas used was argon. The temperature of the heated capillary was maintained at 120 °C. GSH and GSSG were quantified in multi-reaction-monitor (MRM) mode using positive electrospray ionization mass spectrometry. The strongest MRM signals for GSH and GSSG were selected for quantification. Their fragment ions assumed and generated by collision-induced dissociation of the [GSH + H] $^+$ (Fig. 1)and [GSSG + Na]$^+$ions (Fig. 2) were observed in product scans. The settings (precursor ion → fragment ion) for the target analytes were GSH m/z 308.0 → 76 and GSSG m/z 636.8 → 330. The setting for the isotopically labeled internal standard ^{15}N, 2-^{13}C-glycine was m/z 78 → 32 [19, 20]. The samples were delivered using an HPLC pump (Waters 1525 μBinary, MA, USA) equipped with a 20-μl sample loop. The samples were run at 116 μl/min from 0 to 0.23 min, at 20 μl/min from 0.24 to 1.35 min, and at 600 μl/min from 1.36 to 1.7 min. The concentration was calculated using Masslynx software, version 4.0 (Waters, Milford, MA, USA) by combining the intensities of the m/z 308.3 → 76 peak for GSH, the m/z 636.8 → 330 peak for GSSG, and the m/z 78 → 32 peak for the internal standard (^{15}N, 2-^{13}C-glycine) from 0.4 to 1.3 min, as measured as peak areas, for each sample. The serum concentrations were determined using the following formula: GSH = hematocrit × coefficient × Intensity m/z 308.3 → 76/78 → 32 + parameter; GSSG = hematocrit × coefficient × Intensity m/z 636.8 → 330/78 → 32.

All analyses were performed with SPSS 19.0 (SPSS Inc. Chicago, IL, USA). Differences of mean were tested by the one-way ANOVA among three groups and by independent *t* test between two groups. Significance was accepted at a *P* value of ≤0.05. Linear regression of the GSH/glycine-IS peak area ratio vs. the concentration of GSH added, and the ROC Curve of GSH/GSSG ratios to predict G6PD deficiency were done.

Results

MS/MS of GSH and GSSG

Based on the MS results for the product and precursor scans of the GSH (Fig. 1)and GSSG solutions (Fig. 2), we decided to use an MRM of m/z 308.0 → 76 for GSH, m/z 636.8 → 330 for GSSG, and m/z 78 → 32 for isotopically labeled glycine (^{15}N, 2-^{13}C-glycine) as an internal standard. We also combined the intensity of scans as the peak area for each analyte.

Linearity

Calibration curves were obtained by linear regression based on a plot of the GSH/glycine internal standard peak-area ratio(x) vs. the concentration(y) of added GSH (Fig. 3). The concentration range used for the added GSH was 200–4000 μmol/L. The slope was 570 μmol/L, the intercept was 200 μmol/L, and the squared correlation coefficient was 0.994, $p < 0.0001$. We used the formula Y = 762 μmol/L × intensitym/z 308.3 → 76/

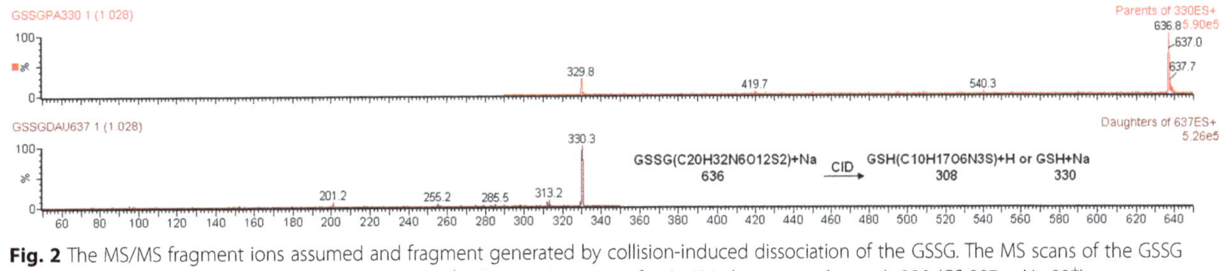

Fig. 2 The MS/MS fragment ions assumed and fragment generated by collision-induced dissociation of the GSSG. The MS scans of the GSSG solution show a peak at m/z 636.8 (GSSG613 + Na23$^+$). The product scan of m/z 636 shows a peak at m/z 330 (GS 307 + Na 23$^+$)

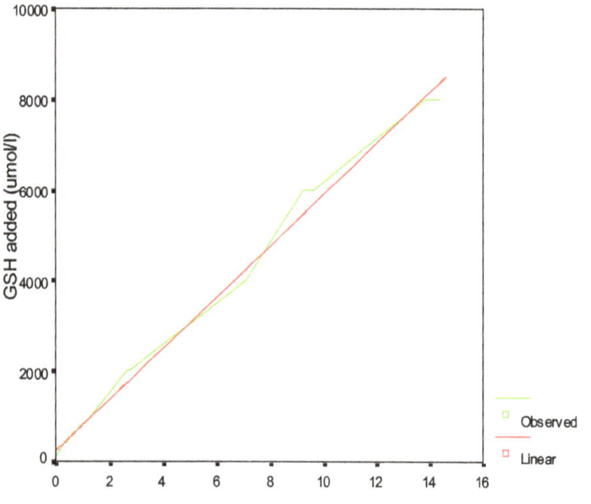

Fig. 3 Linear regression of the GSH/glycine-IS peak area ratio vs. the concentration of GSH added

78 → 32 + 200 μmol/L(hematocrit0.5 is assumed)to calculate the concentrations of GSH in the blood samples. The value used to represent GSH/GSSG was the peak area ratio of these compounds.

Precision, accuracy, and recovery

The recoveries of GSH added DBSs were determined at nine concentrations and were found to be in the range 90 to 126% for GSH in the concentration range 200–4000 μmol/L (Table 1) when examined on the first day (within 24 h) after sample preparation. However, the GSH recovery gradually decreased when the samples were examined on the second day and thereafter (Table 1).

GSH and GSH/GSSG in confirmed G6PD-deficient newborns

The confirmed G6PD-deficient newborns had lower blood levels of GSH and lower GSH/GSSG ratios than the neonatal and parental controls (Table 2). All the blood samples for confirming test contained sodium citrate were prepared in DBS and examined on the first day. The parents should carry the allele conferring G6PD deficiency, and some exhibited decreased, albeit only slightly, G6PD activity, led to the GSH concentrations and GSH/GSSG ratios in the parent group were higher than patient group and lower than the normal control group.

On the ROC Curve for GSH/GSSG ratios predicting G6PD deficiency, the area under the curve was 0.679, $p = 0.003$. GSH/GSSG ratios lower than 30 was used as cut-off value to determine state of oxidative stress, which caused by G6PD-deficiency in newborns, the sensitivity is 91.9%; and 1-speficity is 79.3%.

GSH levels and GSH/GSSG ratios in newborns screening positively for G6PD deficiency

The GSH levels and GSH/GSSG ratios in DBS samples are routinely examined in neonatal disease screening by combining the detection of amino acids and acylcarnitines using MS/MS. These DBS samples were prepared in maternity hospitals without the use of sodium citrate and examined at least three days after collection. The activity of G6PD in the DBS samples was examined on the second day after the GSH levels were examined using MS/MS. The activity of G6PD was positively correlated to the GSH/GSSG ratio ($R = 0.213$, $p < 0.001$ $n = 278$), though no significant positive relationship with the GSH content was observed ($R = 0.027$, $p > 0.05$, $n = 278$). However, there were no significant differences in the mean GSH concentrations and the GSH/GSSG ratios between the G6PD deficiency-positive group and the G6PD deficiency-negative group (Table 3).

Discussion

Human blood contains GSH, and in addition to diet and aging, many pathological conditions influence the GSH concentration [21, 22]. The whole blood and plasma concentrations of GSH differ, and the concentrations

Table 1 Recoveries and precision of GSH measured on the 1st and 3rd days after sample preparation

	Day 1 (n = 6)			Day 3 (n = 6)	
GSH Added (μmol/L)	GSH Measured (μmol/L)	CV %	GSH Recovery (%)	GSH Measured (μmol/L)	GSH Recovery (%)
0	213.2 ± 7.0	3.2		207.7 ± 3.62	
100	211.6 ± 1.4	0.6		208.4 ± 1.12	
200	253.4 ± 9.2	3.6	126.7 ± 4.6	214.7 ± 5.1	107.3 ± 2.6
400	397.9 ± 27.4	6.8	99.5 ± 6.8	257.3 ± 5.7	64.3 ± 1.4
600	584.3 ± 41.3	7.0	97.5 ± 6.9	345.4 ± 17.2	57.5 ± 2.8
800	726.5 ± 13.1	1.8	90.8 ± 1.6	488.6 ± 14.4	61.0 ± 1.8
1000	939.4 ± 6.0	0.6	93.9 ± 0.6	678.9 ± 16.5	67.9 ± 1.6
2000	1748.8 ± 27.4	1.5	87.4 ± 1.4	1574.8 ± 121.9	78.74 ± 6.10
4000	4234.6 ± 6.4	0.2	105.9 ± 0.2	3745.1 ± 488.4	93.6 ± 12.2

Table 2 The GSH content and GSH/GSSG ratios in confirmed G6PD-deficient newborns, neonatal controls, and parental controls

	Number	GSH (μmol/L)	GSH/GSSG
G6PD-deficient newborn	37	242.9 ± 15.9	14.9 ± 7.2
Neonatal control	21	370.0 ± 53.2	46.7 ± 19.6
Parental control	37	287.5 ± 48.2	27.3 ± 16.1
P		0.001	0.001

measured differ within the same group of people depend on the method used [23–26]. We found whole blood GSH concentrations to be 100–500 μmol/L, which is 100 times higher than in plasma and approximately half the GSH concentration found in red blood cells (data not shown). Although consistent with another study [26], the values obtained in this study were slightly lower than those found by some other studies [22, 25]. This discrepancy might have occurred because our samples were collected from neonates or adults with alleles conferring G6PD deficiency; further, we only selected the MRM m/z 308.3 → 76 peak to detect GSH and combined the MRM signals rather than the GSH peak area. This simplified method made it possible to combine the neonatal disease screening system for detecting amino acids and acylcarnitines with MS/MS.

GSH is an unstable molecule. We used labeled glycine (^{15}N, 2-^{13}C-glycine m/z 78 → 32) rather than labeled GSH as an internal standard. The Glycine + H^+fragmentis an ion that is generated by the collision-induced dissociation of GSH, and stable labeled glycine can more accurately reflect unstable GSH levels. The observed recovery of GSH levels decreased gradually after the GSH samples were prepared, which has also been reported by other studies that used reagents to ensure that GSH was not oxidized to GSSG or other GS-X compounds [27]. In our study, the GSH levels in blood that was mixed with sodium citrate (an anticoagulant) were more stable than those in blood collected by newborn heel puncture without the use of anticoagulant. This finding may be one of the reasons why the GSH measured in the neonatal screening DBS sample did not reflect the activity of the G6PD enzyme; indeed, the DBS samples were usually measured at least three days after they were collected.

Table 3 G6PD activity, GSH levels, and GSH/GSSG ratios in test samples from newborns that screened positive or negative for G6PD deficiency

Screening for G6PD deficiency	Number	G6PD activity	GSH (μmol/L)	GSH/GSSG ratio
Positive	12	1.12 ± 0.55	376.6 ± 56.3	44.5 ± 19.5
Negative	623	4.59 ± 1.39	413.6 ± 84.5	52.8 ± 20.9
P		0.001	0.13	0.17

A decrease in the levels of GSH, the reduced form of glutathione, which was accompanied by an increase in the basal level of GSSG, has been correlated to a lower susceptibility of RBCs to osmotic hemolysis [5, 28]. The ratio of GSH/GSSG measured in blood is different from that measured in other tissues and also differs depending on the technique [17, 23, 27]. In our study, the ratio of GSH/GSSG in whole blood was 10–100 times higher than that observed in other reports. One reason for this discrepancy is that we did not use an antioxidant to treat the sample. The GSH/GSSG ratio in the whole blood (with added sodium citrate) of the G6PD deficiency group was lower than that of their parents, and the latter was lower than that of the normal neonatal group. These findings indicate that the ratio of GSH/GSSG can be correlated to the activity of G6PD in blood that contains sodium citrate and is examined on the first day of sample preparation. Therefore, we can use MS/MS to measure GSH/GSSG ratios to confirm G6PD deficiency or predict that patients are more likely to suffer from hemolytic anemia because they already have a lower antioxidant status.

Conclusion

The concentration of GSH and the ratio of GSH/GSSG in the blood, as measured using MS/MS on the first day of sample preparation, are consistent with the G6PD activity and are helpful for diagnosing G6PD deficiency.

Abbreviations

DBS: dry-blood-spot; G6PD: Glucose-6-phosphate dehydrogenase; GSH: reduced glutathione; GSSG: glutathione disulfide; MS/MS: tandem mass spectrometry

Acknowledgements

We are appreciated the staffs of the neonatal screening center and clinical laboratory, who gave us help to do this study.

Funding

This study was supported by the Science and Technology Commission of Shanghai Municipality (134119a4000), which will pay for the article-processing charge. They have no influence on the results.

Authors' contributions

ZG have made substantial contributions to conception and design, acquisition of data, analysis and interpretation of data, drafting the manuscript. GT carried out mass screening for G6PD studies. QW was in charge of diagnosis and treatment for patients with G6PD. YW and HX carried out the molecular genetic studies and screening test and affirming test for G6PD. All authors read and approved the final manuscript.

Competing interests

We have no competing interests in authorship or with other groups and government who support this study.

Author details

[1]Department of general surgery, Shanghai Children's Hospital, Shanghai Jiao Tong University, road, West Lane 1400, number 24. Shanghai, Beijing 200040, China. [2]Neonatal screening center, Shanghai Children's Hospital, Shanghai Jiao Tong University, Shanghai, China. [3]Department of neonatology, Shanghai Children's Hospital, Shanghai Jiao Tong University, Shanghai, China.

References

1. Cappellini MD, Fiorelli G. Glucose-6-phosphate dehydrogenase deficiency. Lancet. 2008;371(9606):64–74.
2. Arese P, Gallo V, Pantaleo A, Turrini F. Life and death of glucose-6-phosphate dehydrogenase (G6PD) deficient erythrocytes - role of redox stress and band 3 modifications. Transfus Med Hemother. 2012;39(5):328–34.
3. van Zwieten R, Verhoeven AJ, Roos D. Inborn defects in the antioxidant systems of human red blood cells. Free Radic Biol Med. 2014;67:377–86.
4. Mason PJ, Bautista JM, Gilsanz F. G6PD deficiency: The genotype-phenotype association. Blood rev. 2007;21(5):267–83.
5. Shimo H, Nishino T, Tomita M. Predicting the kinetic properties associated with redox imbalance after oxidative crisis in G6PD-deficient erythrocytes: a simulation study. Adv Hematol. 2011;2011:398945.
6. Winterbourn CC. Reconciling the chemistry and biology of reactive oxygen species. Nat Chem Biol. 2008;4(5):278–86.
7. Garibotto G, Sofia A, Saffioti S, et al. Interorgan exchange of aminothiols in humans. Am J Physiol Endocrinol Metab. 2003;284(4):E757–63.
8. Dass PD, Bermes EW Jr, Holmes EW. Renal and hepatic output of glutathione in plasma and whole blood. Biochim Biophys Acta. 1992; 1156(1):99–102.
9. Giustarini D, Milzani A, Dalle-Donne I, Rossi R. Red blood cells as a physiological source of glutathione for extracellular fluids. Blood Cells Mol Dis. 2008;40(2):174–9.
10. Kalinina EV, Chernov NN, Novichkova MD. Role of glutathione, glutathione transferase, and glutaredoxin in regulation of redox-dependent processes. Biochemistry (Mosc). 2014;79(13):1562–83.
11. Rossi R, Milzani A, Dalle-Donne I, et al. Different metabolizing ability of thiol reactants in human and rat blood: biochemical and pharmacological implications. J Biol Chem. 2001;276(10):7004–10.
12. Cakir Y, Yildiz D. Efflux of glutathione and glutathione complexes from human erythrocytes in response to vanadate. Blood Cells Mol Dis. 2013;50(1):1–7.
13. Ellison I, Richie JP Jr. Mechanisms of glutathione disulfide efflux from erythrocytes. Biochem Pharmacol. 2012;83(1):164–9.
14. Sakhi AK, Blomhoff R, Gundersen TE. Simultaneous and trace determination of reduced and oxidizedglutathione in minute plasma samples using dual mode fluorescence detection and column switching high performance liquid chromatography. J Chromatogr A. 2007;1142(2):1.
15. Rellán-Alvarez R, Hernández LE, Abadía J, Alvarez-Fernández A. Direct and simultaneous determination of reduced and oxidized glutathione and homoglutathione by liquid chromatography-electrospray/mass spectrometry in plant tissue extracts. Anal Biochem. 2006;356(2):254–64.
16. Zhu P, Oe T, Blair IA. Determination of cellular redox status by stable isotope dilution liquid chromatography/mass spectrometry analysis of glutathione and glutathione disulfide. Rapid Commun Mass Spectrom. 2008; 22(4):432–40.
17. Harwood DT, Kettle AJ, Brennan S, Winterbourn CC. Simultaneousdetermination of reduced glutathione, glutathione disulfide and glutathionesulphonamide in cells and physiological fluids by isotope dilution liquid chromatography-tandem mass spectrometry. J Chromatogr B Analyt Technol Biomed Life Sci. 2009;877(28):3393–9.
18. Yan JB, Xu HP, Xiong C, et al. Rapid and reliable detection of glucose-6-phosphate dehydrogenase (G6PD) gene mutations in Han Chinese using high-resolution melting analysis. J Mol Diagn. 2010;12(3):305–11.
19. Piraud M, Vianey-Saban C, Petritis K, et al. ESI-MS/MS analysis of underivatised amino acids: a new tool for the diagnosis of inherited disorders of amino acid metabolism. Fragmentation study of 79 molecules of biological interest in positive and negative ionisation mode. Rapid Commun Mass Spectrom. 2003;17(12):1297–311.
20. Gong ZH, Tian GL, Huang QW, et al. Quantification of total hexose on dry blood spot by tandem mass spectrometry. Clin Biochem. 2012;45(18):1673–7.
21. Giustarini D, Dalle-Donne I, Lorenzini S, et al. Age-related influence on thiol, disulfide, and protein-mixed disulfide levels in human plasma. J Gerontol A Biol Sci Med Sci. 2006;61(10):1030–8.
22. Moriarty-Craige SE, Jones DP. Extracellular thiols and thiol/disulfide redox in metabolism. Annu Rev Nutr. 2004;24:481–509.
23. Johnson JM, Strobel FH, Reed M, et al. A rapid LC-FTMS method for the analysis of cysteine, cystine and cysteine/cystine steady-state redox potential in human plasma. Clin Chim Acta. 2008;396(1–2):43–8.
24. Squellerio I, Caruso D, Porro B, et al. Direct glutathione quantification in human blood by LC-MS/MS: comparison with HPLC with electrochemical detection. J Pharm Biomed Anal. 2012;71:111–8.
25. Steghens JP, Flourié F, Arab K, Collombel C. Fast liquid chromatography-mass spectrometry glutathione measurement in whole blood: micromolar GSSG is a sample preparation artifact. J Chromatogr B Analyt Technol Biomed Life Sci. 2003;798(2):343–9.
26. Feng CH, Huang HY, Lu CY. Quantitation of the glutathione in human peripheral blood by matrix-assisted laser desorption ionization time-of-flight mass spectrometry coupled with micro-scale derivatization. Anal Chim Acta. 2011;690(2):209–14.
27. Monostori P, Wittmann G, Karg E, Túri S. Determination of glutathione and glutathione disulfide in biological samples: an in-depth review. J Chromatogr B Analyt Technol Biomed Life Sci. 2009;877(28):3331–46.
28. Rossi R, Giustarini D, Milzani A, Dalle-Donne I. Membrane skeletal protein S-glutathionylation and hemolysis in human red blood cells. Blood Cells Mol Dis. 2006;37(3):180–7.

7

Umbilical cord bilirubin as a predictor of neonatal jaundice

Kelsey D. J. Jones[1,2], S E. Grossman[3], Dharshini Kumaranayakam[3], Arati Rao[1,3], Greg Fegan[4] and Narendra Aladangady[1,3*]

Abstract

Background: Hyperbilirubinaemia is a major cause of neonatal morbidity. Early identification of those infants most at risk might allow the development of targeted primary preventative therapy and follow-up. The objective of this study was to assess whether arterial umbilical cord bilirubin (aUCB) level at delivery predicts the development of neonatal jaundice in term deliveries.

Methods: Retrospective analysis of hospital biochemistry records identified term deliveries with recorded aUCB. Infant medical records were reviewed to identify those who developed neonatal hyperbilirubinaemia (requiring treatment according to UK NICE guidelines) with/without a positive direct antiglobulin test (DAT).

Results: Of 1411 term deliveries with a clearly recorded aUCB, 30 infants developed clinically-significant jaundice (2.7%), of whom 8 were DAT + ve (0.6%) mostly due to ABO incompatibility. aUCB strongly predicted the development of DAT + ve jaundice (area under the ROC curve = 0.996), as well as all-cause jaundice (area under the ROC curve = 0.74). However, this effect was critically dependent on maternal blood group. Amongst infants at risk of ABO incompatibility (maternal blood groups O + ve/O-ve, 39.7%) the predictive value of aUCB for all cause jaundice was strengthened (area under the ROC curve = 0.88). Amongst those not at risk (defined maternal blood group not O + ve/O-ve, 51.0%) it disappeared completely (area under the ROC curve = 0.46). A cutoff of 35 μmol/l for mothers with blood group O + ve/O-ve increased the pre-test probability for all-cause jaundice of 4% to a post-test probability of 30%.

Conclusions: For infants of mothers with blood group O, aUCB predicts development of neonatal jaundice. There was no evident utility for infants of mothers with other blood groups. Estimation of aUCB should be considered as a strategy for early identification of those at risk of neonatal haemolytic jaundice.

Keywords: Neonatology, Jaundice, Haematology

Background

Hyperbilirubinaemia is one of the commonest causes of admission to hospital in the neonatal period amongst term babies in all settings [1–3]. Prevention of serious complications depends on effective early treatment, but clinically significant jaundice may not develop until one or more days after delivery. Current practice, which usually promotes early discharge after delivery, may introduce delays in recognition and initiation of medical therapy [4, 5]. Identification of biomarkers that could be measured within a few hours following birth, which robustly predict incident jaundice, would represent a significant advance.

Estimation of umbilical cord blood bilirubin (UCB) at delivery is practicable, cheap and non-invasive. It could be easily integrated with the current trend towards routine umbilical cord blood biochemical evaluation practiced in many centres. Several previous studies have investigated the potential utility of UCB estimation in predicting subsequent hyperbilirubinaemia [6–12]. Results have been inconsistent, and a review by the UK National Institute for

* Correspondence: n.aladangady@nhs.net
[1]Neonatal Unit, Homerton University Hospital NHS Foundation Trust, London, UK
[3]Barts and the London School of Medicine & Dentistry, Queen Mary, University of London, London, UK
Full list of author information is available at the end of the article

Health and Care Excellence (NICE) concluded that it was not a useful index of risk [13].

In this study we exploited the fact that at our institution UCB estimation is routine, and performed a retrospective analysis to assess the potential utility of arterial umbilical cord bilirubin (aUCB) in predicting clinically significant hyperbilirubinaemia, and hyperbilirubinaemia due to neonatal haemolytic disease.

Methods

Homerton University Hospital is an inner-London District General Hospital providing maternity care to one of the most economically deprived areas in the UK. The local population is ethnically diverse, with large Afro-Caribbean, Turkish, and Orthodox Jewish communities. The obstetric unit is a local referral centre with approximately 5000 deliveries annually, 9% of which are below 2.5 kg. The delivery unit combines midwife and obstetric-led care, and is equipped with a GEM4000 whole blood analyzer, which is operated by delivery suite staff and used for umbilical cord gas analysis at delivery. For this project we have exploited the fact that it is departmental policy to perform umbilical cord gas analysis on all obstetric-led deliveries, and that the GEM4000 automatically provides total bilirubin estimation on such samples.

From an electronic database backup of the delivery unit whole blood analyzer, we extracted data on all samples processed in the 9 months from February to November 2010. We used the hospital case number and date of birth to identify and group all samples belonging to a single individual (mother), and used these data to interrogate the electronic patient records of each mother and infant pair.

Because it is well recognised that paired umbilical cord blood samples are frequently mislabelled, we only considered samples to be a true arterial cord blood sample if there was another sample with the same hospital case number processed within 30 min, with a pH that was higher by >0.02. This accounts for the fact that umbilical cord veins are easier to sample than arteries such that where a single or two identical samples are received they are most likely to be venous regardless of how they have been labelled [14].

We recorded clinical and demographic factors including maternal blood group (in the UK all pregnant women are offered prenatal blood group analysis to assess for risk of Rhesus-incompatibility disease), gestation at delivery (estimated by dating ultrasound scan or last menstrual period), the infant's sex and birthweight. We recorded maternal ethnicity because of ethnically-defined differences in some causes of neonatal jaundice (e.g. glucose-6-phosphate dehydrogenase deficiency (G6PD)). Electronic notes and blood test results from the delivery admission and any subsequent readmissions were scanned by two experienced paediatricians (KJ and AR, who were blinded to the aUBC level) in order to identify all infants who developed clinically significant jaundice. This was defined as a single total bilirubin result above the phototherapy treatment threshold on charts from the UK's NICE Guideline on Neonatal Jaundice [13]. We scanned electronic neonatal notes and cross-checked with separate laboratory databases to record positive direct antiglobulin tests (DAT) and low glucose-6-phosphate dehydrogenase levels for each term infant with an arterial cord blood sample.

Single variable logistic regression (for continuous or ordinal variables) or chi-squared (for categorical variables) analyses were performed to screen for association with clinically significant neonatal jaundice, and with DAT-positive (haemolytic) neonatal jaundice. Variables demonstrating significant associations ($p < 0.05$) were included in a multivariable analysis. Receiver operator characteristic (ROC) curves were plotted. Subgroup analyses was performed amongst those mothers with either O-ve or O + ve blood groups (whose infants are at risk of ABO incompatibility haemolytic disease), and mothers with a defined blood group that was neither O-ve or O + ve (whose infants are not at risk of ABO incompatibility). In our setting ABO incompatibility is the commonest cause of haemolytic jaundice. Analysis was performed in Stata version 11.0.

The study was reviewed and approved by the UK National Research Ethics Service (NRES) Committee London – Harrow (reference 11/LO/0796) and received institutional approval from Homerton University Hospitals Research and Development Department.

Results

Over the 9-month period, there were 4069 inborn deliveries, on whom umbilical cord blood analysis had been performed on 2128 (52.2%). Of these, 263 (12.3%) were premature (gestation less than 37 weeks) and 432 (20.3%) did not have an umbilical cord blood result that could clearly be identified as arterial. Medical notes were missing in 22, which left 1411 (66.3%) mother-infant pairs who were included in the analysis.

3.7% of mothers had O-ve blood group, and 36.0% were O + ve (39.7% group O, overall). In terms of self-defined ethnicity, 27.3% of mothers were black (African or Caribbean origin), 7.3% were south Asian, and 6.3% were Middle Eastern. Median birthweight was 3390 g (interquartile range (IQR) 3080 to 3680 g), and median gestation in weeks + days was 40 + 0 (IQR 39 + 0 to 41 + 0, range 37 + 0 to 43 + 0). 52.4% of deliveries were male.

There were 30 episodes of clinically significant jaundice (2.1%). 9 infants were found to be DAT + ve (0.6%) of whom 8 were jaundiced, and there was a single case of G6PD deficiency. One case of DAT + ve jaundice was due to Rhesus incompatibility (O-ve mother), and the rest were due to ABO incompatibility (O + ve mothers).

Gestation and aUCB were both significantly associated with development of clinically significant jaundice ($P = 0.001$ and $P < 0.001$, respectively). Maternal blood group was only significant when dichotomised into those potentially at risk of ABO incompatibility (blood groups O + ve or O-ve) or not (other blood groups) ($P = 0.02$). Apart from blood group, the only variable associated with DAT + ve jaundice was aUCB (P < 0.001), as shown in Fig. 1.

ROC curves demonstrate that amongst all infants, aUCB strongly predicts the development of DAT + ve jaundice (area under the ROC curve = 0.996 (95% CI 0.991 to 0.998); Fig. 2a), as well as all-cause jaundice (area under the ROC curve = 0.75 (95% CI 0.72 to 0.77); Fig. 2a) even when DAT + ve cases are omitted (area under ROC curve = 0.68 (95% CI 0.66 to 0.71); graph not shown).

We separated out infants at risk of ABO incompatibility (i.e. whose mothers were blood groups O + ve or O-ve) from those certainly not (with a recorded blood type not O + ve or O-ve) and considered the groups separately. Amongst 560 (39.7%) infants at risk of ABO incompatibility, aUCB had similar specificity but substantially higher sensitivity for predicting all-cause jaundice than when all infants were considered, with an area under the ROC curve of 0.89 (95% CI 0.86 to 0.91). The area under the ROC curve for DAT + ve jaundice in this group was 0.994 (0.982 to 0.998). Interestingly, the predictive effect was completely lost for those not at risk of ABO incompatibility (720 infants, 51.0%), with an area under the ROC curve of 0.46 (95% CI 0.43 to 0.50; Fig. 2b). Furthermore, considering only those at risk of ABO incompatibility the effect of gestation on risk of all-cause jaundice was no longer significant ($P = 0.06$).

The aUCB cutoff levels and sensitivity and specificity for predicting all-cause and DAT + ve jaundice are presented in Tables 1 and 2. Furthermore, since the rate of clinically significant jaundice, at 2.1% (3.9% in O + ve/ −ve mothers), was similar to that found in other studies in similar settings, we also calculated positive and negative predictive values at the different cutoffs [15–17].

Finally, since all subjects in the study had verifiable arterial and venous samples, we assessed the correlation between arterial and venous bilurubin levels. The correlation coefficient was 0.80 ($P < 0.001$).

Discussion

This study demonstrates that aUCB is potentially useful screening tool for haemolytic jaundice in term infants of mothers with blood groups O + ve or O-ve. Although the study design has several limitations, it is the largest study to date investigating the role of umbilical cord bilirubin in predicting neonatal jaundice in term babies, and identifies a subgroup of infants in whom aUCB screening may have considerable utility. Infants with high aUCB could be subjected to primary preventative measures such as early feeding, prophylactic phototherapy, and enhanced monitoring, with the aim of preventing severe jaundice.

Consideration of umbilical cord bilirubin as an index of risk for neonatal jaundice is not a new idea. It has been an area of interest since the 1950s, and most studies have found it to be a useful predictor to a greater or lesser extent [6]. Comparison and meta-analysis of studies has been complicated by the fact the most have tended to consider aUCB as a categorical instead of continuous variable. Substantial differences in reported sensitivity and specificity values may simply have reflected the use of different arbitrary cutoffs. For example, Knupfer et al. found that

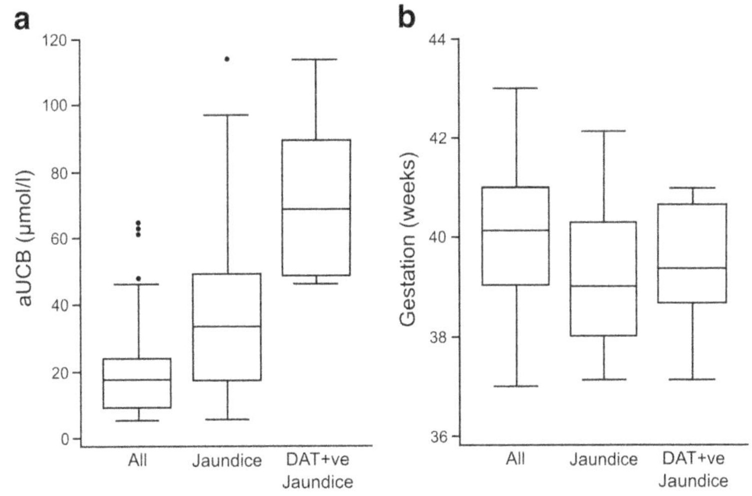

Fig. 1 a shows aUCB levels amongst all infants, infants with all-cause jaundice ($P < 0.001$), and infants with DAT + ve jaundice (P < 0.001). **b** shows gestation amongst all infants, infants with all-cause jaundice ($P = 0.02$), and infants with DAT + ve jaundice ($P = 0.28$)

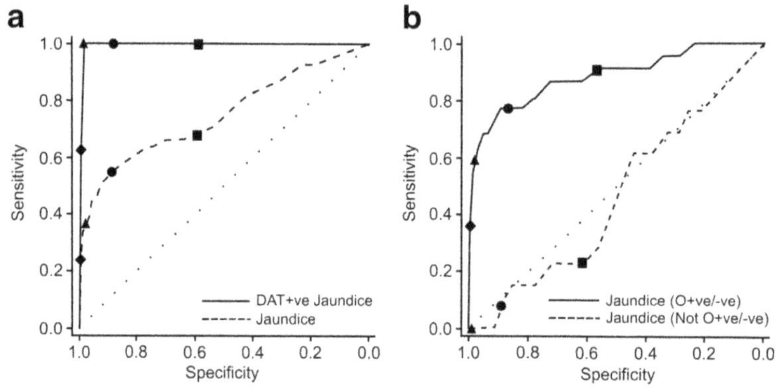

Fig. 2 a shows ROC curves for aUCB predicting all cause jaundice (dashed line) or DAT + ve jaundice (thick line) amongst all infants. **b** shows ROC curves for all-cause jaundice amongst infants at risk of ABO incompatibility (i.e. with maternal blood group O + ve or O-ve, thick line), and amongst those infants not at risk (i.e. documented maternal blood group not O + ve or O-ve, dashed line). In both instances the symbols denote aUCB cutoffs (in μmol/l) as follows: Diamond = 50, Triangle = 40, Circle = 30, Square = 20

using a cutoff of 30μmol/l to predict neonatal hyperbilirubinaemia had very high sensitivity and low specificity of 97% and 41.4% respectively (compared to 88.2% and 55.3% for that cutoff in our study), whereas Carbonell et al. found that an aUCB cutoff of 37μmol/l had low sensitivity but high specificity of 22.2% and of 94.7%, (compared to 44.7% and 95.6% in our study) [8, 10]. Both studies have results not dissimilar to those found in our analysis, even though their reported conclusions appear to be contradictory. In addition, direct comparison between studies may be misleading as most do not make clear whether arterial, venous or a mixture of umbilical samples were analysed. Our data suggest that venous and arterial values are strongly correlated, but that venous levels are consistently lower than arterial, leaving open the possibility of systematic error when comparing between study groups.

A significant advantage of the current study is that infants at risk of the most common cause of haemolytic disease of the newborn in our setting (ABO incompatibility) have been considered separately to those not at risk, and that the number of events in both arms is sufficient to meaningfully compare the two. The data strongly suggest that aUCB should be considered a predictor of jaundice due to haemolytic disease rather than all-cause jaundice, and that umbilical cord bilirubin estimation has no predictive value for jaundice in infants not at risk of haemolysis. This presents a further reason why comparison between studies is problematic, because it suggests the predictive characteristics of aUCB will be partly determined by percentage of the population at risk of haemolytic causes of jaundice, which is subject to geographic variation. Although these results mainly reflect jaundice due to ABO incompatibility, the two infants with haemolysis not caused by ABO also had very high aUCB; the only infant with proven Rhesus-incompatibility disease had the highest aUCB recorded in the study period at 113.9μmol/l, and the infant with G6PD manifesting as early jaundice had an aUCB of 51μmol/l, on the 99th centile of our data.

The study has a number of limitations. Umbilical cord blood specimens were not systematically processed during the study period, with analysis undertaken in only 52% of inborn deliveries. Cord blood analysis was not generally undertaken in deliveries under midwifery-led care, introducing an important bias into our dataset towards complicated pregnancies and deliveries requiring medical intervention. Although these features might

Table 1 aUCB and all-cause jaundice

aUCB (μmol/l)	All subjects						Only O + ve/O-ve Mothers					
	Sens (%)	Spec (%)	PPV (%)	NPV (%)	LR+	LR-	Sens (%)	Spec (%)	PPV (%)	NPV (%)	LR+	LR-
>20	68.4	59.2	4.4	98.6	1.7	0.53	90.9	56.1	7.8	99.3	2.1	0.16
>25	63.2	76.0	6.8	98.7	2.6	0.48	86.4	73.2	11.7	99.2	3.2	0.19
>30	55.3	88.2	11.5	98.6	4.7	0.51	77.3	86.4	18.9	98.9	5.7	0.26
>35	44.7	94.2	17.7	98.4	7.7	0.59	68.2	93.9	31.3	98.6	11.1	0.34
>40	36.8	97.7	30.4	98.2	15.8	0.65	59.1	97.4	48.1	98.3	22.7	0.42
>45	31.6	98.8	42.9	98.1	27.1	0.69	50.0	98.7	61.1	98.0	38.4	0.51
>50	23.7	99.5	56.3	97.9	46.5	0.77	36.4	99.3	66.7	97.4	48.9	0.64

Sens sensitivity, *spec* specificity, *PPV* positive predictive value, *NPV* negative predictive value, *LR+* positive likelihood ratio, *LR-* negative likelihood ratio

Table 2 aUCB and DAT + ve jaundice

aUCB (μmol/l)	All subjects						Only O + ve/O-ve Mothers					
	Sens (%)	Spec (%)	PPV (%)	NPV (%)	LR+	LR-	Sens (%)	Spec (%)	PPV (%)	NPV (%)	LR+	LR-
>20	100	58.8	1.4	100	2.4	0.00	100	55.1	3.1	100	2.2	0.00
>25	100	75.4	2.3	100	4.1	0.00	100	71.9	4.9	100	3.6	0.00
>30	100	87.5	4.4	100	8.0	0.00	100	85.1	8.9	100	6.7	0.00
>35	100	93.7	8.2	100	15.8	0.00	100	92.8	16.7	100	13.8	0.00
>40	100	97.3	17.4	100	36.9	0.00	100	96.6	29.6	100	29.1	0.00
>45	100	98.6	28.6	100	70.2	0.00	100	98.2	44.4	100	55.2	0.00
>50	62.5	99.2	31.3	99.8	79.7	0.38	62.5	98.7	41.7	99.5	49.3	0.30

Sens sensitivity, *spec* specificity, *PPV* positive predictive value, *NPV* negative predictive value, *LR+* positive likelihood ratio, *LR-* negative likelihood ratio

influence the probability of developing neonatal jaundice, it was reassuring to see that the jaundice rate in our sample was in line with previous population-based studies. Furthermore the retrospective data capture is incomplete with substantial gaps, for example maternal blood group is missing in 3.3% of cases. The study presents data from a single centre that is atypical compared to the wider UK population, serving an economically deprived and unusually ethnically diverse catchment area. Although our efforts to identify infants with each of the three outcomes have been thorough, it is difficult to exclude that some who did develop jaundice have been miscategorised as not developing it, which could lead to overestimation of sensitivity. It is disappointing that it was not possible to identify an unambiguous arterial sample in such a high proportion of cases. It may be that future studies focus on venous levels, although occasional inadvertent sampling of the artery will compromise specificity in that case.

In our dataset small changes in aUCB cutoffs may be associated with substantial alterations in sensitivity and specificity for predicting hyperbilirubinaemia. The exact level of an 'ideal' cutoff, will probably be different between different centres serving distinct populations. In our setting, a cutoff of 35 μmol/l for mothers with blood group O + ve or O-ve had a positive predictive value of almost a third for predicting early neonatal jaundice, increasing the pre-test probability of 4% to a post-test probability of 30%.

Conclusion

This study proves the concept that umbilical cord bilirubin is predictive of the development of neonatal jaundice, especially haemolytic jaundice, in infants of O + ve and O-ve mothers. It should prompt re-consideration of the applicability of this practical, cheap and non-invasive approach.

Abbreviations

aUCB: Arterial umbilical cord bilirubin; DAT: Direct Antiglobulin Test; G6PD: Glucose-6-phosphate dehydrogenase deficiency; IQR: Interquartile range; NICE: UK National Institute for Health and Care Excellence; ROC: Receiver operator characteristic; UCB: Umbilical cord bilirubin; UK: United Kingdom

Acknowledgements

We are grateful to Karen Stade and John Gooch of the Homerton University Hospital's Biochemistry Department for assisting with data extraction.

Funding

KDJJ was partly funded by a UK National Institute for Health Research Academic Clinical Fellowship. No other external funding was secured for this study.

Authors' contributions

KDJJ conceptualised and designed the study, supervised data collection, performed data analysis and wrote the first draft of the manuscript. SEG, DK and AR performed data collection and participated in data analysis. GF participated in data analysis and contributed to the first draft of the manuscript. NA contributed to study design, participated in data analysis and contributed to the first draft of the manuscript. All authors edited and approved the final manuscript.

Ethics approval and consent to participate

The study was reviewed and approved by the UK National Research Ethics Service (NRES) Committee London – Harrow (reference 11/LO/0796) and received institutional approval from Homerton University Hospitals Research and Development Department. These approvals incorporated permission to access clinical and laboratory databases as described in the text. Requirement for individual informed consent for participation was waived by the UK National Research Ethics Service (NRES) Committee London – Harrow (reference 11/LO/0796) following review, and was therefore not provided for this retrospective study.

Competing interests

The authors have no conflicts of interest to disclose.

Author details

[1]Neonatal Unit, Homerton University Hospital NHS Foundation Trust, London, UK. [2]Department of Paediatrics, Imperial College, London, UK. [3]Barts and the London School of Medicine & Dentistry, Queen Mary, University of London, London, UK. [4]Swansea Trials Unit, School of Medicine, Swansea University, Swansea, UK.

References

1. Sarici SU, Serdar MA, Korkmaz A, et al. Incidence, course, and prediction of hyperbilirubinemia in near-term and term newborns. Pediatrics. Apr 2004; 113(4):775–80.
2. Escobar GJ, Greene JD, Hulac P, et al. Rehospitalisation after birth hospitalisation: patterns among infants of all gestations. Arch Dis Child. Feb 2005;90(2):125–31.
3. Mwaniki MK, Gatakaa HW, Mturi FN, et al. An increase in the burden of neonatal admissions to a rural district hospital in Kenya over 19 years. BMC Public Health. 2010;10:591.
4. Madden JM, Soumerai SB, Lieu TA, Mandl KD, Zhang F, Ross-Degnan D. Length-of-stay policies and ascertainment of postdischarge problems in newborns. Pediatrics. Jan 2004;113(1 Pt 1):42–9.
5. Grupp-Phelan J, Taylor JA, Liu LL, Davis RL. Early newborn hospital discharge and readmission for mild and severe jaundice. Archives of pediatrics & adolescent medicine. Dec 1999;153(12):1283–8.
6. Ipek IO, Bozaykut A, Cagril SC, Sezer RG. Does cord blood bilirubin level help the physician in the decision of early postnatal discharge? *The journal of maternal-fetal & neonatal medicine: the official journal of the European Association of Perinatal Medicine, the Federation of Asia and Oceania Perinatal Societies, the International Society of Perinatal Obstet.* Aug 2012;25(8):1375–1378.
7. Sun G, Wang YL, Liang JF, Du LZ. [predictive value of umbilical cord blood bilirubin level for subsequent neonatal jaundice]. *Zhonghua er ke za zhi.* Chinese journal of pediatrics. Nov 2007;45(11):848–52.
8. Knupfer M, Pulzer F, Gebauer C, Robel-Tillig E, Vogtmann C. Predictive value of umbilical cord blood bilirubin for postnatal hyperbilirubinaemia. Acta Paediatr. May 2005;94(5):581–7.
9. Bernaldo AJ, Segre CA. Bilirubin dosage in cord blood: could it predict neonatal hyperbilirubinemia? *Sao Paulo medical journal = Revista paulista de medicina.* May 6 2004;122(3):99–103.
10. Carbonell X, Botet F, Figueras J, Riu-Godo A. Prediction of hyperbilirubinaemia in the healthy term newborn. Acta Paediatr. Feb 2001; 90(2):166–70.
11. Rataj J, Kornacka M, Korman E. Usefulness of measuring bilirubin levels in cord blood for predicting hyperbilirubinemia in newborns. Ginekol Pol. Jun 1994;65(6):276–80.
12. Knudsen A. Prediction of the development of neonatal jaundice by increased umbilical cord blood bilirubin. Acta Paediatr Scand. Mar 1989; 78(2):217–21.
13. National Institute for Health and Care Excellence. Jaundice in newborn babies under 28 days [CG98]. 2010; http://www.nice.org.uk/guidance/cg98/resources/jaundice-in-newborn-babies-under-28-days-975756073669.
14. Westgate J, Garibaldi JM, Greene KR. Umbilical cord blood gas analysis at delivery: a time for quality data. Br J Obstet Gynaecol. Dec 1994;101(12): 1054–63.
15. Romagnoli C, Tiberi E, Barone G, et al. Development and validation of serum bilirubin nomogram to predict the absence of risk for severe hyperbilirubinaemia before discharge: a prospective, multicenter study. Ital J Pediatr. 2012;38:6.
16. Usatin D, Liljestrand P, Kuzniewicz MW, Escobar GJ, Newman TB. Effect of neonatal jaundice and phototherapy on the frequency of first-year outpatient visits. Pediatrics. Apr 2010;125(4):729–34.
17. Kuzniewicz MW, Escobar GJ, Newman TB. Impact of universal bilirubin screening on severe hyperbilirubinemia and phototherapy use. Pediatrics. Oct 2009;124(4):1031–9.

An infant formula containing dairy lipids increased red blood cell membrane Omega 3 fatty acids in 4 month-old healthy newborns

Maria Lorella Gianni[1], Paola Roggero[1], Charlotte Baudry[2*], Catherine Fressange-Mazda[3], Claudio Galli[4^], Carlo Agostoni[5], Pascale le Ruyet[2] and Fabio Mosca[1]

Abstract

Background: When breastfeeding is not possible, infants are fed formulas (IF) in which lipids are usually of plant origin. However, the use of dairy fat in combination with plant oils enables a lipid profile closer to breast milk in terms of fatty acid (FA) composition, triglyceride structure, polar lipids and cholesterol contents. The objective of this study was to determine the effect of an IF containing a mix of dairy fat and plant oils on Omega-3 FA content in red blood cells (RBC).

Methods: This study was a monocentric, double-blind, controlled, randomized trial. Healthy term infants were fed formulas containing a mix of dairy fat and plant oils (D), plant oils (P) or plant oils supplemented with ARA and DHA (PDHA). Breastfed infants were enrolled as a reference group (BF). FA in RBC phosphatidylethanolamine was evaluated after 4 months and FA in whole blood were evaluated at enrollment and after 4 months by gas chromatography. Differences between groups were assessed using an analysis of covariance with sex and gestational age as covariates.

Results: Seventy IF-fed and nineteen BF infants completed the protocol. At 4 months, RBC total Omega-3 FA levels in infants fed formula D were significantly higher than in group P and similar to those in groups PDHA and BF. RBC DHA levels in group D were also higher than in group P but lower than in groups PDHA and BF. RBC n-3 DPA levels in group D were higher than in groups P, PDHA and BF. A decrease in proportions of Omega-3 FA in whole blood was observed in all groups.

Conclusions: A formula containing a mix of dairy lipids and plant oils increased the endogenous conversion of Omega-3 long-chain FA from precursor, leading to higher total Omega-3, DPA and DHA status in RBC than a plant oil-based formula. Modifying lipid quality in IF by adding dairy lipids should be considered as an interesting method to improve Omega-3 FA status.

Keywords: Infant nutrition, Infant formula, Lipid quality, Dairy fat, Fatty acids, Omega 3, Red blood cells membrane fatty acids, Erythrocyte membrane fatty acids

* Correspondence: charlotte.baudry@lactalis.fr
^Deceased
[2]Nutrition Department, Lactalis R&D, Retiers, France
Full list of author information is available at the end of the article

Background

Breast milk is considered by the World Health Organization (WHO) as the optimal form of nourishment for infants up to 6 months. Lipids are major components in human milk, providing approximately 50% of total dietary energy. Triacylglycerols in human milk have a specific fatty acid (FA) composition, which can be influenced by maternal dietary habits or by lactation stages. Proportions of saturated and monounsaturated FA are relatively stable whereas proportions of polyunsaturated FA (PUFA) can vary more widely [1]. Among PUFA, human milk provides alpha-linolenic (ALA) and linoleic acids (LA) which are essential fatty acids (EFA). They can be endogenously converted by the newborn into long-chain derivatives of Omega 3 and Omega 6 families, such as docosahexaenoic acid (DHA) and arachidonic acid (ARA), respectively. However, this conversion is considered to be low in humans [2]. Human milk also contains preformed long-chain PUFA (LCPUFA) of both series with DHA representing 0.1–1% of total FA and ARA 0.4–0.9% of total FA [1]. LCPUFA accumulation is very important during both the fetal and postnatal periods in brain and retina [3]. Consequently, bioavailability of ALA, LA, DHA and ARA from breast milk or infant formulas is critical in early life to sustain optimal visual and brain development of the newborn and later-life cognitive functions [4].

Fat sources used in most infant formulas currently marketed are blends of plant oils used to match the FA profile found in human milk. Indeed, since the middle of 20th century, infant formulas have been enriched in EFA-rich plant oils and bovine milk fat has been progressively removed [1]. Infant formulas can also be optionally supplemented with fish, algae or fungus oils providing preformed DHA and ARA. However, lipids of plant oils are not comparable to lipids of human milk in terms of FA diversity, triacylglycerol structure, fat globule composition, complex lipids and cholesterol contents. Although not containing high levels of LCPUFA, the use of dairy lipids in combination with plant oils could provide a lipid composition and structure closer to human milk, thus improving the quality of infant formula fat profile. Indeed, infant formulas provide milk-specific FA and cholesterol only when dairy lipids are used as a fat source in combination with plant oils [1]. Short and medium chain FA, lauric acid, myristic acid and palmitic acid contents in formulas can vary considerably according to the use of palm oil, coconut oil or dairy lipids [1]. Moreover, plant oils do not encounter the specific triglyceride structure with palmitic acid in sn2 position found in breast milk (60–85% of sn2-palmitate) or cow's milk (more than 45%). Therefore, it has been shown that formulas with only plant oils as sources of lipids had less than 15% of palmitic acid in sn2 position whereas formulas containing a blend of dairy lipids and plant oils had 48% of palmitic acid in sn2 position [5]. This triglyceride structure is of particular importance because long-chain saturated FA in the sn2 position are more efficiently digested and absorbed [6].

Dairy lipids specifically contain about 10% of myristic acid and 10% of short and medium chain FA (C4-C10) while plant oils provide much less of these FA. Short-chain FA represent a rapid source of energy for the infant, because they enter directly the portal vein and are known to be completely absorbed and metabolized. Myristic and short/medium chain FA could also increase bioavailability and conversion of n-3 PUFA as demonstrated in vitro [7]. Furthermore, benefits of dairy lipids on the conversion of Omega 3 precursor to long-chain derivatives have been described in several studies. Indeed, in adults, a moderate intake of dairy lipids and rapeseed oil improved plasma DHA levels and blood fluidity [8, 9]. In Omega 3-deficient rats, it has been demonstrated that for a similar ALA content, a blend of dairy lipids and rapeseed oil induced a higher level of brain DHA than a blend of plant oils even if supplemented with preformed DHA [10, 11]. In mice, a diet containing a blend with dairy lipids given from the first day of gestation until adulthood increased DHA levels and neuroplasticity in the brain of the offspring compared with a diet containing only plant oils [12]. In the same mouse model, it has been also demonstrated that a diet containing dairy lipids protected from the adverse effects induced by an early life inflammatory event on neurogenesis and adult spatial memory [13]. Consequently, these data suggest that the use of dairy lipids in combination with plant oils could potentially improve long-chain Omega 3 status and promote the accretion of DHA in the developing brain.

The aim of the present study was to assess the impact of an infant formula containing dairy lipids and plant oils on FA composition in RBC and whole blood, especially on Omega 3 FA content, in 4 month-old healthy infants.

Methods

Study design

This monocentric, double-blind, controlled, randomized trial was conducted in 2012–2013 in the Department of Neonatology of the Fondazione IRCCS Cà Granda Ospedale Maggiore Policlinico, Milano, Italy (NCT01611649). The study was approved by the local Ethical Committee and conducted in accordance with Good Clinical Practice and the principles and rules of the Declaration of Helsinki. Parents or legal caregivers provided written informed consent prior to enrollment of their infants in the study. The study protocol has been previously published [14].

Population

Healthy full-term infants born in the Department of Neonatology were screened for participation in the study. When breastfeeding was not possible (contraindication or mothers not intended to breastfeed), infants were randomly allocated to be fed for 4 months with a formula containing either: a mix of plant oils and dairy fat (D), only plant oils (P) or plant oils supplemented with ARA and DHA (PDHA). Infants whose mothers intended to exclusively breastfeed from birth through at least 4 months were enrolled in a nonrandomized reference group (BF). Inclusion criteria were: gestational age 37 to 42 weeks, birth weight > 2500 g, healthy newborns from normal pregnancy, aged up to 3 weeks when entering the study, no breastfeeding (for the formula-fed groups) or exclusive breastfeeding (for the reference group). Exclusion criteria were: positive family history of allergy to milk proteins, known congenital or postnatal diseases which could interfere with the study and newborns whose parents had planned to move within 6 months after birth.

Study formulas

Study formulas were formulated into powders and were reconstituted at 13.3%. They were manufactured and provided by Milumel®, Lactalis, Craon, France. The 3 tested formulas were packaged in blinded containers labeled only with study details and number of randomization; they were indistinguishable in appearance and texture. Both the investigators and the infants' parents were blind to the group allocation. The randomization schedule was computer-generated and stratified on sex. Compositions of the 3 study formulas were in compliance with the European Directive 2006/141/EC on infant formulas and are detailed in Table 1. The 3 formulas had similar energy and macronutrient contents but they differed by the nature of their lipid sources. Formula D contained a mixture of dairy lipids and plant oils (rapeseed, sunflower, high oleic sunflower); formula P contained only plant oils (palm, rapeseed, sunflower) and formula PDHA contained plant oils (palm, rapeseed, sunflower) supplemented with ARA (0.4%) and DHA (0.2%). Study formulas were consumed straightaway after randomization and were provided for the 4 subsequent months.

Objectives and outcomes

The main objective of this study was to investigate the effect of formula D on the RBC membrane total Omega 3 FA content as compared to formulas P and PDHA and to BF reference group. Total Omega 3 FA levels included ALA, EPA (eicosapentaenoic acid, 20:5n-3), DPA (docosapentaenoic acid, 22:5n-3) and DHA levels. The secondary objective was to evaluate changes between 4 months and enrollment in whole blood FA contents in infants consuming formula D in comparison to formula P and PDHA and BF. Impact of formulas on growth, body composition and gastrointestinal tolerance was also investigated but these data are under publication in another article.

Table 1 Composition of study formulas

		Formula D 100 ml[a]	Formula P 100 ml[a]	Formula PDHA 100 ml[a]
Energy	kJ	275	275	275
	kcal	66	66	66
Protein	g	1.3	1.3	1.3
Carbohydrates	g	8.1	8.1	8.1
Lactose	g	6.8	6.8	6.8
Fat	g	3.1	3.1	3.1
LA	mg	439	549	549
	% TFA	14.2	17.7	17.7
ALA	mg	73	55	55
	% TFA	2.3	1.8	1.8
Ratio LA/ALA		6	10	10
ARA	mg	≤ 0.1		12.4
	% TFA			0.4
DHA	mg			6.2
	% TFA			0.2
Ratio ARA/DHA				2

Composition of tested formulas according to manufacturer data. Formula D contained a mixture of dairy lipids (cream) and plant oils (rapeseed, sunflower and high oleic sunflower); formula P contained only plant oils (palm, rapeseed, sunflower) and formula PDHA contained plant oils (palm, rapeseed, sunflower) supplemented with ARA and DHA)
LA linoleic acid, *ALA* alpha-linolenic acid, *ARA* arachidonic acid, *DHA* docosahexaenoic acid, *TFA* total fatty acids
[a]Reconstituted 13.3%

Measurement of FA levels in RBC membrane

Venous blood samples were drawn after consumption of the allocated formula or breastfeeding for 4 months. Blood was collected on heparin. Plasma was separated by 15-min centrifugation (2200 g at 4 °C) from RBC that were rinsed with saline solution (NaCl 0.9%). Plasma and RBC were stored at − 80 °C for later analysis. RBC total lipids were extracted and phosphatidylethanolamine (PE) was isolated from other phospholipids by thin layer chromatography. FA levels of RBC PE were measured by means of a gas–liquid chromatography (HPLC) by ITERG, Pessac, France. Results are expressed as percentage of total FA.

Measurement of blood FA levels

Whole blood samples were collected using a heel stick at enrollment and after 4 months of consumption of the allocated formula or breastfeeding. FA levels were quantified by means of a gas–liquid chromatography (HPLC) by Oxigenlab, Brescia, Italy. Results are expressed as percentage of total FA.

Sample size

Calculation of sample size for this study has been previously detailed [14]. In order to detect a difference of 20% in the RBC membrane Omega 3 FA levels (basal value of 7.3% and standard deviation of 1.3 [15]) between infants receiving formula D and infants receiving formula P or formula PDHA, at a power of 90% and with an alpha error of 5%, a total of 17 infants per group was necessary. To take into account the multiplicity of comparisons, the calculation was done with an alpha error of 2.5% and a total of 21 infants per group was needed. Considering dropouts, a total of 30 infants per group were enrolled.

Statistical analyses

Statistical analyses were performed using SAS software (SAS Institute Inc., Cary NC, USA) by Soladis, Lyon, France. Continuous variables were expressed as mean and standard deviation. Differences among groups for FA levels were analyzed with an analysis of variance with 3 fixed factors (group, sex, gestational age). Pairwise comparisons were made using post-hoc Tukey's test for multiple comparisons. A p-value < 0.05 was considered significant.

Results

Study population

A total of 117 healthy newborns were enrolled. Of these, 88 were randomized to the formula-fed groups and 29 were enrolled in the breastfed reference group (Fig. 1). A total of 18 (20%) infants from the formula groups and 10 (34%) in the breastfed group withdrew before the end of the study (Fig. 1). Rates of discontinuation were similar in the 3 formula groups (23% in formula D and PDHA; 14% in formula P). Gastrointestinal symptoms (ie. regurgitations, reflux, constipation, colic and flatulence) were the most common reason for study discontinuation in the 3 formula groups: 57% in group D, 75% in group P and 43% in group PDHA. Among the breastfed group, 8 babies were lost to follow-up and breastfeeding was stopped before the next visit for 2 babies.

Baseline characteristics in each group are presented in Table 2. Proportion of boys was similar in the 3 formula groups (53–57%) and was of 38% in the breastfed reference group (Table 2). A high proportion of caesarean births (43–64%) was observed in all groups without any difference between groups (Table 2). Gestational age was around 38 weeks in the 3 formula groups and around 39 weeks in the breastfed group. On average, infants were enrolled in the study at 5–10 days of life (Table 2). At baseline, weight in group P was significantly lower than in breastfed infants ($p = 0.015$) (Table 2). Height, head circumference and body composition were similar in the 4 groups at baseline (all $p > 0.05$) (Table 2). Total Omega 3 and DHA levels in whole blood were similar in the 4 groups at baseline, despite a tendency for higher DHA levels in the BF group but not statistically significant (Table 2).

Mean daily volume of formula consumed was evaluated during a 2 day-period at 1 month and 3 months. Most of formula-fed infants consumed more than 600 ml daily at 1 month (around 95% of infants) and more than 700 ml daily at 3 months (around 82%). No significant differences in formula intake were observed among the 3 formula groups at 1 month ($p = 0.980$) or at 3 months ($p = 0.177$).

RBC membrane FA levels after 4 months

Primary endpoint was total Omega 3 FA levels in PE of RBC membrane after 4 months (Fig. 2). RBC total Omega 3 FA levels were significantly higher in infants fed with formula D (8.6 ± 1.2% TFA) than with formula P (5.7 ± 0.8%

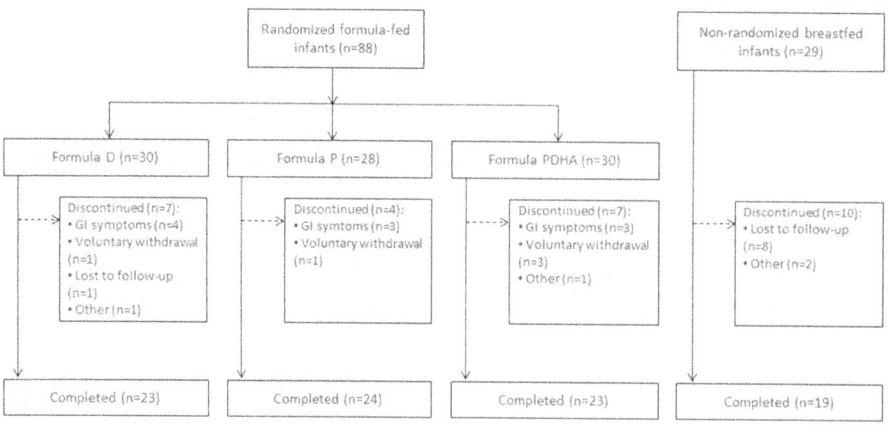

Fig. 1 Flow of study subjects. Formula D contained a mixture of dairy lipids and plant oils; formula P contained only plant oils and formula PDHA contained plant oils supplemented with ARA and DHA. GI (gastrointestinal) symptoms included regurgitation, reflux, constipation, colic and flatulence

Table 2 Infants' characteristics at enrollment

	Formula D $n = 30$	Formula P $n = 28$	Formula PDHA $n = 30$	Breastfed $n = 29$	*p*-value
Sex, no. (%)					
Girls	13 (43.3)	11 (39.3)	14 (46.7)	18 (62.1)	0.329
Boys	17 (56.7)	17 (60.7)	16 (53.3)	11 (37.9)	
Delivery mode, no. (%)					
Natural	11 (36.7)	10 (35.7)	17 (56.7)	14 (48.3)	0.310
Caesarean	19 (63.3)	18 (64.3)	13 (43.3)	15 (51.7)	
Gestational age, weeks, mean (SD)	38.4 (1.2)	38.4 (1.1)	38.3 (1.0)	39.0 (1.0)	0.072
Age at enrollment, days, mean (SD)	6.8 (5.6)	4.9 (4.5)	9.6 (7.9)	8.8 (6.6)	0.076
Weight, g, mean (SD)	3144.2 (448.6)	2942.9 (386.6)^{X}	3156.4 (431.8)	3308.7 (533.9)	0.029
Height, cm, mean (SD)	49.1 (2.2)	48.9 (2.2)	49.7 (1.9)	50.1 (1.8)	0.112
Head circumference, cm, mean (SD)	34.4 (1.2)	34.3 (1.4)	34.7 (1.4)	35.3 (2.0)	0.068
Fat mass, % BW, mean (SD)	10.3 (2.9)	10.8 (3.4)	9.8 (3.5)	11.6 (5.4)	0.321
Total Omega 3 in whole blood, %, mean (SD)	12.9 (3.1)	14.2 (3.6)	13.2 (4.2)	15.0 (4.3)	0.384
DHA in whole blood, %, mean (SD)	3.2 (1.1)	3.6 (1.1)	3.4 (0.9)	4.1 (1.8)	0.057

Formula D contained a mixture of dairy lipids and plant oils; formula P contained only plant oils and formula PDHA contained plant oils supplemented with ARA and DHA. BW: body weight. Comparison of the 4 groups by ANOVA 1 fixed factor (Group) and post-hoc Tukey's adjustments
$^{X}p < 0.05$ vs. BF

TFA; $p < 0.001$) but similar to those of infants fed with formula PDHA (8.8 ± 1.1% TFA; $p = 0.956$) or BF (9.7 ± 1.8% TFA; $p = 0.191$) (Fig. 2). Sum of DHA and n-3 DPA levels accounts for more than 90% of RBC total Omega 3. DHA levels in group D (4.1 ± 0.8% TFA) were significantly higher than in group P (3.4 ± 0.7% TFA; $p = 0.029$) but lower than in groups PDHA (6.8 ± 1.0% TFA) and BF (7.0 ± 1.4% TFA; both $p < 0.001$) (Fig. 2). n-3 DPA levels in group D (3.6 ± 0.6% TFA) were higher than in all the other groups (P: 1.9 ± 0.3; PDHA: 1.6 ± 0.2; BF: 2.2 ± 0.5% TFA; $p < 0.001$ for all) (Fig. 2). In group PDHA, total Omega 3 and DHA levels were similar to breastfed but n-3 DPA levels were significantly lower ($p < 0.001$).

When the BF group was excluded from the statistical comparison, results were similar with significantly higher levels of total Omega 3 and DHA in group D than in group P ($p < 0.001$ and $p = 0.006$, respectively).

RBC membrane compositions for the other FA are presented in Table 3. Total saturated FA were similar in the 3 formula groups. Percentage of MUFA was significantly higher in formula D-fed infants than in formula PDHA ($p < 0.001$) and BF ($p = 0.034$) (Table 3). Total Omega 6 and ARA levels were similar in the 3 formula groups and breastfed BF (Table 3). However, LA levels in formula D-fed infants were similar to formula P-fed ($p = 0.630$) but higher than in formula PDHA-fed ($p < 0.001$) and BF ($p < 0.001$). ALA and EPA levels in formula D-fed infants were significantly higher than in the other groups (all $p < 0.05$).

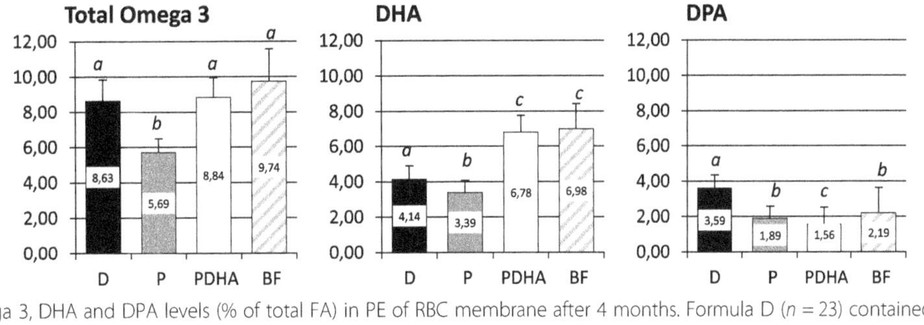

Fig. 2 Total Omega 3, DHA and DPA levels (% of total FA) in PE of RBC membrane after 4 months. Formula D ($n = 23$) contained a mixture of dairy lipids and plant oils; formula P ($n = 24$) contained only plant oils and formula PDHA ($n = 23$) contained plant oils supplemented with ARA and DHA. BF: breastfed reference group ($n = 18$). PE: phosphatidylethanolamine. Comparison of the 4 groups by ANOVA with 3 fixed factors (Sex, gestational age, group) and post-hoc Tukey's adjustments. *a ≠ b ≠ c; p < 0.05*

Table 3 RBC membrane FA levels (% of total FA) after 4 months

	Formula D $n = 23$	Formula P $n = 24$	Formula PDHA $n = 23$	BF $n = 18$	*p*-value
Total SFA	33.4 ± 3.1	34.1 ± 3.6	35.2 ± 2.5	34.7 ± 2.9	0.514
Total MUFA	22.4 ± 2.1^{a}	21.5 ± 1.5$^{a, b}$	20.2 ± 1.4^{b}	21.0 ± 2.1^{b}	< 0.001
Total PUFA	43.7 ± 3.6	44.1 ± 3.7	44.3 ± 2.5	43.9 ± 3.5	0.342
Total Omega 6	35.0 ± 2.7	38.3 ± 3.3	35.4 ± 1.8	34.0 ± 2.5	0.465
18:2(n-6) LA	6.2 ± 0.6^{a}	6.3 ± 0.6^{a}	4.4 ± 0.4^{b}	3.8 ± 0.8^{c}	< 0.001
20:4(n-6) ARA	20.3 ± 1.9	21.6 ± 2.2	22.6 ± 1.5	22.2 ± 1.7	0.747
22:4(n-6)	5.9 ± 1.1	6.9 ± 1.3	6.2 ± 1.1	5.6 ± 1.5	0.261
22:5(n-6) DPA n-6	0.8 ± 0.2	1.1 ± 0.3	0.9 ± 0.2	0.9 ± 0.3	0.359
18:3(n-3) ALA	0.2 ± 0.0^{a}	0.1 ± 0.0^{b}	0.1 ± 0.0^{b}	0.1 ± 0.1^{b}	< 0.001
20:5(n-3) EPA	0.7 ± 0.2^{a}	0.3 ± 0.1^{b}	0.4 ± 0.1^{c}	0.5 ± 0.1^{c}	< 0.001

Formula D ($n = 23$) contained a mixture of dairy lipids and plant oils; formula P ($n = 24$) contained only plant oils and formula PDHA ($n = 23$) contained plant oils supplemented with ARA and DHA. BF: breastfed reference group ($n = 18$). PE: phosphatidylethanolamine
Comparison of the 4 groups by ANOVA with 3 fixed factors (Sex, gestational age, group) and post-hoc Tukey's adjustments
$^{a} \neq {}^{b} \neq {}^{c}$; $p < 0.05$

Changes in whole blood FA levels between enrollment and 4 months

Changes of total Omega 3 and DHA levels (expressed as deltas) in whole blood between 4 months and enrollment are presented in Fig. 3. Percentage of total Omega 3 significantly decreased between 4 months and enrollment in all groups (Fig. 3). The decrease in percentage of Omega 3 in group D ($-6.1 \pm 4.4\%$ TFA) was similar to those in group P ($-9.2 \pm 4.3\%$ TFA; $p = 0.087$), PDHA ($-3.5 \pm 4.2\%$ TFA; $p = 0.144$) and BF ($-5.2 \pm 4.7\%$ TFA; $p = 0.847$) (Fig. 3). However, this decrease was significantly higher in group P than in group PDHA ($p < 0.001$) and BF ($p = 0.15$) (Fig. 3). Proportions of DHA in whole blood also decreased with time in all groups (Fig. 3). The decrease in DHA observed in group D ($-1.8 \pm 1.2\%$ TFA) was similar to those in group P ($-2.5 \pm 1.2\%$ TFA; $p = 0.388$) and BF ($-1.4 \pm 1.9\%$ TFA; $p = 0.639$) but higher than in group PDHA ($-0.4 \pm 0.8\%$ TFA; $p < 0.001$) (Fig. 3). n-3 DPA levels were not evaluated in whole blood.

Discussion

This study demonstrated that 4-month consumption of a formula containing dairy lipids was associated with a higher total Omega 3 level in RBC membrane compared with a formula containing only lipids of plant origin in healthy infants. Total Omega 3 levels reached with a formula containing dairy lipids were similar to those of infants fed with a formula supplemented with DHA and to breastfed infants. Although breast milk remains the best nutritional choice for infants, the results of this study suggest that dairy

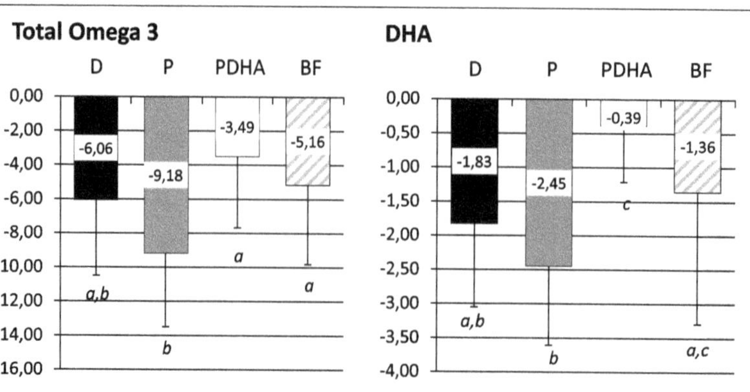

Fig. 3 Changes in total Omega 3 and DHA levels in whole blood between 4 months and enrollment expressed as deltas (% of total FA). Formula D ($n = 23$) contained a mixture of dairy lipids and plant oils; formula P ($n = 24$) contained only plant oils and formula PDHA ($n = 23$) contained plant oils supplemented with ARA and DHA. BF: breastfed reference group ($n = 18$). Comparison of the 4 groups by ANOVA with 3 fixed factors (Sex, gestational age, group) and post-hoc Tukey's adjustments. $a \neq b \neq c$; $p < 0.05$

lipids in infant formulas could stimulate the conversion of Omega 3 FA precursors into long-chain derivatives.

The beneficial effects of dairy lipids on Omega 3 FA conversion have already been described in previous studies in humans [8, 9] or animal models [10–12]. These effects of dairy lipids could be due to several mechanisms resulting from the specific FA composition of dairy fat. Firstly, dairy fat contains high proportions of short and medium chain FA, which are highly oxidized after absorption. Therefore, they may spare ALA from oxidation and consequently favor its partitioning towards desaturation and elongation pathways to form long-chain derivatives. Another mechanism to explain the effects of dairy fat could be a selective gene or post-traductional activation of desaturases and elongases which are the enzymes involved in n-3 conversion. In particular, the dairy lipid-based formula had a higher content of myristic acid than plant oil-based formulas and this FA has been shown to increase delta 6 desaturase activity in vitro [7]. However, these hypothesis would need to be demonstrated.

One limitation of this study was that formulas slightly differed by their LA and ALA contents and by their LA to ALA ratio, which was lower in the formula with dairy lipid (around 6:1) than in formulas with only plant oils (around 10:1). The n-6 to n-3 ratio has been recognized as an important factor driving the conversion of ALA to long-chain derivatives because of the competition between LA and ALA for their desaturation and elongation pathways. This could partly explain the increase in RBC total Omega 3 FA observed with the dairy lipid-based formula. However, previous data in rats showed benefits of dairy lipids versus plant oils on RBC composition and brain DHA accretion for similar ALA contents and LA to ALA ratios in the diets [11].

In this study, the increase in RBC total Omega 3 levels with the dairy lipid-based formula resulted from an increase in all the n-3 FA, with n-3 DPA and DHA representing more than 90% of total Omega 3 in RBC. RBC DHA level after 4 months was higher in infants fed the formula containing dairy lipids than in those fed the formula with only plant oils but remained lower than in infants fed with preformed DHA (formula or breastfed infants). RBC membrane DHA levels in infants fed with a formula supplemented with DHA were significantly higher than those observed in infants fed the similar formula without DHA, suggesting that RBC DHA levels are strongly influenced by the DHA supplementation, as already described in previous studies [16–18].

Results of FA compositions in whole blood showed a decrease in proportions of total Omega 3 and DHA between 4 months and enrollment in all groups, but it was more pronounced in infants fed formula with only vegetable lipids. These results are in concordance with those reported in a previous study showing that the largest postnatal decline in DHA was observed in infants fed nonsupplemented formula [19].

RBC n-3 DPA was the main FA affected by dairy lipids and was increased by 90% compared with the plant oil-based formula while DHA was only increased by 22%. The literature on n-3 DPA is quite limited but available data suggests beneficial health effects of this FA [20]. The preferential accumulation of n-3 DPA in RBC observed in this study could be due to a limited rate of the conversion of n-3 DPA to DHA, mainly in liver, as shown by in vivo studies [20]. On the other hand, n-3 DPA might represent the preferred form of incorporation of n-3 long chain FA in RBC. Indeed, ALA can be elongated and desaturated in a tissue-dependent manner, with a tissue-selective accumulation of its derivatives [21]. For example, in ALA-fed rats, an increase in ALA, EPA and DPA was observed in plasma, liver and heart while an increase in DPA and DHA occurred in the brain [21]. Also, in neonatal baboons who received an oral dose of labeled ALA at 4 weeks of age, the distribution of labeled FA at 6 weeks of age was similar in brain, retina and liver, with DHA being the main form of labeled FA whereas in RBC n-3 DPA predominated [22]. Finally, in rats, RBC n-3 DPA was found to be the most reliable indicator of brain DHA status, more than RBC DHA [11]. Therefore, blood analysis might not reflect the potential elongation seen in other tissue compartments such as brain. As further limitation, through this study we were not able to observe the effects of a formula containing dairy lipids on brain or retina FA composition.

Even if RBC DHA levels represent an interesting parameter to evaluate the effects of dietary interventions, they are not always correlated with functional outcomes. For example, in the DIAMOND study, RBC DHA was positively correlated with visual acuity but not with cognitive parameters in term infants [16, 23]. Consequently, it would be interesting to study the effect of an infant formula containing dairy lipids on functional outcomes in infants to verify previous results obtained in animal models.

Conclusions

This study showed that a formula containing dairy lipid increased RBC total Omega 3 status in healthy term infants, at levels similar to breastfed babies. Breast milk remains the optimal food for infants. However, when breastfeeding is not possible, modifying lipid quality in formula by adding dairy lipids should be considered as an alternative method to improve infants' Omega 3 FA status. However, further investigation would be needed to evaluate the effect of a dairy lipid-based formula (supplemented or not with DHA) on functional outcomes such as visual acuity or cognitive development.

Abbreviations

ALA: Alpha-linolenic acid; ARA: Arachidonic acid; BF: Breastfed; BW: Body weight; DHA: Docosahexaenoic acid; EFA: Essential fatty acid; FA: Fatty acid; formula D: With a mix of plant oils and dairy lipids; formula P: With only plant oils; formula PDHA: With plant oils and supplemented with ARA and DHA; LA: Linoleic acid; PUFA: Polyunsaturated fatty acid; SD: Standard deviation; TFA: Total fatty acids; WHO: World Health Organization

Acknowledgements

We would like to thank participating families, Elisa Garavaglia and Domenica Mallardi for their contribution to this study, Soladis for statistical analysis and Aurélie Lemaitre for study product management.

Funding

This study was funded by Lactalis Nutrition Europe, Torcé, France. Study formulas were provided by Milumel®, Lactalis, Craon, France. Lactalis also contributed to the design of the study and the writing of the manuscript.

Authors' contributions

PR, PLR, CFM and FM formulated the research question and wrote the study protocol. CB, MLG, PR wrote the draft of the manuscript. CA and CG have been involved in revising the manuscript for important intellectual content. All authors reviewed the manuscript and approved the final version.

Competing interests

This study was funded by Lactalis Nutrition Europe, Torcé, France. Study formulas were provided by Milumel®, Lactalis, Craon, France. CB, CFM and PLR are employees of the Lactalis group, France. MLG is a member of the editorial board of BMC Pediatrics.

Author details

[1]Neonatal Intensive Care Unit (NICU), Department of Clinical Science and Community Health, Fondazione IRCCS "Ca' Granda" Ospedale Maggiore Policlinico, University of Milan, Milan, Italy. [2]Nutrition Department, Lactalis R&D, Retiers, France. [3]Lactalis Nutrition Europe, Torcé, France. [4]University of Milan, Milan, Italy. [5]Pediatric Intermediate Care Unit, Department of Clinical Science and Community Health, Fondazione IRCCS "Ca' Granda" Ospedale Maggiore Policlinico, University of Milan, Milan, Italy.

References

1. Delplanque B, Gibson R, Koletzko B, Lapillonne A, Strandvik B. Lipid quality in infant nutrition: current knowledge and future opportunities. J Pediatr Gastroenterol Nutr. 2015;61:8–17.
2. Uauy R, Mena P, Wegher B, Nieto S, Salem N. Long chain polyunsaturated fatty acid formation in neonates: effect of gestational age and intrauterine growth. Pediatr Res. 2000;47:127–35.
3. Guesnet P, Alessandri J-M. Docosahexaenoic acid (DHA) and the developing central nervous system (CNS) - implications for dietary recommendations. Biochimie. 2011;93:7–12.
4. Innis SM. Fatty acids and early human development. Early Hum Dev. 2007; 83:761–6.
5. González HF, Vicentin D, Giumelli O, Vazzano M, Tavella M. Profile of triacylglycerols and percentage of palmitic acid at the sn-2 in breast milk substitutes. Arch Argent Pediatr. 2012;110:227–30.
6. Innis SM. Dietary triacylglycerol structure and its role in infant nutrition. Adv Nutr. 2011;2:275–83.
7. Jan S, Guillou H, D'Andrea S, Daval S, Bouriel M, Rioux V, et al. Myristic acid increases delta6-desaturase activity in cultured rat hepatocytes. Reprod Nutr Dev. 2004;44:131–40.
8. Dabadie H, Peuchant E, Bernard M, LeRuyet P, Mendy F. Moderate intake of myristic acid in sn-2 position has beneficial lipidic effects and enhances DHA of cholesteryl esters in an interventional study. J Nutr Biochem. 2005; 16:375–82.
9. Dabadie H, Motta C, Peuchant E, LeRuyet P, Mendy F. Variations in daily intakes of myristic and alpha-linolenic acids in sn-2 position modify lipid profile and red blood cell membrane fluidity. Br J Nutr. 2006;96:283–9.
10. Delplanque B, Du Q, Agnani G, Le Ruyet P, Martin JC. A dairy fat matrix providing alpha-linolenic acid (ALA) is better than a vegetable fat mixture to increase brain DHA accretion in young rats. Prostaglandins Leukot Essent Fatty Acids. 2013;88:115–20.
11. Du Q, Martin J-C, Agnani G, Pages N, Leruyet P, Carayon P, et al. Dairy fat blends high in α-linolenic acid are superior to n-3 fatty-acid-enriched palm oil blends for increasing DHA levels in the brains of young rats. J Nutr Biochem. 2012;23:1573–82.
12. Dinel AL, Rey C, Bonhomme C, Le Ruyet P, Joffre C, Laye S. Dairy fat blend improves brain DHA and neuroplasticity and regulates corticosterone in mice. Prostaglandins Leukot Essent Fatty Acids. 2016;109:29–38.
13. Dinel AL, Rey C, Baudry C, Fressange-Mazda C, Le Ruyet P, Nadjar A, et al. Enriched dairy fat matrix diet prevents early life lipopolysaccharide-induced spatial memory impairment at adulthood. Prostaglandins Leukot Essent Fatty Acids. 2016;113:9–18.
14. Giannì ML, Roggero P, Baudry C, Ligneul A, Morniroli D, Garbarino F, et al. The influence of a formula supplemented with dairy lipids and plant oils on the erythrocyte membrane omega-3 fatty acid profile in healthy full-term infants: a double-blind randomized controlled trial. BMC Pediatr. 2012;12:164.
15. Auestad N, Montalto MB, Hall RT, Fitzgerald KM, Wheeler RE, Connor WE, et al. Visual acuity, erythrocyte fatty acid composition, and growth in term infants fed formulas with long chain polyunsaturated fatty acids for one year. Ross pediatric lipid study. Pediatr Res. 1997;41:1–10.
16. Birch EE, Carlson SE, Hoffman DR, Fitzgerald-Gustafson KM, Fu VLN, Drover JR, et al. The DIAMOND (DHA Intake And Measurement Of Neural Development) study: a double-masked, randomized controlled clinical trial of the maturation of infant visual acuity as a function of the dietary level of docosahexaenoic acid. Am J Clin Nutr. 2010;91:848–59.
17. Visentin S, Vicentin D, Magrini G, Santandreu F, Disalvo L, Sala M, et al. Red blood cell membrane fatty acid composition in infants fed formulas with different lipid profiles. Early Hum Dev. 2016;100:11–5.
18. Miller MR, Seifert J, Szabo NJ, Clare-Salzler M, Rewers M, Norris JM. Erythrocyte membrane fatty acid content in infants consuming formulas supplemented with docosahexaenoic acid (DHA) and arachidonic acid (ARA): an observational study. Matern Child Nutr. 2010;6:338–46.
19. Guesnet P, Pugo-Gunsam P, Maurage C, Pinault M, Giraudeau B, Alessandri JM, et al. Blood lipid concentrations of docosahexaenoic and arachidonic acids at birth determine their relative postnatal changes in term infants fed breast milk or formula. Am J Clin Nutr. 1999;70:292–8.
20. Kaur G, Cameron-Smith D, Garg M, Sinclair AJ. Docosapentaenoic acid (22: 5n-3): a review of its biological effects. Prog Lipid Res. 2011;50:28–34.
21. Barceló-Coblijn G, Murphy EJ. Alpha-linolenic acid and its conversion to longer chain n-3 fatty acids: benefits for human health and a role in maintaining tissue n-3 fatty acid levels. Prog Lipid Res. 2009;48:355–74.
22. Su HM, Bernardo L, Mirmiran M, Ma XH, Nathanielsz PW, Brenna JT. Dietary 18:3n-3 and 22:6n-3 as sources of 22:6n-3 accretion in neonatal baboon brain and associated organs. Lipids. 1999;34(Suppl):S347–50.
23. Drover JR, Hoffman DR, Castañeda YS, Morale SE, Garfield S, Wheaton DH, et al. Cognitive function in 18-month-old term infants of the DIAMOND study: a randomized, controlled clinical trial with multiple dietary levels of docosahexaenoic acid. Early Hum Dev. 2011;87:223–30.

9

Sonographic evaluation of adrenal size in neonates (23 to 41 weeks of gestation)

Shigeo Iijima

Abstract

Background: Fetal adrenal gland size is known to have a positive correlation with both gestational age and estimated body weight. In contrast, some clinical observations suggest that maturation of the adrenal stress response occurs after 30 weeks of gestation. In this study, adrenal gland size at birth in extremely preterm to term neonates was investigated using ultrasonography to evaluate the adrenal developmental pattern and the impact of prematurity and perinatal factors.

Methods: The area of the right adrenal gland was measured in the first 3 h of life in 350 neonates and corrected for birth weight (BW) to determine the corrected adrenal area index (cAI). The neonates were subdivided into three groups: group 1 (before 30 weeks of gestation), group 2 (30 to 36 weeks), and group 3 (after 37 weeks). Differences in the cAI among the 3 groups were compared to estimate the impact of perinatal factors.

Results: The adrenal gland size was measurable in all neonates with gestational age ranging from 23 to 41 weeks. Right adrenal gland area was highly correlated with BW ($r = 0.75$, $p < 0.01$). cAI showed a significant negative correlation with gestational age in group 1 ($r = -0.67$, $p < 0.01$), whereas it showed no correlation with gestational age in both groups 2 and 3. As for the impact of perinatal parameters on cAI, only gestational age in group 1 and only fetal distress in group 2 were correlated with cAI. In group 3, perinatal parameters such as fetal distress and low Apgar score were correlated with cAI.

Conclusions: The present study demonstrated that the developmental pattern of fetal adrenal gland was different before and after 30 weeks of gestation, suggesting that the magnitude of adrenal stress response might mature after 30 weeks of gestation.

Keywords: Adrenal gland, Size, Adrenal gland area, Ultrasonography, Neonate

Background

With the advent of ultrasonography (US), many authors have studied the sonographic appearance and measurement of normal fetal adrenal gland in utero [1–4]. These studies showed that fetal adrenal gland size is positively correlated with both gestational age and estimated body weight. In neonates, US has been shown to provide a useful method of evaluating the appearance of the adrenal glands to diagnose pathologies such as adrenal hemorrhage and hyperplasia [5, 6]. However, regarding postnatal adrenal size, some authors reported sonographic evaluation in the late 1980s, but the focus was solely on the change in size postnatally, based on marked involution of the fetal zone component during the early weeks and months of extra-uterine life [7, 8].

During the last two decades, the advances in the field of US have enabled higher resolution display and precise quantitative measurement of the organ dimensions.

Recently, it has been recognized that some very preterm infants develop acute profound primary circulatory failure that responds to glucocorticoid therapy, and a relationship between hypotension and relative adrenal insufficiency in preterm infants has been discussed [9, 10]. Previous findings demonstrated that preterm infants born before 30 weeks of gestation have a higher risk for the development of, not only chronic lung disease, but also early adrenal insufficiency in comparison to infants born after 30 weeks of gestation [5, 11].

Correspondence: sige_pd@yahoo.co.jp
Department of Neonatology, Toho University Medical Center, Tokyo, Japan

The objective of the present study was to demonstrate adrenal gland size in extremely preterm to term neonates in a specially designed prospective study, and to compare adrenal gland size between preterm and term infants to estimate the impact of prematurity and perinatal factors.

Methods

The author prospectively assessed the relationship between neonatal adrenal gland size, as measured by 2-dimensional (2D) US, and perinatal factors. Written informed parental consent was obtained.

Patients

Neonates admitted immediately after birth to the neonatal intensive care unit (NICU) at Toho University Medical Center between April 1, 2009, and March 31, 2011, were eligible for the study. Exclusion criteria were as follows: 1) outborn; 2) major congenital anomalies; 3) evident intrauterine infections (e.g. cytomegalovirus infection); and 4) parental refusal of participation.

Sonographic evaluation of the adrenal gland

All ultrasonographic scans were performed by an experienced operator (the author), using a Toshiba SSA-660A (Toshiba, Tokyo, Japan) ultrasound machine with a 7-MHz sector transducer within the first 3 h of life. With the infant in the supine position, longitudinal images of the adrenal glands were taken and the adrenal area was measured. The techniques for locating the adrenal glands and measuring the adrenal area were previously described (Fig. 1) [12]. Some researchers previously reported less variability in right than in left adrenal gland [8, 12, 13]. Therefore, only the right adrenal was used for all measurements to minimize technical errors that could influence the results.

Sonographic data analyses

It was previously described that fetal adrenal gland size was positively correlated with estimated body weight in ultrasonographic studies [1–4]. Moreover, in the previous study, we demonstrated that the adrenal area at birth was positively correlated with birth weight (BW) [12]. Therefore, a corrected adrenal area index (cAI) was calculated as the ratio of adrenal area to BW (mm^2/kg) to investigate the correlation with gestational age (GA) and perinatal parameters. Based on the previous finding that preterm infants born before 30 weeks of gestation have a higher risk of developing adrenal insufficiency compared with those born after 30 weeks of gestation [5, 11], infants were subdivided into three groups: preterm infants born before 30 weeks of gestation (group 1), preterm infants born between 30 and 36 weeks of gestation (group 2), and term infants born after 37 weeks of gestation (group 3). Differences in the cAI among the 3 groups were analyzed.

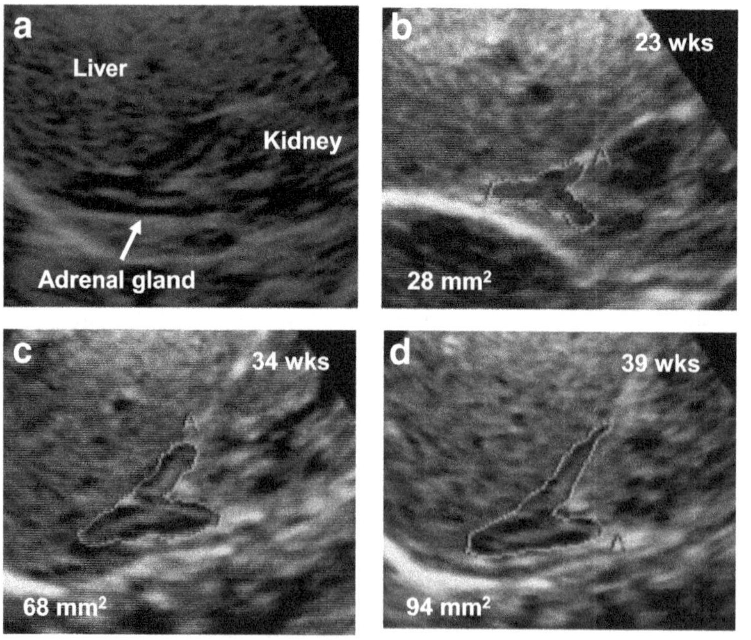

Fig. 1 (**a**) Ultrasonographic scan of the right adrenal region of a representative neonate obtained immediately after birth by the longitudinal antero-lateral approach. Sonographic appearances of the right adrenal gland of a representative in each group: (**b**) group 1: a neonate born at 23 weeks of gestation, (**c**) group 2: a neonate born at 34 weeks of gestation, and (**d**) a neonate born at 39 weeks of gestation. The border of the adrenal gland was traced manually to calculate the adrenal gland area

Clinical parameters

Collected maternal data included complications during pregnancy and conditions surrounding delivery, such as premature rupture of membranes (PROM), preeclampsia, use of antenatal steroids, fetal distress, and mode of delivery (cesarean section or not). Collected infant data included GA, BW, sex, Apgar score, and small for gestational age (SGA). The GA at birth was determined by maternal history based on the last menstrual period and obstetric examination with ultrasonography. PROM and preeclampsia were diagnosed clinically by the attending obstetrician. Fetal distress was diagnosed by intrapartum fetal heart rate irregularities, meconium staining of amniotic fluid, and abnormal fetal movement. The Apgar score was assessed at 1 and 5 min, and low 1-min Apgar score was defined if the Apgar score at 1 min was 6 or lower. SGA was defined as both BW and birth length below the 10th percentile for GA based on standards of birth size for Japanese neonates [14].

Statistical analysis

All statistical analyses were conducted using the Statistical Package for Social Sciences, version 18 (SPSS, Tokyo, Japan) for Windows. The Kolmogorov-Smirnov test was used for data normality testing. Data were presented as median (interquartile range) and percentage. The relation between continuous variables was investigated by the Pearson's and Spearman's rank correlation coefficients. Differences between both groups were compared using the Mann-Whitney U test, and Kruskal-Wallis one-way analysis of variance on ranks was used to compare the overall differences among the 3 groups. A p value < 0.05 was considered statistically significant.

Results

A total of 374 neonates were admitted to our NICU during the study period between April 2009 and March 2011, and 350 of these neonates met the inclusion criteria. Among the excluded 24 infants, 17 were outborn, 5 had major congenital anomalies, and the parents of 2 did not agree to participate. Two infants had intrauterine cytomegalovirus infection with severe brain anomaly and were excluded because of the presence of major congenital anomalies. There was no infant whose adrenals were not ultrasonographically examined in the first 3 h of life. In the enrolled 350 consecutive neonates (male/female ratio, 172:178), the median GA was 36.3 weeks, with an interquartile range (IQR) of 33.5 to 38.4 weeks, and the median BW was 2156 g, with an IQR of 1744 to 2847 g. Among the subjects, none was subsequently diagnosed with congenital adrenal hyperplasia, adrenal hemorrhage, or primary adrenal tumor (e.g. neuroblastoma).

Sonographic appearance

The adrenal gland was identified in a suprarenal location in all neonates (100%), without difficulties. However, the right adrenal was consistently easier to identify in its entirety than was the left. The glands were visualized in the configuration of a "V" or "Y" with a characteristic echogenicity of a thin, central hyperechoic stripe surrounded by a thicker hypoechoic rim. The appearance of the adrenal gland was not different by gestational age (Fig. 1). The central hyperechogenic area was not identified only in the cases whose gestational age was 23 weeks.

Measurement of right adrenal gland area

In all subjects, the median adrenal gland area was 71.0 mm^2, with IQR of 35.3 to 94.0 mm^2. As for the correlations between the adrenal area and BW, a strong correlation was observed between BW and adrenal area ($r = 0.75$, $p < 0.001$).

The data on cAI were compared among the 3 groups. cAI was significantly higher in group 1 than in groups 2 and 3, and there was no difference between groups 2 and 3 (Table 1). Next, the cAI was plotted against GA in each group (Fig. 2). As a result, two different patterns of the relationship were observed between group 1 and the other groups. The cAI was negatively correlated with gestational age in group 1 ($r = -0.67$, $p < 0.001$), whereas it was not correlated to gestational age in groups 2 ($r = -0.14$, $p = 0.07$) or 3 ($r = 0.05$, $p = 0.49$).

Influence of perinatal parameters on adrenal area index

Clinical and sonographic data of the 3 groups are summarized in Table 1. As for the comparison of adrenal sonographic data among the 3 groups, differences were significant for all perinatal parameters except for SGA and fetal distress. However, for the intragroup correlation study, only gestational age in group 1 and only fetal distress in group 2 were correlated with cAI. In group 3, perinatal parameters such as fetal distress, Apgar score, and low 1-min Apgar score were associated with cAI (Table 2). In this subgroup, cAI was greater in neonates with 1-min Apgar score 0-3 (median: 44.3 mm^2/kg) than in those with 1-min Apgar score 7-10 (median: 33.0 mm^2/kg) ($p < 0.01$); cAI was also greater in neonates with 1-min Apgar score 0-3 than in those with 1-min Apgar score 4-6 (median: 36.2 mm^2/kg) ($p = 0.04$) (Fig. 3).

Discussion

The measurement of neonatal adrenal gland has been the subject of only a few previous ultrasonographic studies, with the latest report published in the early 1990s [7, 8, 13]. Various methods of measuring the adrenal size using US have been described because of the irregular shape of the gland. These include measurements of adrenal length, width, and circumference [7, 8, 13, 15–17]. In the present

Table 1 Clinical characteristics and adrenal size of the study population (*n* = 350)

	Group 1 (*n* = 41) Gestational age < 30 wk	Group 2 (*n* = 154) Gestational age 30 - 36 wk	Group 3 (*n* = 155) Gestational age > 36 wk	*P* value
Neonatal characteristics				
Gestational age, wk	27.3 (25.2–29.1)	34.6 (33.2–35.7)	39.0 (37.7–39.9)	< 0.01
Birth weight, g	849 (622–1206)	1970 (1670–2203)	2886 (2264–3260)	< 0.01
Sex, male: female	10: 31	85: 69	77: 78	< 0.01
1-min Apgar score	6 (3–7)	8 (7–9)	8 (8–9)	< 0.01
5-min Apgar score	7 (6–8.5)	9 (9–9)	9 (8–9)	< 0.01
Low 1-min Apgar score, *n* (%)	29 (71)	23 (15)	28 (18)	< 0.01
Small for gestational age, *n* (%)	13 (32)	34 (22)	36 (23)	0.34
Maternal characteristics				
Maternal preeclampsia, *n* (%)	12 (29)	23 (15)	5 (0.3)	< 0.01
Premature rupture of the membrane, *n* (%)	16 (39)	56 (36)	22 (14)	< 0.01
Antenatal steroids, *n* (%)	31 (76)	67 (44)	0 (0)	< 0.01
Tocolysis, *n* (%)	26 (63)	99 (64)	0 (0)	< 0.01
Fetal distress, *n* (%)	10 (24)	22 (14)	34 (22)	0.12
Cesarean section, *n* (%)	29 (71)	98 (64)	52 (34)	< 0.01
Adrenal size of the neonates				
Adrenal area at birth, mm^2	47.0 (37.0–53.5)	64.0 (51.0–76.3)	93.0 (75.0–112.0)	< 0.01
Corrected adrenal area index at birth, mm^2/kg	51.1 (38.1–65.2)	33.3 (26.8–40.0)	33.9 (28.4–38.7)	< 0.01

Values are presented as median (interquartile range) or number (percentage). Low 1-min Apgar score was defined if the Apgar score at 1 min was 6 or lower

study, the adrenal area measurements were chosen. The author found only one study about the evaluation of adrenal size by adrenal area, which was conducted in the 1980s [8]. In addition to the multipart shape of the gland, insufficient resolution of the US device at that time resulted in difficulty in obtaining accurate information on the anatomical size of the glands. With the advent of the resolution and trace technology of US, it was possible to measure the adrenal area with higher accuracy than in the past. Therefore, as a measurement parameter to estimate the actual adrenal size, adrenal area might be preferable to adrenal length or width. Previously, we evaluated adrenal

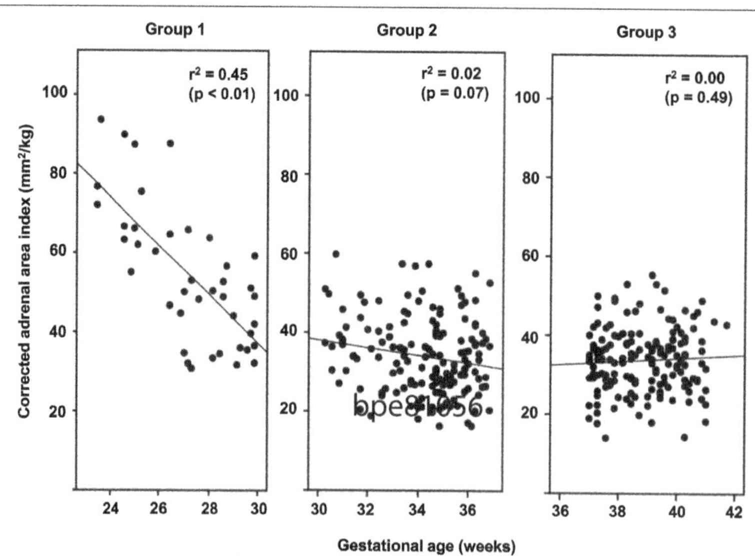

Fig. 2 Scatter plots showing the correlations between the corrected adrenal gland area index and gestational age in each group. Group 1: preterm infants born before 30 weeks of gestation, group 2: preterm infants born between 30 and 36 weeks of gestation, group 3: term infants born after 37 weeks of gestation

Table 2 Correlation between corrected adrenal area index and perinatal parameters in each group

	Group 1		Group 2		Group 3	
	CC	*P* value	CC	*P* value	CC	*P* value
Neonatal characteristics						
Gestational age	−0.67	< 0.01	−0.15	0.07	0.06	0.49
Male sex	−0.31	0.05	0.08	0.33	0.06	0.49
1-min Apgar score	0.30	0.06	−0.06	0.47	−0.24	< 0.01
5-min Apgar score	−0.31	0.05	−0.11	0.18	−0.12	0.15
Low 1-min Apgar score	0.35	0.02	0.07	0.38	0.24	< 0.01
Small for gestational age	0.07	0.67	0.01	0.96	−0.08	0.31
Matemal characteristics						
Maternal Preeclamsia	−0.16	0.33	−0.02	0.81	−0.05	0.56
Premature rupture of the membrane	0.12	0.45	0.13	0.10	0.10	0.21
Antenatal steroids	0.06	0.73	0.14	0.10	–	–
Tocolysis	0.16	0.29	0.07	0.39	–	–
Fetal distress	−0.02	0.89	0.21	0.01	0.21	< 0.01
Cesarean section	−0.15	0.34	0.03	0.67	0.04	0.64

Group 1: Gestational age < 30 weeks (n = 41); Group 2: gestational age 30-36 weeks (n = 154); Group 3: gestational age > 36 weeks (n = 155). Low 1-min Apgar score was defined if the Apgar score at 1 min was 6 or lower. *CC*, Correlation coeficient

size by measurements of the adrenal area and demonstrated that the adrenal area could be measured in all neonates born after 23 weeks of gestation [12]. In the present study, although the author evaluated a larger number of subjects than in the previous study, the right adrenal gland was seen and measured in the assessment, without difficulty, in all study subjects.

In the present study, cAI was calculated to investigate the correlation with GA. A peculiar pattern was found between cAI in preterm infants with a GA below 30 weeks and in those with a GA above 30 weeks. cAI was negatively correlated with GA up to 30 weeks, whereas it remained almost constant from 30 weeks to term. Previously, Kangaloo et al. demonstrated in their

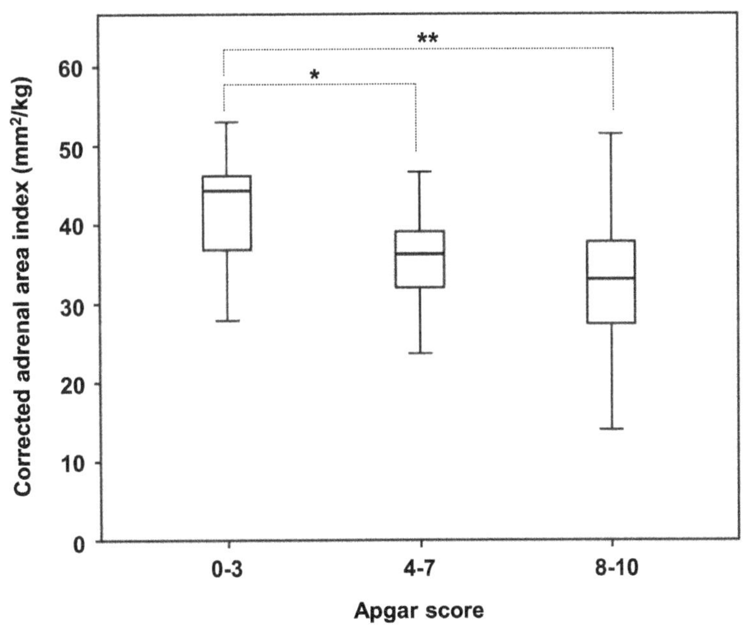

Fig. 3 Box and whisker plot showing the results of corrected adrenal gland area index for the 155 term infants with 1-min Apgar score of 0-3, 4-7, and 8-10. Each box ranges from the 25th percentile at the lower edge to the 75th percentile at the upper edge. The median is shown as a line across the box. The two adjacent values below and above the box are: the largest value is below the upper inner limit and the smallest value is above the lower inner limit

ultrasonographic study that the length of the adrenal gland was directly correlated with GA up to 32 weeks of gestation, after which no significant increase in the length of the gland occurred to full term [13]. There might be some functional differences in fetal adrenal gland around 30 weeks of gestation. In the present study, however, the intergroup and intragroup comparisons among the 3 groups could not identify any significant perinatal factors that could explain why the correlation patterns between cAI and GA differed between before and after 30 weeks of gestation.

The fetal adrenal gland develops and exhibits a marked change in size, structure, and function during the fetal and perinatal periods. The fetal adrenal cortex consists of three compartments: the relatively large, inner fetal zone (FZ), the outer definitive zone (DZ), and the intermediate transitional zone (TZ). The FZ mainly produces androgens, the DZ produces mineralocorticoids, and the TZ contains enzymes for cortisol production [18]. The fetal adrenal cortex grows rapidly from approximately 10 weeks of gestation to term almost entirely owing to the enlargement of the FZ. Subsequently, the adrenal size almost equals that of fetal kidneys by 20 weeks of gestation, and the weight doubles between 20 and 30 weeks [19]. In contrast, the DZ growth occurs owing to hyperplasia by 10 to 12 weeks of gestation. Subsequently, the TZ cells, which differentiate from the definitive cortex, have the capacity to synthesize cortisol. By 30 weeks of gestation, the DZ and TZ begin maturation into the zona glomerulosa and the zona fasciculata, respectively [19]. Fetal adrenal size exhibits disproportionality relative to body weight throughout the entire growth process. The present study plainly showed that fetal adrenal growth might greatly change after 30 weeks of gestation.

Considering adrenal functions, Bolt et al. showed in their study that the cortisol response to adrenocorticotropic hormone stimulation in infants born before 30 weeks of gestation was significantly lower than in more mature infants [20]. Moreover, Heckmann et al. demonstrated that the severity of illness did not have a significant influence on cortisol production rates in preterm infants born before 30 weeks of gestation, and they concluded that cortisol production rates in such immature infants might reflect inadequate stress reaction [21]. Grofer et al. demonstrated a maturation of the adrenal stress response in infants born after 30 weeks of gestation by showing a positive association between severity of illness and cortisol production rate in those infants, unlike in more immature infants [22]. The hormonal demands of growth and maturation in premature infants need to be balanced with those of acute critical stress. However, this process is not yet complete in a preterm infant born before 30 weeks of gestation. Fetal mechanisms regulating glucocorticoid homeostasis might persist after birth to protect such immature infant from excessive glucocorticoids [23]. Recently, relative adrenal insufficiency has been discussed in the preterm infant born before 30 weeks of gestation [24]. This could be explained by the above-mentioned immature adrenal function of such preterm infants. It is thought that the developmental process of fetal adrenal function might support the change of the cAI shown in the present study. A limitation of this study is that the data collected about the mode of delivery included only whether cesarean section (CS) was performed or not, rather than including all the details. Especially in extremely preterm delivery, CS is often performed after the onset of labor. Turan et al. have suggested that the premature onset of labor has a relationship with fetal adrenal gland enlargement [4]. Therefore, the result may be influenced by the fact that the delivery occurs before or after the onset of labor.

In this study, especially in term neonates, there were significant correlations between cAI and both fetal distress and low 1-min Apgar score, that is, adrenal enlargement was associated with a clinical history of perinatal distress. A similar sonographic feature has been previously reported by some investigators [25–27]. Their histological studies postulated that adrenal enlargement was caused by adrenal congestion. Perinatal stress like asphyxia causes a redistribution of cardiac output to preserve blood flow to the more vital organs such as the brain, heart, and adrenal glands, and the consequent congestion may increase the pressure within the capillary network [27]. As hypoxic events cause damage to endothelial cells and impair vascular autoregulation, hemorrhage or infarction can occur in these organs, and probably in the adrenal gland [27]. However, the pathophysiology is not fully understood. Further investigations to demonstrate the causal relationship between perinatal asphyxia and adrenal size are warranted.

Conclusions

The present study demonstrated that the developmental pattern of fetal adrenal gland was different before and after 30 weeks of gestation. In addition, the adrenal area relative to body weight correlated with perinatal asphyxia after 30 weeks of gestation. The results in the present study suggest that the magnitude of adrenal stress response might mature after 30 weeks of gestation.

Abbreviations

2D: 2-dimensional; BW: Birth weight; cAI: Corrected adrenal area index; DZ: Definitive zone; FZ: Fetal zone; GA: Gestational age; IQR: Interquartile range; NICU: Neonatal intensive care unit; PROM: Premature rupture of membranes; SGA: Small for gestational age; TZ: Transitional zone; US: Ultrasonography

Acknowledgments

The author would like to extend his thanks to the NICU doctors working at the Perinatal Center of Toho University Medical Center.

Funding
The authors received no specific funding for this research.

Authors' contributions
SI conceived the study; collected, analyzed, and interpreted the data; and prepared the first draft of the manuscript. The author has read and approved the final version of the manuscript.

Competing interests
The authors declare that they have no competing interests.

References

1. Rosenberg ER, Bowie JD, Andreotti RF, Fields SI. Sonographic evaluation of fetal adrenal glands. AJR. 1982;139:1145–7.
2. Jeanty P, Chervenak F, Grannum P, Hobbins JC. Normal ultrasonic size and characteristics of the fetal adrenal glands. Prenat Diagn. 1984;4:21–8.
3. Lewis E, Kurtz AB, Dubbins PA, Wapner RJ, Goldberg BB. Real-time ultrasonographic evaluation of normal fetal adrenal glands. J Ultrasound Med. 1982;1:265–70.
4. Turan OM, Turan S, Funai EF, Buhimschi IA, Copel JA, Buhimschi CS. Fetal adrenal gland volume: a novel method to identify women at risk for impending preterm birth. Obstet Gynecol. 2007;109:855–62.
5. Velaphi SC, Perlman JM. Neonatal adrenal hemorrhage: clinical and abdominal sonographic findings. Clin Pediatr (Phila). 2001;40:545–8.
6. Al-Alwan I, Navarro O, Daneman D, Daneman A. Clinical utility of adrenal ultrasonography in the diagnosis of congenital adrenal hyperplasia. J Pediatr. 1999;135:71–5.
7. Oppenheimer DA, Carroll BA, Yousem S. Sonography of the normal neonatal adrenal gland. Radiology. 1983;146:157–60.
8. Scott EM, Thomas A, McGarrigle HHG, Lachelin GCL. Serial adrenal ultrasonography in normal neonates. J Ultrasound Med. 1990;9:279–83.
9. Watterberg KL. Adrenal insufficiency and cardiac dysfunction in the preterm infant. Pediatr Res. 2002;51:422–5.
10. Ng PC, Lee CH, Lam CW, Ma KC, Fork TF, Chan HIS, et al. Transient adrenocortical insufficiency of prematurity and systemic hypotension in very low birthweight infants. Arch Dis Child Fetal Neonatal Ed. 2004;89:F119–26.
11. Watterberg KL, Scott SM. Evidence of early adrenal insufficiency in babies who develop bronchopulmonary dysplasia. Pediatr. 1995;95:120–5.
12. Iijima S, Uga N, Ohzeki T. Postnatal changes in adrenal size in very low birth weight infants: sonographic evaluation for the prediction of late-onset glucocorticoid-responsive circulatory collapse. Am J Perinatol. 2010;27:485–91.
13. Kangaloo H, Diament MJ, Gold RH, Barrett C, Lippe B, Geffner M, et al. Sonography of adrenal glands in neonates and children: changes in appearance with age. J Clin Ultrasound. 1986;14:43–7.
14. Ogawa Y, Iwamura T, Kuriya N, Nishida H, Takeuchi H, Takada H, et al. Birth size standards by gestational age for Japanese neonates. J Jpn Soc Perin Neon Med. 1998;34:624–32. (in Japanese)
15. Sivit CJ, Hung W, Taylor GA, Catena LM, Brown-Jones C, Kushner DC. Sonography in neonatal congenital adrenal hyperplasia. AJR Am J Roentgenol. 1991;156:141–3.
16. Bryan PJ, Caldamone AA, Morrison SC, Yulish BS, Owens R. Ultrasound findings in the adreno-genital syndrome. J Ultrasound Med. 1988;7:675–9.
17. Hauffa BP, Menzel D, Stolecke H. Age-related changes in adrenal size during the first year of life in normal newborns, infants and patients with congenital adrenal hyperplasia due to 21-hydroxylase deficiency: comparison of ultrasound and hormonal parameters. Eur J Pediatr. 1988;148:43–9.
18. Winter JSD. Fetal and neonatal adrenocortical physiology. In: Polin RA, Fox WW, Abman H, editors. Fetal and neonatal physiology. 3rd ed. Philadelphia: WB Saunders; 2003. p. 1915–26.
19. Mesiano S, Jaffe RB. Developmental and functional biology of the primate fetal adrenal cortex. Endocrine Rev. 1997;18:378–403.
20. Bolt RJ, Van Weissenbruch MM, Popp-Snijders C, Sweep FG, Lafeber HN, Delemarre-van de Waal HA. Maturity of the adrenal cortex in very preterm infants is related to gestational age. Pediatr Res. 2002;52:405–10.
21. Heckmann M, Hartmann MF, Kampschulte B, Gack H, Bödeker R-H, Gortner L, et al. Cortisol production rates in preterm infants in relation to growth and illness: a noninvasive prospective study using gas chromatography-mass spectrometry. J Clin Endocrinol Metab. 2005;90:5737–42.
22. Grofer B, Bodeker RH, Gortner L, Heckmann M. Maturation of adrenal function determined by urinary glucocorticoid steroid excretion rates in preterm infants of more than 30 weeks of gestational age. Neonatology. 2010;98:200–5.
23. Beitins IZ, Bayard F, Ances IG, Kowarski A, Migeon CJ. The metabolic clearance rate, blood production, interconversion and transplacental passage of cortisol and cortisone in pregnancy near term. Pediatr Res. 1973;7:509–19.
24. Watterberg KL. Adrenocortical function and dysfunction in the fetus and neonate. Semin Neonatol. 2004;9:13–21.
25. Cohen EK, Daneman A, Stringer DA, Soto G, Thorner P. Focal adrenal hemorrhage: a new US appearance. Radiology. 1986;161:631–3.
26. Nissenbaum M, Jequier S. Enlargement of adrenal glands preceding adrenal hemorrhage. J Clin Ultrasound. 1989;16:349–52.
27. Koplewitz BZ, Daneman A, Cutz E, Hellmann J. Neonatal adrenal congestion: a sonographic-pathologic correlation. Pediatr Radiol. 1998;28:958–62.

10

Prevalence and determinants of essential newborn care practices in the Lawra District of Ghana

Mahama Saaka*, Fusena Ali and Felicia Vuu

Abstract

Background: There was less than satisfactory progress, especially in sub-Saharan Africa, towards child and maternal mortality targets of Millennium Development Goals (MDGs) 4 and 5. The main aim of this study was to describe the prevalence and determinants of essential new newborn care practices in the Lawra District of Ghana.

Methods: A cross-sectional study was carried out in June 2014 on a sample of 422 lactating mothers and their children aged between 1 and 12 months. A systematic random sampling technique was used to select the study participants who attended post-natal clinic in the Lawra district hospital.

Results: Of the 418 newborns, only 36.8% (154) was judged to have had safe cord care, 34.9% (146) optimal thermal care, and 73.7% (308) were considered to have had adequate neonatal feeding. The overall prevalence of adequate new born care comprising good cord care, optimal thermal care and good neonatal feeding practices was only 15.8%.

Mothers who attained at least Senior High Secondary School were 20.5 times more likely to provide optimal thermal care [AOR 22.54; 95% CI (2.60–162.12)], compared to women had no formal education at all. Women who received adequate ANC services were 4.0 times (AOR = 4.04 [CI: 1.53, 10.66]) and 1.9 times (AOR = 1.90 [CI: 1.01, 3.61]) more likely to provide safe cord care and good neonatal feeding as compared to their counterparts who did not get adequate ANC. However, adequate ANC services was unrelated to optimal thermal care. Compared to women who delivered at home, women who delivered their index baby in a health facility were 5.6 times more likely of having safe cord care for their babies (AOR = 5.60, CI: 1.19–23.30), $p = 0.03$.

Conclusions: The coverage of essential newborn care practices was generally low. Essential newborn care practices were positively associated with high maternal educational attainment, adequate utilization of antenatal care services and high maternal knowledge of newborn danger signs. Therefore, greater improvement in essential newborn care practices could be attained through proven low-cost interventions such as effective ANC services, health and nutrition education that should span from community to health facility levels.

Keywords: Essential newborn care, Newborn danger signs, Neonate feeding, Optimal thermal care, Safe cord care, Lawra District

* Correspondence: mmsaaka@gmail.com
University for Development Studies, School of Allied Health Sciences, P O Box, 1883 Tamale, Ghana

Background

Many countries especially in sub-Saharan Africa were unable to achieve the Millennium Development Goals (MDGs) 4 and 5. In particular, the set target of reducing under-five mortality rates by two-thirds as of 2015 was not met because there was little reduction in neonatal mortality (NMR). Many countries are reported to have made little or no progress towards the child survival target, and that some countries in sub-Saharan Africa had even witnessed a deterioration in child survival rates [1].

Suboptimal newborn care practices still persist and neonatal mortality rates have been resistant to change and now contribute about 40% of all under-five deaths world-wide [2]. In Ghana, neonatal mortality is estimated at 29 /1000 live births and 68% of all deaths among children under age five years take place before a child's first birthday, with 48% occurring during the first month of life [3]. Though there has been a decline of 29% in neonatal mortality since 1993 in Ghana, the decrease was at a slower pace than infant and child mortality. Consequently, the contribution of neonatal deaths to infant deaths had increased from 53% in 1998 to 71% in 2014 [3].

World leaders have launched a renew effort to reduce child mortality under the Sustainable Development Goals (SDGs). One major target of the SDGs is to "end preventable deaths of newborns and children under 5 years of age, with all countries aiming to reduce neonatal mortality to at least 12 per 1,000 live births and under-5 mortality to at least 25 per 1,000 live births by 2030" [4]. To achieve this target, it is important for mothers to adopt essential newborn care practices. To help reduce newborn morbidity, mortality and promote healthy newborn care practices, the World Health Organization (WHO) recommended a package of essential newborn care practices some of which include clean cord care (that is, cutting and tying of the umbilical cord with a sterilized instrument and thread), thermal care (drying and wrapping the newborn immediately after delivery and delaying the newborn's first bath for at least 24 h or several days to reduce hypothermia risk), and initiating breastfeeding within the first hour of birth [5].

It has been estimated globally that over two-thirds of newborns could be saved through existing maternal and child health programmes that relate to cord care to decrease sepsis, temperature control and initiation of early breastfeeding [6–10].

In Ghana, skilled assistance during delivery has increased from 40% in 1988 to 74% in 2014. Facility-based deliveries have increased from 42% in 1993 to 73% in 2014. Despite this modest improvement, more than one-quarter of births occur at home especially in rural areas. In the Upper West Region where this study was conducted, delivery in a health facility was 63% of births [3].

Deliveries at home are usually without the support of skilled birth attendants (SBA). Under such circumstances, babies may not receive the recommended immediate newborn care practices and so become more vulnerable to infection-related risks [11]. There is evidence that suggests that most neonatal deaths in developing countries occur at home, and attended by unskilled health practitioners [2]. However, very little is documented on the traditional newborn care practices in the Lawra District of Ghana where a significant number of deliveries still take place at home. It is in view of this that this study was undertaken. The main aim was to describe the prevalence and determinants of essential newborn care practices.

Methods

Study setting

The study was carried out in the Lawra District hospital. The Lawra District lies in the North-West corner of the upper West Region of Ghana. The total area of the District is 1051.2 km^2. The District has two hospitals located in Lawra and Nandom. They provide clinical and public health services as well as serve as a referral centres for the sub-districts. There are 10 sub-districts which provide primary health care services.

Apart from agriculture, which engages about 80% of the population, there are small scale enterprises such as petty trading, artisanal works, small-scale industry enterprises, hotel/restaurants/chop bar and transport services. There are also those employed as public servants, although wages are low. The dominant economic activity is agriculture which does not yield the required returns necessary for meaningful standards of living. The result is wide spread poverty among the people with severe impact on women and children.

The study design, population, sampling

A cross-sectional study was carried out in June 2014 on a sample of 422 lactating mothers and their children. The primary study population comprised women of reproductive age (15 to 49 years) who have delivered a live baby within the past 12 months prior to the conduct of this study. The 12-month limit was set with the intention of mitigating recall bias by the mother. A systematic random sampling technique was used to select the study participants who attended post-natal clinic in the Lawra District Hospital. The list of mothers contained in the attendance register for mothers who sought post-natal care served as the sampling frame. A sampling interval was calculated by dividing the total number of mothers (800) by the required sample size of 422. A random number between 1 and the sampling interval was selected to be the starting point of the sample extraction. Subsequently, the study participants were selected by adding the sampling interval to the number corresponding to the previous mother chosen on the list. This process was continued until the required number was obtained.

A sample size of 384 was required to ensure that the estimated prevalence of the main outcome variable (coverage of essential new born care practices) was within plus or minus 5% of the true prevalence at 95% confidence level. An additional 10% to adjust for unexpected events (e.g. damaged/incomplete questionnaire) was factored in the sample size determination and so the sample size was 422.

Data collection

A structured questionnaire was administered through face to face interview to obtain information from respondents. The questionnaire comprised different sections including socioeconomic and demographic information, birth preparedness, knowledge of women about newborn danger signs, care during pregnancy and delivery (Additional file 1).

Dependent and independent variables

The women were asked questions on essential newborn care practices including a) type of instrument used to cut the umbilical cord b) whether the newborn was dried and wrapped soon after delivery, c) the number hours or days after birth the newborn was first bathed d) the temperature of the water used in bathing e) whether any pre-lacteal food or drink was given, and f) the number of hours or days after birth breastfeeding was initiated g) whether colostrum was fed to the baby h) whether exclusive breast feeding was practiced.

Three composite indices of essential newborn care practices (safe cord care, optimal thermal care and good neonatal feeding practices) were the main outcome measures used in the study.

Safe cord care was defined as use of a clean cutting instrument to cut the umbilical cord plus clean thread to tie the cord plus no substance applied to the cord. Optimal thermal care was defined as baby wrapped within 10 min of birth plus first bath after 6 or more hours plus using warm water to bath the baby. A child was considered to have received good neonatal feeding, he/she should be breast feeding at the time of the study, initiated breastfeeding within the first 1 hour after birth, not being fed with prelacteals, fed with colostrum and avoidance of bottle-feeding. If one or more of the conditions were not met, then the feeding practice was described as inadequate or bad.

The independent variables included socio-demographic factors, maternal age, educational attainment, ethnicity, religion etc. Socio-economic status (SES) was measured as household wealth index. Principal components analysis (PCA) was used to quantify a proxy measure of SES based on ownership of specified durable goods (television, radio, car, mobile telephone, etc.) and housing characteristics (access to electricity, source of drinking water, type of toilet facilities, type of flooring material and type of cooking fuel) [12]. Utilization of antenatal care services and maternal knowledge on newborn danger signs were also assessed as explanatory variables.

Data analysis

Descriptive and inferential statistics were done using the predictive analytic software (PASW) for Windows version 18.0 and statistical significance was taken when $p < 0.05$. Chi-square statistics were performed to compare the levels of each of the dependent variables with the explanatory variables. A multiple logistic regression was used to identify socio-demographic, mothers' knowledge of specific newborn danger signs, attendance at delivery by skilled birth attendant, antenatal and delivery care factors that were associated with the three newborn care practices (that is, safe cord care, optimal thermal care and good neonatal breastfeeding). Explanatory variables which were significant at bivariate analysis at a p-value of 0.05 or less were fed into the regression model after confirming the absence of multi-collinearity between these independent variables.

Ethical considerations

The study protocol was approved by the Scientific Review and Ethics Committee of the School of Allied Health Sciences, University for Development Studies, Ghana.

Informed consent was also obtained after needed information and explanation. In situations, where the respondent could not write or read, verbal informed consent was sought from all the study participants before the commencement of any interview. Data were analyzed and presented anonymously.

Results

In all 422 women were recruited for the study, but due to incomplete responses to questionnaires, the valid responses obtained from respondents was 418, giving a response rate of 99.1%.

Socio-demographic characteristics of study sample

The 418 respondents were mothers who were residents in rural settings. The mean age was 28.5 (SD 5.6) years with a range of 16–49 years. The details of the sample characteristics including maternal educational level, marital status, religion of mothers, occupation of mothers, and maternal age distribution are shown in Table 1. About 29 (6.9%) of the mothers had no formal education and 75 (17.9%) attained tertiary level of education. The majority of the mothers 333 (79.7%) were married. Most of the mothers 239 (57.2%) were Christians.

Table 1 Socio-demographic and reproductive characteristics of respondents ($N = 418$)

Age category	Frequency *n* (%)
Under 20 years	14 (3.3)
20–34 years	349 (83.5)
At least 35 years	55 (13.2)
Religion	
Christianity	239 (57.2)
Islam	179 (42.8)
Marital Status	
Married	333 (79.7)
Single	81 (19.4)
Divorced	1 (0.2)
Widowed	3 (0.7)
Educational Level	
None	29 (6.9)
Primary	54 (12.9)
JHS	113 (27.0)
SHS/Vocational/Technical	147 (35.2)
Tertiary	75 (17.90
Occupational Level	
Unemployed	69 (16.5)
Petty trader	182 (43.5)
Farmer	18 (4.3)
Civil / Public Servant	50 (12.0)
Others	99 (23.7)
Maternal Knowledge of dangers of newborn care signs	
1–3	229 (54.8)
At least 4	189 (45.2)
Total	418 (100.0)
Gravidity	
Primigravidae	166 (39.7)
Secundigravidae	132 (31.6)
Multigravidae	120 (28.7)
Parity	
Primiparous	211 (50.5)
Secundiparous	111 (26.6)
Multiparous	96 (23.0)
Timing of first ANC visit	
First trimester	372 (89.0)
Second trimester	41 (9.8)
Third trimester	5 (1.2)

Most 182 (43.5%) of the mothers were petty traders and only 18 (4.3%) mothers were farmers. More than half 263 (62.9%) of the infants were females.

Coverage of essential newborn care practices

Of the 418 respondents, 215 (51.4%) reported their babies were wrapped 5 min after delivery and 12(2.9%) were wrapped between 30 and 60 min after birth. In 85.4% of the deliveries, scissors were used to cut the cord and 39.7% (166) of the babies were bathed within 1–6 h of delivery. Shea- butter was commonly applied to the umbilical stump in 60.3% (252) of the babies and 51.4% were wrapped immediately after delivery. The main reasons given by mothers for applying substances to the cord stump were to prevent infection and aid healing (Table 2).

Three composite indices of essential newborn care practices (safe cord care, optimal thermal care and good neonatal feeding practices) were created. The coverage of these composite newborn care measures was generally low. Of the 418 newborns, only 36.8% (154) were judged to have had safe cord care, 34.9% (146) optimal thermal care, and 73.7% (308) were considered to have had adequate neonatal feeding. The overall prevalence of adequate newborn care comprising good cord care, optimal thermal care and good neonatal feeding practices was only 15.8% (Table 3).

Women who were classified as high ANC content had a significantly higher prevalence of good infant feeding compared to women who received low ANC content (75.5% versus 58.7%) (Chi-squared = 6.0, $p = 0.014$). Similarly, women whose ANC attendance was adequate were more likely to provide optimal thermal care (37.9% versus 10.9%) (Chi-squared = 13.2, $p < 0.001$). Adequate ANC attendance was also associated with safe cord care ($\chi 2 = 15.0$, $p < 0.001$).

Determinants of essential newborn care practices

We tested whether the composite newborn care practices (safe cord care, optimal thermal care and good neonatal feeding) were related to socio-demographic factors, socio-economic status, and adequacy of antenatal services and mothers' knowledge of specific newborn danger signs.. The predictors were common for the newborn care practices. Overall, the findings show that good neonatal feeding practices, optimal thermal care and good cord care were commonly adopted among women aged 25–34 years, women who had adequate ANC attendance (that is, ANC early initiated in first trimester and at least 4 ANC visits), and those who could mention at least 4 danger signs of the newborn (Tables 4, 5, 6).

In logistic regression analysis, the main predictors of essential new born care practices were maternal educational attainment, maternal age, and adequacy of antenatal care (ANC) attendance and maternal knowledge of newborn danger signs.

Maternal age at interview showed an independent association with essential newborn care practices. Compared to women aged at least 35 years, women under 20 years

Table 2 Newborn Care Practices ($N = 418$)

New born care practice	Frequency *n* (%)
Instrument used to cut the umbilical cord	
New blade	48 (11.5)
Any available blade	5 (1.2)
Scissors	357 (85.4)
Others	8 (1.9)
Total	418 (100)
Material used to clamp tie cord	
Thread	18 (4.3)
Cord tie	14 (3.3)
Cord clamp	385 (92.1)
Others	1 (0.2)
Total	418 (100.0)
What was applied to cord	
Nothing	12 (2.9)
Shea butter	252 (60.3)
Spirit	147 (35.2)
Shea butter with powder	3 (0.7)
String	1 (0.2)
Others	3 (0.7)
Total	418 (100.0)
Time baby was wrapped	
Immediately (< 5 min)	215 (51.4)
5–10 min	155 (37.1)
30–60 min	12 (2.9)
Unknown	36 (8.6)
Total	418 (100.0)
Timing of newborn's first bath	
Soon after birth	29 (6.9)
1–6 h	166 (39.7)
More than 6 h but less than 24 h	148 (35.4)
More than 24 h	4 (1.0)
Can't tell	71 (17.0)
Total	418 (100.0)
Reasons for applying substances to the cord stump	
Prevent infection	109 (26.1)
To aid healing	281 (67.2)
Keep it dry	4 (1.0)
Prevent water from entering the stomach	8 (1.9)
Midwifes advised me to used	8 (1.9)
Not Applicable	8 (1.9)
Total	418 (100.0)

were 6.6 times more likely to provide safe cord care to their babies (AOR = 6.57, CI: 1.71–25.31), $p = 0.006$. Compared to women aged at least 35 years, their counterparts aged 20–34 years were 3.3 times (AOR = 3. 28 [CI: 1.34, 8.04]), 2.0 times (AOR = 2.02 [CI: 1.11, 3.70]) and 7.3 times (AOR = 7.31 [CI: 1.65, 32.44]) more likely to provide optimal thermal care, good neonatal feeding and overall adequate new born care practices respectively (Table 7). Compared to women who delivered at home, women who delivered their index baby in a health facility were 5.6 times more likely to have safe cord care for their babies (AOR = 5.60, CI: 1.19–23.30).

Table 3 Composite measures of newborn care practices

New born care practice	Frequency *n* (%)
Safe cord care	
No	264 (63.2)
Yes	154 (36.8)
Total	418 (100.0)
Optimal thermal care	
No	272 (65.1)
Yes	146 (34.9)
Total	418 (100.0)
Good neonatal feeding	
No	110 (26.3)
Yes	308 (73.7)
Total	418 (100.0)
Adequate total neonatal care	
No	352 (84.2)
Yes	66 (15.8)
Total	418 (100.0)

Women who received adequate ANC services were 4.0 times (AOR = 4.04 [CI: 1.53, 10.66]) and 1.9 times (AOR = 1.90 [CI: 1.01, 3.61]) more likely to provide safe cord care and good neonatal feeding as compared to their counterparts who did not get adequate ANC. However, adequate ANC services was unrelated to optimal thermal care.

Compared to primiparous women, multiparous women were 2.7 times (AOR = 2.67 [CI: 1.41, 5.05]) more likely to provide optimal thermal care whilst secondi-parous were 2 times (AOR = 2.05 [CI: 1.08, 3.89]) more likely to provide overall adequate new born care.

Mothers who attained at least Senior High Secondary School were 20.5 times more likely to provide optimal thermal care [AOR 22.54; 95% CI (2.60–162.12)], compared to women had no formal education at all.

Maternal knowledge of at least four key newborn danger signs was significantly associated with increased probability of providing good neonatal feeding to babies (AOR = 2.0, 95% CI: 1.26–3.17). Furthermore, mothers who could recall at least 4 new born danger signs were at least 2 times more likely to provide overall adequate

Table 4 Predictors of good cord care (Bivariate analysis)

Variable	N	Good cord care? No n (%)	Yes n (%)	Test statistic
Age (years)				
Under 20 years	14	5 (35.7)	9 (64.3)	Chi-square (χ^2) = 11.6, $p = 0.003$
20–34 years	349	215 (61.6)	134 (38.4)	
At least 35 years	55	44 (80.0)	11 (20.0)	
Adequacy of ANC attendance				
No	46	41 (89.1)	5 (10.9)	Chi-square (χ^2) = 15.0, $p < 0.001$
Yes	372	223 (59.9)	149 (40.1)	
Knowledge of dangers of newborn care signs				
1–3	229	156 (68.1)	73 (31.9)	Chi-square (χ^2) = 5.4, $p = 0.02$
At least 4	189	108 (57.1)	81 (42.9)	
Mothers' education				
None	29	25 (86.2)	4 (13.8)	Chi-square (χ^2) = 14.0, $p = 0.001$
Low	167	115 (68.9)	52 (31.1)	
High	222	124 (55.9)	98 (44.1)	

new born care practices than their counterparts who knew less than 4 new born danger signs.

Discussion

This study is the first that has assessed the prevalence and determinants of newborn care practices in the Lawra District of Ghana. Though some studies conducted in Ghana have highlighted on optimal thermal care and clean delivery practices for newborns [13–15], issues regarding neonatal feeding practices have received less attention. Furthermore, this present study has used composite indices which give a better reflection of safe

Table 5 Relationship between optimal thermal care and socio-demographic/antenatal care factors ($N = 418$)

Variable	N	Optimal thermal care? No n (%)	Yes n (%)	Test statistic
Age (years)				
Under 20 years	14	10 (64.3	5 (35.7)	Chi-square (χ^2) = 10.1, $p = 0.006$
20–34 years	349	216 (61.9)	133 (38.1)	
At least 35 years	55	46 (83.6)	9 (16.4)	
Total				
Mothers education				
None	29	24 (82.8)	5 (17.2)	Chi-square (χ^2) = 45.4, $p < 0.001$
Low	167	131 (78.4)	36 (21.6)	
High	222	113 (50.9)	109 (49.1)	
Religion of mother				
Christianity	239	167 (69.9)	72 (30.1)	$\chi^2 = 5.7$, $p = 0.02$
Islam	179	105 (58.7)	74 (41.3)	
Knowledge of newborn danger signs				
1–3	229	165 (72.1)	64 (27.9)	$\chi^2 = 10.9$ $p = 0.001$
At least 4	189	107 (56.6)	82 (43.4)	
Adequacy of ANC attendance				
No	46	41 (89.1)	5 (10.9)	Chi-square (χ^2) = 13.2, $p < 0.001$
Yes	372	231 (62.1)	141 (37.9)	

Table 6 Relationship between good neonatal feeding and socio-demographic/antenatal care factors ($N = 418$)

Variable	N	Good neonatal feeding? No n (%)	Yes n (%)	Test statistic
Age (years)				
Under 20 years	14	5 (35.7)	9 (64.3)	Chi-square (χ^2) = 6.2, $p = 0.05$
20–34 years	349	85 (24.4)	264 (75.6)	
At least 35 years	55	22 (40.0)	33 (60.0)	
Adequacy of ANC attendance				
No	46	19 (41.3)	27 (58.7)	Chi-square (χ^2) = 5.9, $p = 0.014$
Yes	376	91 (24.5)	281 (75.5)	
Mothers' education				
None	29	10 (34.5)	19 (65.5)	$\chi^2 = 5.5$, $p = 0.06$
Low	167	52 (31.1)	115 (68.9)	
High	222	48 (21.6)	174 (78.4)	
Knowledge of newborn danger signs				
1–3	229	74 (32.3)	155 (67.7)	$\chi^2 = 9.4$ $p = 0.002$
At least 4	189	36 (19.0)	153 (81.0)	

cord, optimal thermal care and neonatal feeding. The findings of our study remain relevant because they confirm that of earlier studies and also fill a knowledge gap by showing that using single practice indicators could be less informative in the magnitude of essential newborn practices. For example, optimal thermal care as assessed in the present study included summing up scores for wrapping the baby within 10 min of birth, delaying for at least 6 h and using warm water. A study that uses only one of these indicators will present a different situation from one that uses a combination of these variables.

Prevalence of essential newborn care practices

Three composite newborn care practices (safe cord care, optimal thermal care, and good neonatal breastfeeding) were investigated and the coverage of these was found to be generally low. These composite variables give a better reflection of safe cord, optimal thermal care and neonatal feeding. The three newborn care practices were associated with socio-demographic, antenatal and delivery care factors.

As in other studies, safe cord care was defined as use of a clean cutting instrument to cut the umbilical cord plus clean thread to tie the cord plus no substance applied to the cord [16–18]. Cord cutting with safe instruments such as new razor blades and scissors was commonly practiced (96.9%) but then when one takes a closer and more holistic approach to safe cord care (that is using composite indicators), only 36.8% actually received that. This means assessing the situation using single practice indicators could be misleading. Poor cord care was driven mainly by putting substances on the cord.

Most mothers applied various things like shea-butter, methylated spirit, shea-butter mixed with powder to the cord stump. The reasons given for applying substances to the cord stump include hastening the healing process, prevent cord stump from smelling and infections and also to prevent water from entering into newborn's stomach. Since these substances are coming from unsterile sources the likelihood of contamination is high and may thus be harmful to newborns. Similar findings have been reported in the Asante Akim North District in Southern Ghana [19] and in Bangladesh where unhygienic cord care practices were prevalent [20].

Optimal thermal care (defined as baby wrapped within 10 min of birth plus first bath after six or more hours plus using warm water to bath the baby) is an essential intervention for the survival of the newborn especially during the first 24 h of birth. Though most babies were wrapped soon after delivery and were also bathed with hot water, poor thermal care was caused mainly by early bathing. In this study, 46.7% of the newborns were given a bath in less than 6 hours of delivery. Apart from exposing newborns to hypothermia, early bathing removes maternal bacteria and the vernix caseosa (a potent inhibitor of *Escherichia coli*) [21], and eliminates the crawling reflex [22]. Aside its role as a protective barrier from liquids while in the uterus, vernix serves as an antioxidant, skin cleanser, moisturizer, temperature regulator, and a natural, safe antimicrobial for the new baby post-delivery [5, 23]. These are some of the reasons why WHO recommended delay bathing up to at least 24 h.

Table 7 Determinants of safe cord care, optimal thermal care and good neonatal feeding

Variable	AOR (95% CI) safe cord care	AOR (95% CI) optimal thermal care	AOR (95% CI) good neonatal feeding	AOR (95% CI) [a]Overall adequacy of new born care practices
Maternal Age (years)				
≥ 35	Reference	Reference	Reference	Reference
Under 20 years	6.57 (1.71, 25.31)**	3.65 (0.79, 16.86)	2.22 (0.55, 9.0)	7.41 (0.85, 64.91)
20–34 years	2.01 (0.98, 4.12)	3.28 (1.34, 8.04) **	2.02 (1.11, 3.70)*	7.31 (1.65, 32.44)**
Adequacy of ANC attendance				
No	Reference	Reference	Reference	Reference
Yes	4.04 (1.53, 10.66)**	2.74 (1.01, 7.55)	1.90 (1.01, 3.61)*	Not significant
Place of delivery				
Home	Reference	Reference	Reference	Reference
Health facility	5.60 (1.19, 26.30)**	Not significant	Not significant in final model	Not significant in final model
Mother could recall at least 4 new born danger signs?				
1–3	Reference	Reference	Reference	Reference
At least 4	Not significant in final model	Not significant	2.00 (1.26, 3.17) **	2.51 (1.41, 4.47)**
Maternal Educational level				
No education	Reference	Reference	Reference	Reference
Low (Primary to JHS)	Not significant in final model	6.76 (0.85, 53.89)	Not significant in final model	Not significant in final model
High (At least SHS)	Not significant in final model	20.54 (2.60, 162.12)**	Not significant in final model	Not significant in final model
Type of religion				
Christianity	Reference	Reference	Reference	Reference
Islam	Not significant in final model	1.72 (1.09, 2.72)*	Not significant in final model	Not significant
Parity				
Primiparous	Reference	Reference	Reference	Reference
Secundiparous	Not significant	1.19 (0.70, 2.02)	Not significant	2.05 (1.08, 3.89)*
Multiparous	Not significant	2.67 (1.41, 5.05)**	Not significant	2.04 (0.97, 4.30)

AOR (95% CI): Adjusted odds ratio at 95% confidence level
*significant at $p < 0.05$; **significant at $p < 0.01$; ***significant at $p < 0.001$
[a]Overall adequacy of new born care practices was defined to comprise safe cord care, optimal thermal care and good neonatal feeding

This notwithstanding, many societies have some reasons why babies are bathed early after delivery.

For a normal uncomplicated vaginal birth in a health facility, it is recommended that healthy mothers and newborns should receive care in the facility for at least 24 h after birth [5]. In Ghana, women who deliver in health facilities are detained for a minimum of 6 h and not 24 h. Women who for some reasons deliver at home do not even wait for the 6 h before bathing the newborn. This is why in our study, we limited waiting period to at least 6 h. Early bathing of the baby is a cultural practice and so asking for a waiting time of 24 h appears to be something that is impossible at least for now. Our data showed that only 4 (1%) of the newborns in our sample will have received optimal thermal care if the 24-h cutoff was used instead of 6 h.

In an intervention trial in Ghana that used home visits to promote positive behavior change regarding thermal care, only 41% of mothers delayed bathing for more than 6 h in the intervention areas compared to 29% in the comparison areas [24].

The timing of bathing the newborn appears inconsistent as reported in some earlier studies conducted in Ghana [13, 15]. Whereas some mothers reported bathing their newborns shortly after delivery, others mentioned waiting until later in the day but the exact waiting period has not been more than a few hours after delivery. As reported in one of these studies, early bathing was commonly practiced in Ghana as a measure to reduce body odour in later life, shaping the baby's head, and to make the baby sleep and feel clean [15].

Some studies conducted on thermal practices in many countries including Ghana, Tanzania, Uganda and India have reported strong cultural beliefs in the benefits of early bathing [15, 25–30], which largely promotes the practice. The practice of early bathing is rooted in the firm belief that the birth process is dirty and that the baby is dirty after birth. This is particularly the case if there is an obvious sign of vernix which is regarded as dirty.

The problem of early bathing of the newborn appears to be widespread across the world. A study in Nepal reported that newborn babies are considered dirty since they came out of their mother's womb, so almost all newborn babies are bathed within the first hour of birth [31]. Another study conducted in low socioeconomic settlements of Karachi, Pakistan, revealed that newborns were bathed immediately after delivery as the vernix was considered "dirty looking" and it was felt it should be removed [32].

A composite index comprising good neonatal feeding showed that more than 70% of respondents practiced adequate feeding behaviours. For example, timely initiation of breastfeeding (TIBF) rate was 97%.

There are a number of benefits associated with early initiation of breastfeeding including stimulation of breast milk production and the release of oxytocin, which helps the contraction of the uterus and reduces post-partum blood loss [33].

The analysis from this study showed that the expected essential newborn care practices are not available to a greater proportion of the newborns. Poor newborn care practices together with poor maternal care and staff shortages in rural health facilities are major contributing factors of newborn mortality in developing countries [34]. The fact that a greater number of newborns are not getting adequate care suggests the need to extend these essential newborn care practices to the rural areas through rigorous training of community health workers in newborn care practices and sustained educational campaigns by the Ghana Health Service and other health related non-governmental agencies.

It is important to note that about 50% of newborn deaths occur within 24 h of birth [2].

Furthermore, though hypothermia contributes to neonatal morbidity and mortality in low-income countries [35, 36], yet the Ghana National Newborn Strategy and Action Plan (2014–2018) is silent on the specifics on the WHO recommendation on delay bathing of the newborn. The preventive basic essential newborn care specified in the action plan document mentioned drying and provision of warmth through skin to skin contact with the mother. The intervention package for the newborn in this strategy and action plan appears to focus on complication of prematurity and low birth weight, adverse intrapartum events including birth asphyxia and infection.

Predictors of essential newborn care practices

In logistic regression analysis, the main predictors of essential new born care practices were maternal educational attainment, maternal age, and adequacy of antenatal care (ANC) attendance and maternal knowledge of newborn danger signs. Adequacy of antenatal care in particular was a consistent determinant of safe cord care, optimal thermal care and good neonatal feeding.

Maternal education of secondary school level or higher was one of the strongest socio-demographic factors that determined safe cord care, optimal thermal care practice and good neonatal feeding. This association has been reported from several countries including India and Nepal [37, 38].

The educational attainment of the mother was positively associated with the adequacy level of ANC attendance ($\chi2 = 59.1$, $p < 0.001$) and maternal knowledge of newborn danger signs ($\chi2 = 16.7$, $p < 0.001$). The effect of maternal education on essential newborn care practices was therefore mediated through ANC attendance and knowledge of newborn dangers.

We observed very strong association between use of antenatal and delivery care and the newborn care practices. This may be explained by the fact that when pregnant women make contact with health workers during ANC, they are provided with health information and made aware of proper newborn care practices. Clean cord care practice and thermal care have found to be positively associated with receiving antenatal care [37].

Mothers' knowledge of newborn care danger signs

Poor knowledge of newborn danger signs delays care seeking and ultimately greater risk of death and so early detection of neonatal danger signs is an important step towards improving newborn survival [39, 40]. Overall, the mothers' knowledge of newborn care issues was not satisfactory in the sample population. In our study sample, only 45.2% of the mothers knew at least four newborn danger signs out of the seven. Knowledge on critical newborn danger signs other than high body temperature, diarrhoea, excessive crying was inadequate and similar findings have earlier been reported in the Asante Akim North District Ghana [19].

The low mothers' knowledge of newborn care practices reported in the present study confirmed what has been reported in some other developing countries including Sri Lanka, Kenya, Uganda and Nepal had unsatisfactory level of knowledge in the recognition of newborn danger signs [34, 41–44]. Available evidence from the literature shows that the maternal knowledge is an important intermediate factor that may lead to good practices and child survival outcomes child survival outcomes [34, 41].

Though maternal knowledge of newborn danger signs was positively associated with the odds of optimal thermal care, only a small proportion of mothers were knowledgeable in newborn danger signs. This means the majority of the women lacked adequate knowledge of good newborn care practices, so their newborn practices were likely to be adversely affected. The low knowledge levels of mothers may be due to inadequate messages received on newborn care practices at the ANC. This calls for strengthening of focused health education on newborn care practices especially during prenatal care to mitigate these problems. By integrating health education on newborn care practices into routine antenatal care services, it may increase a woman's knowledge and the ability to practice safe newborn care behaviours.

Conclusions

The analysis from this study showed that the expected essential newborn care practices are not getting to a greater proportion of the newborns. Early bathing, non-immediate drying and application of substances to cord stump were commonly practiced. This may be depriving newborns of basic protections against infection and death.

Overall, the findings show that good neonatal feeding practices, optimal thermal care and overall adequate newborn care practices were commonly adopted by women aged 20–34 years. The results also showed that essential newborn care practices are positively associated with high maternal educational attainment, adequate utilization of antenatal care services and high maternal knowledge of newborn danger signs.

Policy implications and recommendations

Greater improvement in essential newborn care practices could be attained through modifiable proven low-cost interventions such as effective ANC services, health and nutrition education that should span from community to health facility levels.

Of the three-composite essential newborn services indicators, optimal thermal care was the least provided to babies. Unfortunately, uptake of adequate ANC services in this study population was unrelated to optimal thermal care. This finding has important implications for the implementation of focused ANC to improve essential newborn care practices, especially that of thermal care. Therefore, ANC interventions should lay emphasis on the promotion and provision of thermal care for all newborns to prevent hypothermia (that is, immediate drying, warming, skin to skin, delayed bathing).

Limitations of the study

There are some limitations of the findings of this study. The recall period was limited to the past 1 year in order to avoid recall bias over a longer period of time. This notwithstanding, some amount of recall bias cannot be completely ruled out. During the interviews, the women had to recall a number of events including antenatal care visits and neonatal practices. So, recall bias and misclassification might happen. In order to reduce misclassification errors, the women were required to present their antenatal records booklet for confirmation of verbal information provided.

Our design was a cross sectional study and as with all such studies, the strength of causality is weak. The cross-sectional nature of the data limits our ability to draw any causal conclusions on the relationships found in the current study. Despite these limitations, our results have shed more light on critical areas of newborn care practices that need urgent pragmatic intervention.

Abbreviations

ANC: Antenatal care; AOR: Adjusted odds ratio; MDGs: Millennium Development Goals; NMR: Neonatal mortality; PASW: Predictive analytic software; SBA: Skilled birth attendants; SDGs: Sustainable Development Goals; SES: Socio-economic status; TIBF: Timely initiation of breastfeeding

Acknowledgements

The authors would like to gratefully acknowledge with gratitude the effort of the data collection teams, without their participation, the quality of the data presented in this report would not have been possible. Their commitment to improving maternal and newborn health is commendable.
We very much appreciate the input and support received from the Lawra District Health Management team (DHMT) that granted the research team audience. We also fully appreciate the involvement of all the women and community leaders whose co-operation led to a successful data collection experience.

Authors' contribution

MS conceived the idea and designed the study, coordinated data collection, performed analysis, interpretation of data and drafted the manuscript. FV coordinated the collection of data from the field, designed the study, interpreted data analysis and critical review and obtained funding. FA helped in the data collection, instrument development, assisted in data collection and manuscript writing, and critically commented on the draft manuscript. All authors gave final approval of the version to be published.

Competing interest

The authors declare that they have no competing interests.

Ethics approval and consent to participate

The study protocol was approved by the Scientific Review and Ethics Committee of the School of Allied Health Sciences, University for Development Studies, Ghana.
Written approval was obtained from the local health authorities in the district where the study was conducted. All participants were informed about the purpose of the study and their right to decline participation in the study was explained by the data collectors. Informed consent was also obtained after needed information and explanation. In situations, where the respondent could not write or read, verbal informed consent was sought from all the study participants before the commencement of any interview. The Ethics Committee approved the verbal consent sought from the participants.

References

1. Countdown Coverage Writing Group, Countdown to 2015 Core Group, Bryce J, Daelmans B, Dwivedi A, Fauveau V, Lawn JE, Mason E, Newby H, Shankar A, et al. Countdown to 2015 for maternal, newborn, and child survival: the 2008 report on tracking coverage of interventions. Lancet. 2008;371:1247–58.
2. Lawn JE, Cousens S, Zupan J. 4 million neonatal deaths: when? Where?Why? Lancet. 2005;365(9462):891–900.
3. Ghana Statistical Service (GSS), Ghana Health Service (GHS), ICF International: 2015. Ghana demographic and health survey 2014. Rockville: GSS, GHS, and ICF International; 2015.
4. United Nations: Sustainable Development Goals (SDGs). United Nations sustainable development summit 2015, vol. 2015. New York: United Nations.
5. WHO. WHO recommendations on postnatal care of the mother and newborn. Geneva: World Health Organization; 2013.
6. Gary LD, Bhutta ZA, Cousens S, Taghreed A, Walker N, de Bernis L. Team ftLNSS: evidence-based, cost-effective interventions: how many newborn babies can we save? Lancet. 2005;365:977–88.
7. Lawn J, Kerber K. Opportunities for Africa's newborns: practical data, policy and programmatic support for newborn care in Africa. PMNCH: Cape Town, South Africa; 2006.
8. The Partnership for Maternal NaCH. A global review of the key interventions related to reproductive, maternal, newborn and child health. Geneva: The Partnership for Maternal, Newborn and Child Health; 2011.
9. WHO. Neonatal & Perinatal Mortality; country, regional and global estimate. Geneva: World Health Organization; 2006.
10. McCall EM, Alderdice F, Halliday HL, Jenkins JG, Vohra S. Interventions to prevent hypothermia at birth in preterm and/or low birthweight infants. Cochrane Database Syst Rev. 2010:3(3).
11. WHO. Protecting, promoting and supporting breast-feeding: the special role of maternity services, a joint WHO/UNICEF statement. Geneva: World Health Organization/UNICEF; 2002.
12. Vyas S, Kumaranayake L. Constructing socio-economic status indices: how to use principal components analysis. Health Policy Plan. 2006;21:459–68.
13. Moyer CA, Aborigo RA, Logonia G, Affah G, Rominski S, Adongo PB, Williams J, Hodgson A, Engmann C. Clean delivery practices in rural northern Ghana: a qualitative study of community and provider knowledge, attitudes, and beliefs. BMC Pregnancy and Childbirth. 2012;12:50.
14. Hill Z, Tawiah-Agyemang C, Okeyere E, Manu A, Fenty J, Kirkwood B. Improving hygiene in home deliveries in rural Ghana: how to build on current attitudes and practices. Pediatr Infect Dis J. 2010;29(11):1004–8.
15. Hill Z, Tawiah-Agyemang C, Manu A, Okeyere E, Kirkwood B. Keeping newborns warm: beliefs, practices and potential for behaviour change in rural Ghana. TMIH. 2010;15(10):1118–24.
16. Osuchukwu EC, Ezeruigbo CSF, Eko JE. Knowledge of standard umbilical cord management among mothers in Calabar south local government area, cross river state Nigeria. Int J Nurs Sci. 2017;7(3):57–62.
17. Saaka M, Aryee P, Kuganab-lem R, Ali M, Masahudu AR. The effect of social behaviour change communication package on maternal knowledge on obstetric danger signs among mothers in east Mamprusi District of Ghana. Glob Health. 2017;13(19)
18. Afolaranmi TO, Hassan ZI, Akinyemi OO, Sule SS, Malete MU, Choji CP, Bello DA. Cord care practices: a perspective of contemporary African setting. Front Public Health. 2018;6(10) https://doi.org/10.3389/fpubh.2018.00010.
19. Marah A. Assessing household practices that influence neonatal survival in the Asante-Akim North District of Ashanti region - Ghana. Kumasi, Ghana: Kwame Nkrumah University Science and Technology; 2011.
20. Awasthi S, Verma T, Agarwal M: Danger signs of neonatal illnesses: perceptions of caregivers and health workers in northern India 2006. Available at: http://www.who.int/entity/bulletin/volumes/84/10/05-029207.pdf. Accessed on 20th Dec 2013.
21. Tollin M, Bergsson G, Kai-Larsen Y, Lengqvist J, Sjövall J, Griffiths W, et al. Vernix caseosa as a multicomponent defense system based on polypeptides, lipids and their interactions. Cell Mol Life Sci. 2005;62:2390–9.
22. Righard L, Alade M. Effect of delivery room routines on success of first breastfeed. Lancet. 1990;336:1105–7.
23. World Health Organization. Essential newborn care: a report of a technical working group. Geneva: WHO; 1996.
24. Kirkwood BR, Manu A, ten Asbroek AH, Soremekun S, Weobong B, Gyan T, Danso S, Amenga-Etego S, Tawiah-Agyemang C, Owusu-Agyei S, et al. Effect of the Newhints home-visits intervention on neonatal mortality rate and care practices in Ghana: a cluster randomised controlled trial. Lancet. 2013;381(9884):2184–92.
25. Waiswa P, Kemigisa M, Kiguli J, Naikoba S, Pariyo GW, Peterson S. Acceptability of evidence-based neonatal care practices in rural Uganda – implications for programming. BMC Pregnancy Childbirth. 2008;8:21.
26. Iyengar SD, Iyengar K, Martines JC, Dashora K, Deora KK. Childbirth practices in rural Rajasthan, India: implications for neonatal health and survival. J Perinatol. 2008;28:S23–30.
27. Kesterton AJ, Cleland J. Neonatal care in rural Karnataka: healthy and harmful practices, the potential for change. BMC Pregnancy Childbirth. 2009;9:20.

28. Shamba D, Schellenberg J, Penfold S, Mashasi I, Mrisho M, Manzi F, Marchant T, Tanner M, Mshinda H, Schellenberg D, et al. Clean home delivery in rural southern Tanzania: barriers, influencers and facilitators. J Health Popul Nutr. 2013;1:1107–870.
29. Baqui AH, Williams EK, Darmstadt GL, Kiran TU, Panwar D, Sharma RK, Ahmed S, Sreevasta V, Ahuja R, Santosham M, et al. Newborn care in rural Uttar Pradesh. Indian J Pediatics. 2007;74:241–7.
30. Shamba D, Schellenberg J, Hildon ZJL, Mashasi I, Penfold S, Tanner M, Marchant T, Hill Z. Thermal care for newborn babies in rural southern Tanzania: a mixed-method study of barriers, facilitators and potential for behaviour change. BMC Pregnancy and Childbirth. 2014;14:267.
31. Yadav S. Newborn care: traditional practices in Nepal. Student BMJ. 2007;15: 293–336.
32. Fikree FF, Tazeen SA, Jill MD, Rahbar MH. Newborn care practices in low socioeconomic settlements of Karachi, Pakistan. Social Science Direct and Medicine. 2005;60:911–21.
33. Gartner LM, Morton J, Lawrence RA, Naylor AJ, O'Hare D, Schanler RJ, Eidelman AI. Breastfeeding and the use of human milk. Pediatrics. 2005; 115(2):496–506.
34. Sharan M. Determinants of safe motherhood and newborn care behaviors in rural India. Johns Hopkins University. 2004;
35. Darmstadt GL, Bhutta ZA, Cousens S, Adam T, Walker N, Bernis L. Evidence based, cost-effective interventions: how many newborn babies can we save? Lancet. 2005;365:977–88.
36. Kumar V, Shearer JC, Kumar A, Darmstadt GL. Neonatal hypothermia in low resource settings: a review. J Perinatol. 2009;29:401–12.
37. Baqui AH, Williams EK, Dramstadt GL, Kumar V, Kiran TU, Panwar D, et al. Newborn care in rural Uttar Pradesh. Indian J Pediatr. 2006;74(3):241–7.
38. Ministry of Health and Population (MoHP), New ERA, Macro International Inc. Nepal demographic and health survey 2006. Kathmandu, Nepal: Ministry of Health and Population, New ERA, Macro International Inc; 2007.
39. Choi Y, El Arifeen S, Mannan I, Rahman SM, Bari S, et al. Can mothers recognize neonatal illness correctly? Comparison of maternal report and assessment by community health workers in rural Bangladesh. Tropical Med Int Health. 2010;15(6):743–53.
40. Hill Z, Kendall C, Arthur P, Kirkwood B, Adjei E. Recognizing childhood illnesses and their traditional explanations: exploring options for care-seeking interventions in the context of the IMCI strategy in rural Ghana. Tropical Med Int Health. 2003;8(7):668–76.
41. Senarath U, Fernando D, Vimpani G, Rodrigo I. Factors associated with maternal knowledge of newborn care among hospital-delivered mothers in Sri Lanka. Trans R Soc Trop Med Hyg. 2007;101(8):823–30.
42. Obimbo E, Musoke RN, Were F. Knowledge, attitudes and practices of mothers and knowledge of health workers regarding care of the newborn umbilical cord. East Afr Med J. 1999;76(8):425–9.
43. Tuladhar S. The determinants of good newborn care practices in the rural areas of Nepal. Australia: University of Canterbury; 2010.
44. Sandberg J, Odberg Pettersson K, Asp G, Kabakyenga J, Agardh A. Inadequate knowledge of neonatal danger signs among recently delivered women in southwestern rural Uganda: a community survey. PLoS One. 2014;9(5):e97253.

11

Atypical CHARGE associated with a novel frameshift mutation of *CHD7* in a Chinese neonatal patient

Yan-ping Xu[1*], Li-ping Shi[1] and Jiajun Zhu[2*]

Abstract

Background: CHARGE syndrome is an autosomal dominant malformation disorder caused by heterozygous loss of function mutations in the chromatin remodeler *CHD7*, which has been estimated to occur in 1:10,000 births worldwide. It is a genetic disorder closely resembles other pattern of anomalies. Genetic testing should be pointed out as a useful method for clinical diagnosis.

Case presentation: A female infant was the second child born to a 33-year-old, gravida 3, para 2 mother. The infant was born at 37 + 4 weeks of gestation with a birth weight of 2440 g (− 1.1 S.D.). Clinical examination showed atypical CHARGE syndrome, with choanal atresia, a heart defect, and sensorineural deafness. Genomic DNA was extracted from peripheral venous blood sample using molecular biological technique. We used the Illumina TruSigt One sequencing panel on the MiSeq next- generation sequencing (NGS) platform for mutation screening and found a novel frameshift mutation in chromodomain helicase DNA binding protein 7 (*CHD7*; c.4656dupT). This mutation results in a new reading frame ending in p.(Ile1553fs). At the first month of age, the patient had a posterior nostril plasty operation by nasal endoscope. At the second month of age, she had patent ductus arteriosus ligation surgery. At the 4th month of age, she was discharged from the hospital.

Conclusions: Our findings further reveal that patients should not be rejected for CHD7 mutational analysis even if they do not fulfill CHARGE syndrome Verloes criteria.

Keywords: CHARGE syndrome, Choanal atresia, CHD7

Background

CHARGE syndrome is a complex genetic disorder, which has been estimated to occur in 1:10,000 births worldwide and shows various clinical manifestations, causing multiple birth defects and sensory deficits [1]. The pattern of anomalies now associated with CHARGE syndrome was first recognized in 1979 by Hittner et al. [2] and Hall [3]. The major clinical features of CHARGE syndrome (OMIM 214800) are ocular **C**oloboma, congenital **H**eart defects, choanal **A**tresia, **R**etardation of growth, **G**enital hypoplasia, and **E**ar abnormalities. CHARGE syndrome closely resembles other pattern of anomalies, so genetic testing should be emphasized as a useful method in clinical diagnosis. Of all the clinically diagnosed CHARGE patients, 67 to 90% have been shown to have pathogenic mutations in the gene encoding chromodomain helicase DNA binding protein 7 (*CHD7*, OMIM *608892), which is located on chromosome 8q12.1. Detailed information on the variant in *CHD7* gene reported so far, approximately 70% are nonsense or frameshift, 10% are splice site, 15% are missense, and 5% are whole-gene or chromosomal deletion, exonic deletion and chromosomal rearrangement [4]. Only a few studies have been reported that mutation in *EFTUD2* (OMIM 603892) at chromosome 17q21 may also cause CHARGE like syndrome [5, 6]. Here, we presented a novel monoallelic frameshift mutation of *CHD7*, NM_017780.3 (c.4656dupT) in a Chinese patient with CHARGE syndrome.

* Correspondence: xuyanping726@hotmail.com; xuyanping726@zju.edu.cn; jiajunzhu@zju.edu.cn
[1]NICU, Children's Hospital, Zhejiang University School of Medicine, Hangzhou 310053, China
[2]Department of Neonatology, Women's Hospital, Zhejiang University School of Medicine, Hangzhou 310006, China

Case presentation

We describe the case of a female infant. She was the second child born to a 33-year-old, gravida 3, para 2 mother. The patient was born polyhydramnios by cesarean section at 37 + 4 weeks of gestation with a birth weight of 2440 g (− 1.1 S.D.), a length of 50 cm (+ 0.80 S.D.) and an occipitofrontal circumference of 36 cm (+ 2.0 S.D.). The 1- and 5-min Apgar scores were 8 and 8, respectively. Shortly after birth, she required nasal continuous positive airway pressure (nCPAP) and presented with dyspnea. During the following days, she developed dyspnea continually and needed oxygen to maintain 90–95% saturation. Parenteral nutrition was started on day 1 and breast milk was given 12 h after birth by oral tube. Her parents were nonconsanguineous and her mother had a healthy 13-year-old child. She denied any family history of neonatal disease. Prenatal examination was not found abnormal. Additionally, she denied that she had consumed alcohol, drugs, tobacco, or any other toxic substances during her pregnancy.

On admission to our unit, the patient was 3 days old and weighed 2400 g. Clinical examination showed choanal atresia, bilateral low-set ears, triple restriction and systolic murmur, but coloboma was not observed. Her motor development was almost normal. The patient presents feeding difficulties by nasogastric tube. Her white blood cell count was 12.07 × 109/L (neutrophils, 0.50; lymphocytes, 0.24), and her platelet count was 160.00 × 109/L and CRP < 1 mg/L. The alanine aminotransferase level was 14 U/L, aspartate aminotransferase level was 43 U/L, and gamma-glutamyltransferase level was 68 U/L. On the seventh day of age, her thyroid functional parameters were TSH 5 mIU/L, T3 1.83 nmol/L and T4 123.94 nmol/L, and at the first month of age, thyroid functional parameters were TSH > 100 mIU/L, T3 1.57 nmol/L and T4 35.93 nmol/L. Thus, oral Euthyrox (Levothyroxine sodium tablets) was administered. Newborn screening for metabolic disorders and severe combined immunodeficiency was normal. A chest radiograph showed haziness in both lung fields suggestive of wet lung (Fig. 1b). Two-dimensional and color-Doppler assessment was revealed an atrioventricular septal defect (6.8 mm + 2.2 mm), patent ductus arteriosus (3.6 mm) and pulmonary hypertension (Fig. 1e). A craniocerebral ultrasound showed bilateral lateral ventricle dilatation (Fig. 1d). The auditory brainstem response (ABR) test showed bilateral severe hearing impairment (ABR > 99 dBnHL). Following radiologic testing by computed tomography showed bilateral choanal atresia and insufficient inflatable structure of both semi-circular canals. (Fig. 1c). No clinical characteristics of CHARGE syndrome were detected in the patient's parents. Chromosomal analysis indicated a 46 XX normal female karyotype.

The patient required mechanical ventilation with endotracheal intubation at 4 days of age. On 17 days of age, she was extubated to nCPAP with FiO2 < 25%. On

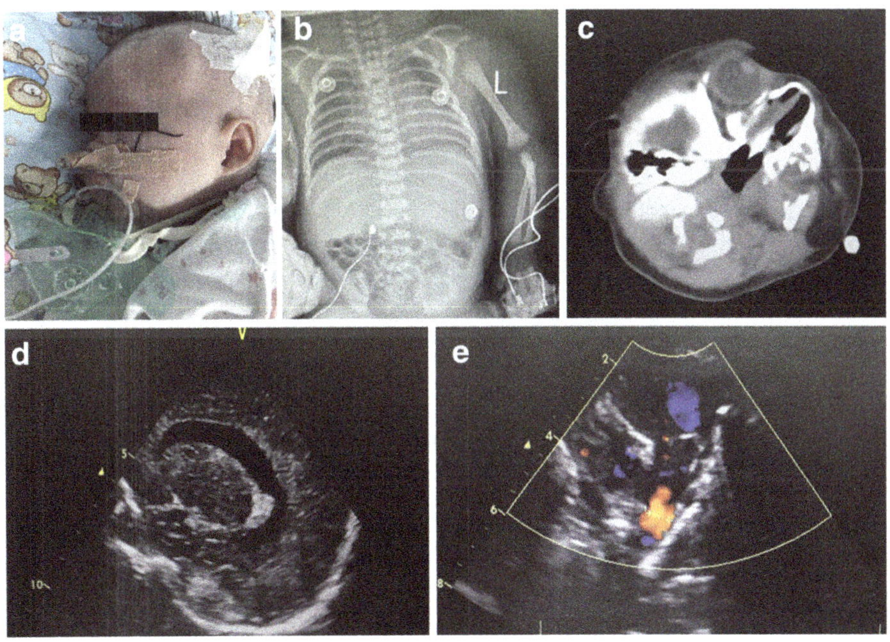

Fig. 1 **a** Patient did posterior nostril plasty operation by nasal endoscope and put silicone tube in one month. **b** Chest radiograph at 3 days. **c** Computed tomography revealed bilateral choanal atresia and semi-circular canals as an insufficient inflatable structure. **d** Craniocerebral ultrasound showed bilateral lateral ventricle dilatation. **e** Echocardiography showed atrioventricular septal defect (6.8 mm + 2.2 mm) and patent ductus arteriosus (3.6 mm)

20 days of age, she needed an oxygen mask. Ampicillin was discontinued when the blood culture from birth was sterile at 72 h. At the first month of age, the patient had a posterior nostril plasty operation by nasal endoscope and had a silicone tube in one month for transition the postoperative (Fig. 1a). At the second month of age, she had patent ductus arteriosus ligation surgery. At the 4th month of age, she was discharged from the hospital. Clinical features summarized in Table 1.

Molecular analysis of the disease-associated genes *CHD7* and *EFTUD2* were performed using the Illumina TruSigt One sequencing panel (Illumina, San Diego, CA, USA) on the MiSeq NGS platform for mutation screening methods (Sinopath Diagnosis, Beijing, China) [7]. Genomic DNA was extracted from peripheral venous blood and informed consent was obtained from the parents. The study was approved by the ethics committee of Zhejiang University Children's Hospital. To identify presumably pathogenic single-nucleotide variants, we used NextGene V2.3.4 (Softgenetics, State College, PA, USA) compared with the UCSC database. We excluded sequence variants with a minor allele frequency > 0.05, in the Human Genetic Variation Database (http://www.genome.med.kyoto-u.ac.jp/SnpDB/) and the NHLBI Grand Opportunity Exome Sequencing Project (ESP6500, http://evs.gs.washington.edu/EVS/). This analyses identified a monoallelic (thymine) insertion in *CHD7*, NM_017780.3 (*CHD7* c.4656dupT), which was confirmed by Sanger sequencing. This mutation leads to a reading frameshift mutation starting from isoleucine, with the new reading frame ending p.(Ile1553fs) (Fig. 2). As shown in Fig. 2, the mutation is located in exon 20, and this mutation was not present in the Human Gene Mutation Database (http://www.hgmd.org/) or ClinVar (http://www.ncbi.nlm.nih.gov/clinvar/),[8] suggesting that it is novel. This heterozygous frameshift mutation was not detected in the patient's parents, suggesting that it is a de novo mutation.

Discussion and conclusions

Applying the scoring scheme by Verloes, a patient can be assigned to atypical CHARGE syndrome, if they have one major criterion (choanal atreisia) and three minor criteria (heart malformation, deafness and external ear malformations) [9]. Low set ears are not a typical feature of CHARGE syndrome. Abnormal outer ears always like cup-shaped in the typical CHARGE syndrome. The aetiology remains unknown. In the second screening of thyroid function (at the age of 1 mo), the patient was diagnosed with hypothyroidism. It has been reported that four patients had hypothyroidism combined with CHARGE syndrome: two had central hypothyroidism with a low response to the thyrotropin-releasing hormone loading test, while the others had primary hypothyroidism and received thyroxine replacement. Some cases also had Growth Hormone Deficiency (GHD) and used growth hormone therapy [10]. This is a reason for the presentation of development delay and growth retardation. However, the concentration of growth hormone was not assessed in the neonatal period, and we could not determine the precise frequency of GHD in our patient. Typical features of CHARGE syndrome is well diagnosed, but the atypical part of the disease is difficult to identify. A person with subtle symptoms can pass their mutations on to offspring who is associated with a more severe phenotype. It is important to provide such patients with accurate prognostic information and genetic counseling. Additionally, compared to children or adults, features of CHARGE syndrome in neonates are atypical and less, so analysis of disease-associated genes including *CHD7* and *EFTUD2* should be done in infants, who do not completely meet the major clinical criteria. We identified a monoallelic c.4656dupT insertion of *CHD7*, leading to a novel frameshift mutation and an early stop codon, which resulted in a truncated CHD7 protein. *CHD7* genomic structure spans 188 kb and consists of 38 exons, the first of which is noncoding.*CHD7* expression remains ubiquitous in later stages of fetal development. Problems appear early in the first trimester and specifically occur between the third and ninth weeks postconception [12, 13]. At multiple stages of embryonic development indicate that CHD7 is localized to specific in both tissue and stage affected for CHARGE syndrome including the developing eye, ear and olfactory system [4]. Sangar sequencing of CHD7 gene was used to detect mutations (point mutation, small deletions and/or insertions in exons) in infants who were suspected of CHARGE syndrome. However, the method may miss some cases. The technique of multiplex ligation dependent probe amplification was used as supplement to detect small exonic deletions. Studies showed that deficit in exon 7 of CHD7 gene was related to CHARGE syndrome [11, 12]. Chai M found that *CHD7* is required for epigenetic activation of superenhancers and central nervous system-specific enhancers. Furthermore, they found that *CHD7*, through its interactions with superenhancer elements, acts as a regulatory hub in the orchestration of the spatiotemporal dynamics of transcription factors to regulate human neuroepithelial and central nervous system lineage identities [14]. Okuno H found that the expression of genes associated with cell migration was altered in CHARGE iPSC-NCCs compared to control iPSC-NCCs. Their results support the historical inference that CHARGE syndrome patients exhibit defects in neural crest migration [15]. Our case had a *CHD7* frameshift mutation at exon 20 leading to an early stop codonpredicting the loss of about 50% of the protein. Further studies are needed to delineate the roles of *CHD7* in enhancer-mediated transcriptional

Table 1 Clinical features and mutation of patients with mutation in the CHD7 gene

Sex	Age	Coloboma	Choanal atresia	Cleft lip and/or palate	SCC hypoplasia	Deafness	Feeding difficulties	Structural brain anomalies	Genital hypoplasia	Growth retardation	Heart defect	Kidney anomalies	IUGR	Classfication	Mutation
F	3 d	–	+	–	–	+	+	–	–	–	+	–	–	Atypical CHARGE	*CHD7* c.4656dupT

SCC semicircular canal

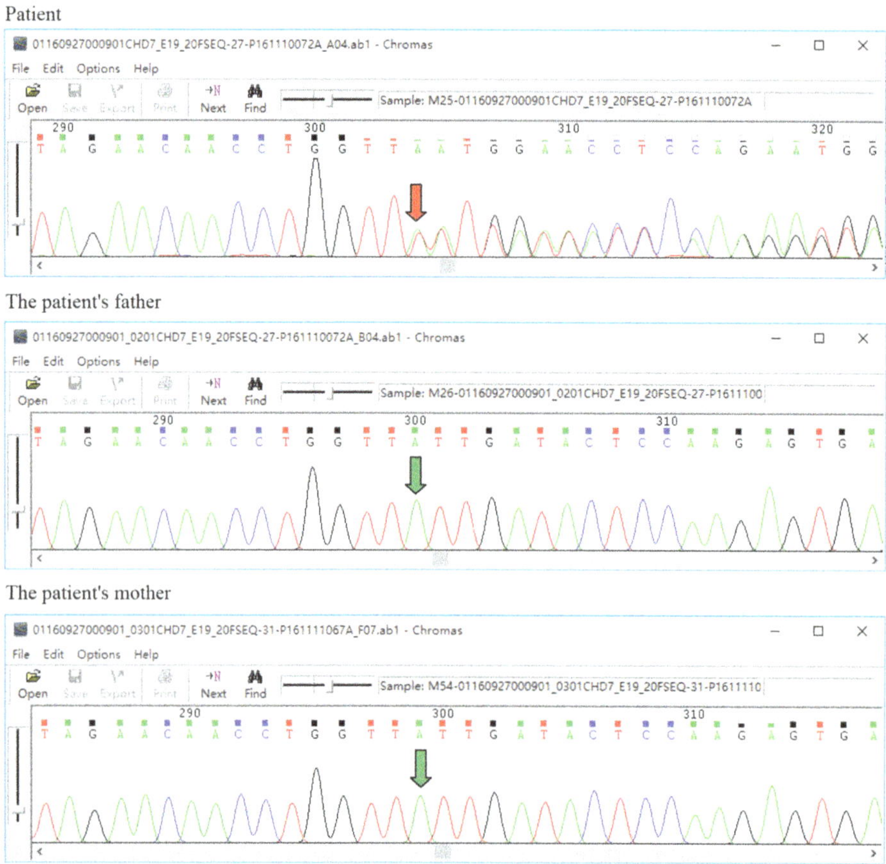

Fig. 2 Results of monoallelic frameshift mutation in *CHD7*, NM_017780.3 (*CHD7* c.4656dupT), this mutation causes a frameshift starting from isoleucine, with the new reading frame ending p.(Ile1553fs)

regulation in CHARGE syndrome in tissues of various development stages and their tissue expression sites. Genetic counseling was important for parents, even before we confirmed the diagnosis of CHARGE syndrome, because it could give them the information of the disease, realize the meaning of further genetic research, and provide the support to family. Most infants with CHARGE syndrome may develop abnormal, with motor and/or language problems, because of multiple sensory deficits. It is essential for family to early refer to rehabilitative therapist. Intelligence Quotients are various in the infants with CHARGE syndrome [16]. In conclusion, we report a case of atypical CHARGE syndrome, with the clinical features of choanal atresia, a heart defect, and sensorineural deafness, caused by a novel frameshift mutation in exon 20 of *CHD7*, with the new reading frame ending p. (Ile1553fs). Additional screening of atypical cases will be facilitated by molecular diagnosis. It should be emphasized that patients should not be rejected for *CHD7* analysis if they do not fulfill all the major criteria of CHARGE syndrome Verloes criteria.

Abbreviations
CHD7: chromodomain helicase DNA binding protein 7; nCPAP: nasal continuous positive airway pressure

Acknowledgments
We would like to thank all the staff in the NICU Department of Children's Hospital, Zhejiang University School of Medicine for their help in the resolution of the case.

Funding
This work was supported by the National Natural Science Foundation of China (No. 81200460) and Zhejiang Provincial Natural Science Foundation of China (Y14H040018). The design of the study, analysis and the fee for publication is supported by National Natural Science Foundation of China. Collection and interpretation of data is supported by Zhejiang Provincial Natural Science Foundation of China.

Authors' contributions
All authors have read and approved the manuscript. They have contributed to the article as follows: YX: contributed to conception, carried out the data collection, and drafted the initial manuscript. LS: helped with the resolution of the clinical management of the patient and reviewed and revised the manuscript and approved the final manuscript as submitted. JZ contributed to clinical management of the patient, obtained the patient consent form, interpretation of data and approved the final manuscript as submitted.

Competing interests
The authors declare that they have no competing interests.

References

1. Jongmans MC, Admiraal RJ, van der Donk KP, et al. CHARGE syndrome: the phenotypic spectrum of mutations in the CHD7 gene. J Med Genet. 2006; 43(4):306–14.
2. Hittner HM, Hirsch NJ, Kreh GM, Rudolph AJ. Colobomatous microphthalmia, heart disease, hearing loss, and mental retardation–a syndrome. J Pediatr Ophthalmol Strabismus. 1979;16(2):122–8.
3. Hall BD. Choanal atresia and associated multiple anomalies. J Pediatr. 1979; 95(3):395–8.
4. Zentner GE, Layman WS, Martin DM, Scacheri PC. Molecular and phenotypic aspects of CHD7 mutation in CHARGE syndrome. Am J Med Genet A. 2010; 152A(3):674–86.
5. Lehalle D, Gordon CT, Oufadem M, et al. Delineation of EFTUD2 haploinsufficiency-related phenotypes through a series of 36 patients. Hum Mutat. 2014;35(4):478–85.
6. Luquetti DV, Hing AV, Rieder MJ, et al. "Mandibulofacial dysostosis with microcephaly" caused by EFTUD2 mutations: expanding the phenotype. Am J Med Genet A. 2013;161A(1):108–13.
7. Mamanova L, Coffey AJ, Scott CE, et al. Target-enrichment strategies for next-generation sequencing. Nat Methods. 2010;7(2):111–8.
8. Kohmoto T, Shono M, Naruto T, et al. A novel frameshift mutation of CHD7 in a Japanese patient with CHARGE syndrome. Hum Genome Var. 2016;3: 16004.
9. Palumbo O, Palumbo P, Stallone R, Palladino T, Zelante L, Carella M. 8q12. 1q12.3 de novo microdeletion involving the CHD7 gene in a patient without the major features of CHARGE syndrome: case report and critical review of the literature. Gene. 2013;513(1):209–13.
10. Shoji Y, Ida S, Etani Y, et al. Endocrinological characteristics of 25 Japanese patients with CHARGE syndrome. Clin Pediatr Endocrinol. 2014;23(2):45–51.
11. Lee B, Duz MB, Sagong B, et al. Revealing the function of a novel splice-site mutation of CHD7 in CHARGE syndrome. Gene. 2016;576(2 Pt 2):776–81.
12. Vatta M, Niu Z, Lupski JR, et al. Evidence for replicative mechanism in a CHD7 rearrangement in a patient with CHARGE syndrome. Am J Med Genet A. 2013;161A(12):3182–6.
13. Verloes A. Updated diagnostic criteria for CHARGE syndrome: a proposal. Am J Med Genet A. 2005;133A(3):306–8.
14. Chai M, Sanosaka T, Okuno H, et al. Chromatin remodeler CHD7 regulates the stem cell identity of human neural progenitors. Genes Dev. 2018;32(2): 165–80.
15. Okuno H, Renault MF, Ohta S, et al. CHARGE syndrome modeling using patient-iPSCs reveals defective migration of neural crest cells harboring CHD7 mutations. Elife. 2017;28:6.
16. Hefner MA, Fassi E. Genetic counseling in CHARGE syndrome: diagnostic evaluation through follow up. Am J Med Genet C Semin Med Genet. 2017; 175(4):407–16.

Ursodeoxycholic acid versus phenobarbital for cholestasis in the Neonatal Intensive Care Unit

Tamorah Lewis[1*], Simisola Kuye[2] and Ashley Sherman[1]

Abstract

Background: Although neonates and young infants with cholestasis are commonly treated with either phenobarbital or ursodeoxycholic acid (ursodiol), there is no evidence that phenobarbital is effective for this indication. Our objective was to compare the effectiveness of ursodiol and phenobarbital for the treatment of cholestasis in a diverse NICU population.

Methods: This is a retrospective cohort study including infants with cholestasis who were admitted to a Level IV NICU between January 2010 and December 2015. Drug courses of phenobarbital and ursodiol were identified within the medical record, and medical, demographic, and drug information were extracted. The primary outcome was reduction in direct bilirubin.

Results: Sixty-eight infants provided a total of 112 courses of drug therapy for comparison. Diverse medical diagnoses were captured in the patient cohort. Ursodiol was significantly more effective in reducing direct bilirubin than was phenobarbital (− 1.89 vs + 0.76 mg/dL; − 33.33 vs + 13.0 umol/L, *p*-value 0.03), even after controlling for baseline cholestasis severity, intrauterine growth restriction status, and lipid lowering therapy (− 2.16 vs + 0.27 mg/dl; − 36.94 vs + 4.62 umol/L, *p*-value 0.03). There was no improvement in direct bilirubin in the majority of infants treated with phenobarbital.

Conclusions: Phenobarbital, as compared to ursodiol, has limited efficacy for the reduction of direct bilirubin in neonates and young infants with cholestasis. Given new data regarding the potential neurotoxicity of phenobarbital in the developing brain, providers may choose to avoid phenobarbital in the treatment of cholestasis in infants.

Keywords: Neonate, Cholestatic jaundice, Ursodiol, Phenobarbital, Neonatal intensive care unit

Background

Hepatic cholestasis is the result of impaired balance between bile acid uptake and efflux. Abnormal hepatic accumulation of bile salts leads to disruption of cell membranes and cellular organelles resulting in necrosis, inflammation, and fibrosis. Cholestasis is commonly encountered in the neonatal intensive care unit (NICU) as a result of multiple medical conditions, including extreme prematurity, growth restriction, and sepsis [1]. Additionally, congenital anomalies of the gastrointestinal tract requiring surgery and other medical conditions requiring prolonged parenteral nutrition are associated with cholestasis. Given the known hepatotoxic effects of bile salt stasis, physicians often treat cholestasis with multiple modalities, including IV lipid limiting [2] and the medications ursodiol (ursodeoxycholic acid) or phenobarbital.

Ursodiol is the only drug approved by the Food and Drug Administration for use in adult cholestatic conditions. Ursodiol protects injured cholangiocytes against the toxic effects of bile acids and stimulates bile acid secretion via calcium-dependent mechanisms. Additionally, it directly modulates transcription of transporters and inhibits bile-acid induced hepatocyte apoptosis [3,

* Correspondence: trlewis@cmh.edu
[1]Department of Pediatrics, Children's Mercy Hospital, University of Missouri Kansas City School of Medicine, 2401 Gillham Rd, Kansas City, MO 64108, USA
Full list of author information is available at the end of the article

4]. Ursodiol is proven effective at treating parenteral nutrition-associated cholestasis in small cohorts of infants [5, 6], but is not used as prophylaxis in high-risk neonates [7, 8].

Phenobarbital acts via the nuclear receptor called constitutive androstane receptor (CAR), controlling hepatocellular metabolizing enzymes and transporters. Phenobarbital improves cholestasis in a small cohort of majority adult patients with anatomic abnormalities, including primary biliary cirrhosis, sclerosing cholangitis, and intrahepatic biliary hypoplasia [9], but there is no evidence that it is effective at treating neonatal cholestasis. There is recent concern that phenobarbital carries more risk than previously appreciated. Specifically, animal models of the developing brain have shown that phenobarbital leads to neuronal apoptosis [10, 11] and long-term behavioral toxicity [12].

Given the limited evidence for efficacy and increased evidence for toxicity with phenobarbital, we aimed to compare the two drugs ursodiol and phenobarbital for effectiveness in treatment of cholestasis in a diverse cohort of infants. We hypothesized that ursodiol would be more effective at reducing direct bilirubin (DBili), a surrogate marker for hepatic cholestasis. Our primary outcome was change in direct bilirubin, with a secondary outcome of direct bilirubin at the end of drug therapy.

Methods

This retrospective cohort study was approved by the Children's Mercy Institutional Review Board prior to data extraction. Eligible infants between January 2010 and December 2015 were identified using the variable "highest direct bilirubin" in the Children's Hospitals Neonatal Database (CHND), and all children admitted to the Children's Mercy Intensive Care Nursery with a documented direct bilirubin > 3.0 mg/dl (51.34 umol/) were identified to eliminate cases of mild cholestasis. Infants were randomly selected from this list, without knowledge of drug treatment or bilirubin changes, for inclusion in the study cohort. Infants included in the study were treated with ursodiol and/or phenobarbital per standard clinical care in the NICU, at the discretion of the neonatologist at the time of treatment. There is no protocol which dictates drug treatment for cholestasis, but most practitioners use phenobarbital while an infant is not enterally fed and ursodiol when on feeds. Because we could not extract important study data from outside charts, infants were excluded if they were transferred to our NICU already on medication for cholestasis, or if they were discharged to another NICU on cholestasis medications.

Study variables

Because many infants were exposed to more than one course of medication treatment for cholestasis, we defined the research unit as a course of medication administration, e.g. ursodiol for 25 days. All relevant variables were then extracted for that medication course, including direct bilirubin levels when the medication was started and stopped. If the direct bilirubin was measured a few days before stopping the medication, we used the date of the last bilirubin measurement as the stop date. If drug treatments overlapped, we only used data until the day before the second drug was added in order to exclude overlapping drug effect. Medication courses were excluded if they were less than 1 week long because we felt that a meaningful change in cholestasis could not be appreciated with such a short treatment course.

Demographic data (gestational age, race, gender, birthweight), major medical diagnoses, and drug data (daily dose, length of therapy) were collected from the charts of eligible infants. Data about potential confounding variables including nutrition (lipid lowering treatment, age when enteral nutrition achieved) were extracted from each patient chart. Lipid lowering refers to the practice of decreasing parenteral intralipid administration from 3 mg/kg/day to 1 mg/kg/day and is used as first line treatment of TPN-associated cholestasis in the NICU where this study was performed. Some infants with cholestasis with not be treated with lipid lowering if they have relative contraindications such as poor growth or inability to tolerate higher glucose infusion rates or protein to supplement calories lost in lipid lowering.

Statistical analysis

To calculate sample size, we assumed based on clinical experience that ursodiol would have a much larger effect on improving direct bilirubin than would phenobarbital (average improvement in DBili 3 mg/dL; 51.34 umol/L vs 0.3 mg/dL; 5.13 umol/L), with a standard deviation of 4 mg/dL (68.45 umol/L). Using a two-sided significance value of .05 and a two group t-test, an N of 35 in each group provides 80% power to detect a difference.

Two analyses were performed. The first analysis included only the first course of drug therapy to eliminate any carryover effect from treatment with a prior medication for cholestasis. The second analysis included all drug courses, and included a variable to account for prior drug therapy within a 14-day window. Categorical variables were compared between the two drug treatment groups using Chi-squared analysis. Continuous variables were compared between the two drug groups using Wilcoxon rank sums analysis. Univariate analysis of the primary outcome of change in direct bilirubin was performed using analysis of variance (ANOVA), and multivariate analysis was performed using mixed effect regression modeling. We controlled for confounders including direct bilirubin at start of therapy (baseline severity), intrauterine growth restriction (IUGR), and lipid lowering (a commonly used alternative treatment for cholestasis). Although these variables were not statistically significantly different between the drug groups, there is biological plausibility that these clinical confounders could affect the scientific comparison. All statistical analyses were performed using SAS version 9.4.

Two infants with extreme phenotypes were excluded: (1) a preterm, IUGR infant with congenital diaphragmatic hernia who died on extracorporeal membrane oxygenation (ECMO) at day 14 with a direct bilirubin of 48 who was treated with phenobarbital, and (2) a full-term infant with congenital leukemia who developed cholestasis as a chemotherapy side effect in whom anti-cholestatic medications were used prophylactically.

Results

Data on 68 infants were extracted to obtain 68 first courses of drug therapy for comparison and 112 total courses of drug therapy for comparison. 49% of patients had one eligible drug course, 40% had two eligible courses, and 11% had more than two eligible courses. The primary medical diagnoses of the patients in the cohort are listed in Table 1.

The gestational ages, gender, race, and IUGR status did not differ significantly between the two patient groups (Table 2). There were similar rates of treatment with lipid lowering at drug start and similar lengths of drug treatment. Doses of phenobarbital and ursodiol were within standard of care ranges. All doses of phenobarbital were given intravenously and all doses of ursodiol were given enterally. The direct bilirubin at start of drug therapy was similar between the two groups. For the first course only analysis, 29% of infants were on 70/kg feeds and 16% of infants were on 140/kg feeds in the phenobarbital group. 89% of infants were on 70/kg feeds and 62% of infants were on 140/kg feeds in the ursodiol group. For the all courses analysis, 43% of infants were on 70/kg feeds and 30% of infants were on 140/kg feeds in the phenobarbital group. 86% of infants were on 70/kg feeds and 60% of infants were on 140/kg feeds in the ursodiol group.

The results of the drug comparisons are displayed in Table 3. In the primary analysis using the first course of drug therapy only, ursodiol was significantly more effective in reducing direct bilirubin than was phenobarbital (– 1.89 vs + 0.76 mg/dl; – 33.33 vs + 13.0 umol/L, *p*-value .03), even after controlling for baseline cholestasis severity, IUGR status, and lipid lowering therapy (– 2.16 vs + 0.27 mg/dl; – 36.94 vs + 4.62 umol/L, *p*-value .03). In the analysis including all treatment courses, ursodiol was again significantly more effective in reducing direct bilirubin than was phenobarbital (– 3.96 vs + 0.28 mg/dl; – 67.73 vs + 4.79 umol/L, *p*-value <.01). Figure 1 is a spaghetti plot of change in direct bilirubin for (a) first courses, and (b) all drug courses.

Table 1 Patient cohort medical diagnoses

Diagnosis	N (68)	ECMO
Preterm, Uncomplicated	11	
Preterm, Sepsis	7	1
Preterm, Spontaneous Intestinal Perforation	2	
Surgical NEC	12	
Medical NEC	7	
Congenital Heart Disease[a]	6	
Congenital Diaphragmatic Hernia (CDH)	4	2
Malrotation ± Bowel Atresia	4	
Gastroschisis / Omphalocele	3	
Other	12	2

Other: 1 Biliary atresia, 3 fullterm with pneumonia/sepsis (2 on ECMO), 3 hepatitis / liver failure of unknown etiology, 1 congenital CMV, 1 homocystinuria, 1 undiagnosed genetic syndrome with multiple anomalies, 1 panhypopituitarism with multiple anomalies, 1 preterm with congenital lung malformation

[a]one with documented medical NEC. NEC = necrotizing enterocolitis

Table 2 Patient variables by drug (first course of drug therapy)

	Phenobarbital (*N* = 37)	Ursodiol (*N* = 31)	*p*-value
Gestational Age at Birth (%)			0.7628
22–28 weeks	38	45	
28–34 weeks	40	32	
> 34 weeks	22	23	
Male (%)	57	71	0.2261
Race (%)			0.1439
Caucasian	58	61	
African American	20	32	
Other	22	7	
IUGR (%)	19	32	0.2058
On Restricted Lipids at start of drug therapy (%)	46	39	0.5479
Length of Drug Course [a]	17 (13,38)	17 (12,32)	0.4557
Dose (mg/kg/day) [a]	4.48 (3.84, 5.05)	27.43 (22.39,29.00)	n/a
Direct Bilirubin at start of drug therapy			0.8458
mg/dL[b]	7.1 (3.98)	6.9 (4.92)	
umol/L [b]	121.1 (68.1)	118.0 (84.2)	

[a]: Median (lower quartile, upper quartile); [b]: Mean (SD). IUGR = in utero growth restriction

Table 3 Cholestasis outcomes by drug treatment

	Phenobarbital	Ursodiol	*p*-value
Univariate analysis (first course only)			
Change in direct Bilirubin			0.03
mg/dl	+ 0.76	−1.89	
umol/L	+ 13.0	−32.3	
Direct Bili at end of drug therapy			0.02
mg/dl	7.84	4.98	
umol/L	134.1	85.2	
Adjusted for direct Bilirubin at start of drug therapy			
Change in direct Bilirubin			
First course			0.01
mg/dl	+ 0.81	−1.95	
umol/L	+ 13.85	- 33.35	
All Courses			<0.01
mg/dl	+ 0.66	−3.63	
umol/L	+ 11.29	−62.08	
Direct Bili at end of drug therapy (mg/dl)			
First course			0.01
mg/dl	7.79	5.03	
umol/L	133.24	86.03	
All Courses			<0.01
mg/dl	8.27	3.98	
umol/L	141.45	68.07	
Adjusted for direct Bilirubin at start of drug therapy, IUGR and limited lipids			
Change in direct Bilirubin			
First course			0.03
mg/dl	+ 0.27	−2.16	
umol/L	+ 4.62	−36.94	
All Courses‡			< 0.01
mg/dl	+ 0.28	−3.96	
umol/L	+ 4.79	−67.73	
Direct Bili at end of drug therapy (mg/dl)			
First Course			0.03
mg/dl	7.25	4.83	
umol/L	124.0	82.61	
All Courses[a]			< 0.01
mg/dl	7.89	3.65	
umol/L	134.95	62.43	

The first course analysis compares 37 phenobarbital to 31 ursodiol courses. The all course analysis compares 46 phenobarbital to 66 ursodiol courses. [a]The all course analysis was also adjusted for a binary variable accounting for previous phenobarbital or ursodiol exposure in prior 14 days

Discussion

This is the first study comparing effectiveness of ursodiol vs phenobarbital for the treatment of cholestasis in infants. In a real world NICU population, our results show that phenobarbital, on average, causes no improvement in direct bilirubin. Ursodiol is associated with more improvement in direct bilirubin and a lower direct bilirubin at the end of drug therapy. Although it is not typical to compare an IV formulation (phenobarbital) to an enteral formulation of another drug (ursodiol), we feel this comparison is meaningful because these are the two drugs used to treat cholestasis in the NICU in clinical care and the formulations in which they are given for the same diagnosis. A randomized controlled trial of these off-label, off patent medications is unlikely to occur, and thus a comparative cohort study is the current best evidence we can provide.

Ursodiol is the standard of care drug for cholestasis management, and comparing this to phenobarbital, a drug used without evidence of efficacy, is the only way to ascertain phenobarbital's utility for this indication. Many clinicians use phenobarbital for cholestasis when an infant is critically ill and not yet enterally fed or on low percent of enteral feeds, while awaiting the ability to use ursodiol once the infant has improved enteral feeding tolerance. T our knowledge, this is the first data which shows a lack of efficacy of phenobarbital in the treatment of neonatal cholestasis, and suggests that clinicians may consider avoiding phenobarbital treatment and waiting for sufficient enteral feeds to start ursodiol as the treatment of choice.

Despite lack of evidence, clinicians still use phenobarbital to treat neonatal and infant cholestasis. In a retrospective cohort study of neonates receiving phenobarbital for neurologic treatment (5 mg/kg/day), 66% of phenobarbital-treated infants developed cholestasis, as opposed to 33% of untreated controls [13], providing indirect evidence for lack of utility in cholestasis. In studies of drug-augmented hepatobiliary scintigraphy, results are mixed in regards to phenobarbital efficacy. When 50 infants with non-excreting phenotype on HIDA scan were randomized to phenorarbital, ursodiol or placebo, there was no increase in biliary excretion with any treatment [14]. In a direct comparison of the two drugs, the specificities of diagnosis of biliary atresia on drug-augmented scintigraphy were 80% for phenobarbital and 96.6% for ursodiol [15].

In addition to lack of efficacy, there is animal data which supports the role of phenobarbital as a neurotoxin. Normal rat pups equivalent in developmental age to human newborns were exposed to phenobarbital and areas of brain were examined for injury at 24 h. As compared to control, phenobarbital-treated rats had significantly increased levels of neuronal apoptosis in multiple brain regions [10]. In a different study, normal rat pups exposed to a single dose of phenobarbital at human newborn equivalent age exhibited impaired physiologic maturation in synaptogenesis among surviving neurons, suggesting

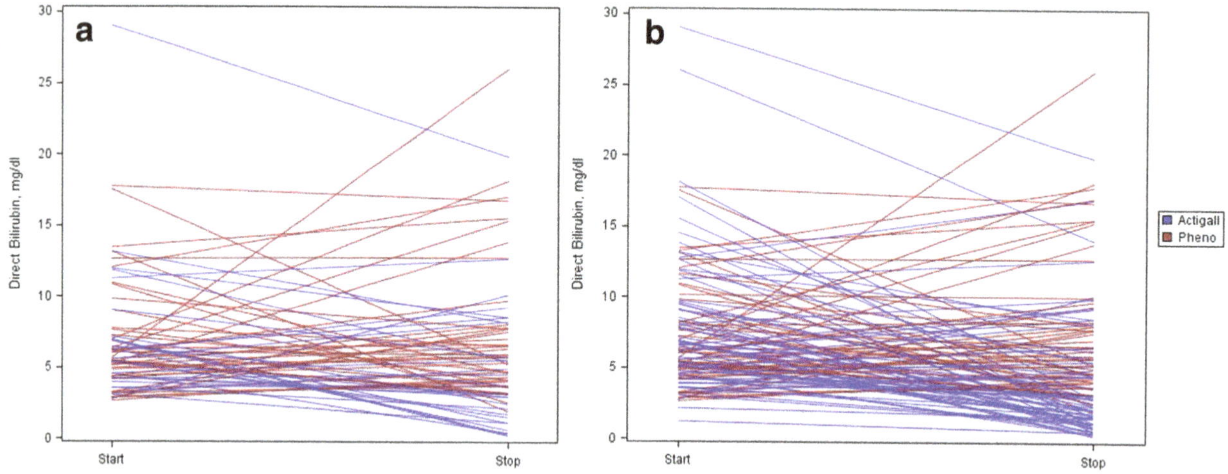

Fig. 1 Change in Direct Bilirubin by Drug Treatment. **a** First Course Only: Direct Bilirubin improved in 37% of phenobarbital courses and 70% of ursodiol courses. **b** All Drug Courses: Direct Bilirubin improved in 39% of phenobarbital courses and 77% of ursodiol courses

that early life exposure can potentially impact cognitive and behavioral outcomes [16]. Rats with a single exposure to phenobarbital during a critical window of brain development showed schizophrenia-like behavioral abnormalities as adults, suggesting that early neuronal injury and disordered synaptogenesis can predispose to psychiatric illness [17]. When used for cholestasis, phenobarbital is dosed daily for multiple days (median of 17 days in our cohort), and this prolonged dosing during a critical period of brain development may place infants at risk for neuronal abnormalities.

As with all retrospective cohort studies, our study has some limitations. First, since other markers of hepatic injury (AST/ALT, GGT, and hepatic ultrasound) are not closely followed clinically in many infants with cholestasis, direct bilirubin was the only universally available marker of cholestasis available as a surrogate marker of disease. Second, most infants with cholestasis in our cohort were treated with multiple courses of medications for cholestasis. To account for the effects of a prior drug course influencing the clinical results of a subsequent drug course, we did a primary analysis comparing only first courses of drug therapy. Third, given the critically ill condition of the patient population, most infants are not enterally fed initially and are treated with intravenous phenobarbital until on sufficient enteral feeds to tolerate ursodiol (an enterally dosed medication). This is the reality of the care of these infants and is reflected in the study results. We understand that enteral feedings could have confounded the association between ursodiol therapy and improvement in direct bilirubin because enteral feeds are themselves associated with improvement in cholestasis. Although enteral feeds likely augment the improvement of direct bilirubin seen with ursodiol, it seems unlikely that this accounts for the entire difference we observed between the two medications.

Strengths of this research include the diversity of medical diagnoses among the patients included in the cohort, making the results widely generalizable for NICU patients. Additionally, the narrow range of phenobarbital and ursodiol daily doses minimized the effect of drug dosing variability on the outcome. Lastly, we were able to account for the other main treatment modality for cholestasis, IV lipid limiting, in the comparative analysis.

There are potential new drugs for the treatment of cholestasis, such as obethicolic acid, a farnesoid C receptor (FXR) agonist, which regulates a wide variety of genes critical to bile acid synthesis and transport. FXR agonism decreases synthesis of bile acids in hepatocytes and increases transport of bile acids out of the cells, overall reducing the cytotoxic injury to hepatocytes. This drug was FDA approved this drug in May 2016 for the treatment of primary biliary cholangitis in combination with ursodiol. The pharmacokinetics, safety and efficacy of this drug have not been studies in neonates.

Conclusion

In conclusion, our study is the first to show that phenobarbital, when dosed over many days, does not significantly improve cholestasis in infants as compared to ursodiol. The burgeoning evidence for neurotoxicity in the developing brain associated with phenobarbital use may steer a treating clinician towards the use of ursodiol as the drug of choice for treatment of cholestasis in neonates.

Abbreviations
ALT: Alanine aminotransferase; ANOVA: Analysis of variance; AST: Aspartate aminotransferase; CAR: Constutuitive androstane receptor; CDH: Congenital diaphragmatic hernia; DBili: Direct bilirubin; dL: deciliter; ECMO: Extracorporeal membrane oxygenation; GGT: Gamma glutamyl transferase; IUGR: In utero growth restriction; IV: Intravenous; NEC: Necrotizing enterocolitis; NICU: Neonatal intensive care unit

Authors' contributions
TL – conception and design of project, data collection, analysis and data interpretation, drafting of manuscript and final approval of versions. SK – conception and design of the project, data collection, drafting of manuscript and final approval of versions. AS – design of project, analysis and data interpretation, drafting of manuscript and final approval of versions.

Competing interests
The authors declare that they have no competing interests.

Author details
[1]Department of Pediatrics, Children's Mercy Hospital, University of Missouri Kansas City School of Medicine, 2401 Gillham Rd, Kansas City, MO 64108, USA. [2]School of Medicine, University of Missouri Kansas City, Kansas City, MO, USA.

References
1. Champion V, Carbajal R, Lozar J, Girard I, Mitanchez D. Risk factors for developing transient neonatal cholestasis. J Pediatr Gastroenterol Nutr. 2012;55:592–8.
2. Jakobsen MS, Jorgensen MH, Husby S, Andersen L, Jeppesen PB. Low-fat, high-carbohydrate parenteral nutrition (PN) may potentially reverse liver disease in long-term PN-dependent infants. Dig Dis Sci. 2015;60:252–9.
3. Paumgartner G, Beuers U. Ursodeoxycholic acid in cholestatic liver disease: mechanisms of action and therapeutic use revisited. Hepatology. 2002;36: 525–31.
4. Beuers U. Drug insight: mechanisms and sites of action of ursodeoxycholic acid in cholestasis. Nat Clin Pract Gastroenterol Hepatol. 2006;3:318–28.
5. Chen CY, Tsao PN, Chen HL, Chou HC, Hsieh WS, Chang MH. Ursodeoxycholic acid (UDCA) therapy in very-low-birth-weight infants with parenteral nutrition-associated cholestasis. J Pediatr. 2004;145:317–21.
6. Al-Hathlol K, Al-Madani A, Al-Saif S, Abulaimoun B, Al-Tawil K, El-Demerdash A. Ursodeoxycholic acid therapy for intractable total parenteral nutrition-associated cholestasis in surgical very low birth weight infants. Singap Med J. 2006;47:147–51.
7. Heubi JE, Wiechmann DA, Creutzinger V, Setchell KD, Squires R Jr, Couser R, Rhodes P. Tauroursodeoxycholic acid (TUDCA) in the prevention of total parenteral nutrition-associated liver disease. J Pediatr. 2002;141:237–42.
8. Arslanoglu SS. Ursodeoxycholic acid treatment in preterm infants: a pilot study for the prevention of cholestasis associated with total parenteral nutrition. J Pediatr Gastroenterol Nutr. 46:228–31.
9. Bloomer JR, Boyer JL. Phenobarbital effects in cholestatic liver diseases. Ann Intern Med. 1975;82:310–7.
10. Kaushal S, Tamer Z, Opoku F, Forcelli PA. Anticonvulsant drug-induced cell death in the developing white matter of the rodent brain. Epilepsia. 2016; 57:727–34.
11. Bittigau P, Sifringer M, Genz K, Reith E, Pospischil D, Govindarajalu S, Dzietko M, Pesditschek S, Mai I, Dikranian K, et al. Antiepileptic drugs and apoptotic neurodegeneration in the developing brain. Proc Natl Acad Sci U S A. 2002; 99:15089–94.
12. Gutherz SB, Kulick CV, Soper C, Kondratyev A, Gale K, Forcelli PA. Brief postnatal exposure to phenobarbital impairs passive avoidance learning and sensorimotor gating in rats. Epilepsy Behav. 2014;37:265–9.
13. Gleghorn EE, Merritt RJ, Subramanian N, Ramos A. Phenobarbital does not prevent total parenteral nutrition-associated cholestasis in noninfected neonates. JPEN J Parenter Enteral Nutr. 1986;10:282–3.
14. Malik D, Khan SH, Ali SW, Rather TA, Pakala R, Hassan MU, Yadav N, Pasupula M. Comparison of phenobarbitone and ursodeoxycholic acid in drug-augmented hepatobiliary scintigraphy for excluding the diagnosis of obstructive cholestasis in neonatal cholestasis syndrome. Nucl Med Commun. 2015;36:827–32.
15. Nemat Khorasani E, Mansouri F. Application of ursodeoxycholic acid in hepatobiliary scintigraphy for neonatal hyperbilirubinemia: comparison with phenobarbital. Iranian J Nuclear Med. 2009;17:20–5.
16. Forcelli PA, Janssen MJ, Vicini S, Gale K. Neonatal exposure to antiepileptic drugs disrupts striatal synaptic development. Ann Neurol. 2012;72:363–72.
17. Bhardwaj SK, Forcelli PA, Palchik G, Gale K, Srivastava LK, Kondratyev A. Neonatal exposure to phenobarbital potentiates schizophrenia-like behavioral outcomes in the rat. Neuropharmacology. 2012;62:2337–45.

13

Illness recognition and appropriate care seeking for newborn complications in rural Oromia and Amhara regional states of Ethiopia

Y. Amare[1*], S. Paul[2] and L. M. Sibley[3]

Abstract

Background: Ethiopia has made significant progress in reducing child mortality but newborn mortality has stagnated at around 29 deaths per 1000 births. The Maternal Health in Ethiopia Partnership (MaNHEP) was a 3.5-year implementation project aimed at developing a community-oriented model of maternal and newborn health in rural Ethiopia and to position it for scale up. In 2014, we conducted a case study of the project focusing on recognition of and timely biomedical care seeking for maternal and newborn complications. In this paper, we detail the main findings from one component of the case study – the narrative interviews on newborn complications.

Methods: The study area, comprised of six districts in which MaNHEP had been implemented, was located in the two most populous federal regions of Ethiopia, Oromia and Amhara. The final purposive sample consisted of 16 cases in which the newborn survived to 28 days of life, and 13 cases in which the newborn died within 28 days of life, for a total sample size of 29 cases. Narrative interview were conducted with the main caregiver and several witnesses to the event. Analysis of the data included thematic content analysis and the determination of care seeking pathways and levels and timeliness of biomedical care seeking.

Results: Mothers and other witnesses do recognize certain symptoms of newborn illness which they often mentioned in clusters. The majority considered the symptoms to be serious and in some case hopeless. Perceived causes were mostly natural. Forty-one percent of care seekers sought timely biomedical care in the neonatal period. Surprisingly, perceived severity did not necessarily trigger care seeking. Facilitators of biomedical care seeking included accessibility of health facilities and counseling by health workers, whereas barriers included perceived vulnerability of newborns, post-partum restrictions on movements, hopelessness, wait-and-see atttitudes, poor communication and physical inaccessibility of health facilities.

Conclusions: Symptom recognition and care seeking patterns indicate the need to strengthen focused locally relevant health messages which target mothers, fathers and other community members, to further enhance access to health care and to improve referral and quality of care.

Keywords: Newborn complications, Symptom recognition, Care seeking, Illness narratives

* Correspondence: yaredamare@yahoo.com
[1]Consultancy for Social Development, P.O. Box – 70196, Addis Ababa, Ethiopia

Background

Globally, 2.6 million newborns died in 2016. In Ethiopia, as in much of the developing world, the death rate among children under 5 years of age has declined at a higher rate than among newborns which has remained around 29 deaths per 1000 live births in 2016. [1] Consequently, 48% of deaths in children under 5 in Ethiopia occur in the neonatal period. [2] The most important causes of newborn death globally are pre-term birth complications (36%), intra-partum related events (24%), sepsis or meningitis (16%) and congenital abnormalities (11%). [2] Low levels of facility delivery, poor newborn care practices and limited care seeking for complications are underlying factors behind high rates of newborn morbidity and care seeking.

The Maternal Health in Ethiopia Partnership (MaNHEP) was a 3.5-year implementation project funded by the Bill & Melinda Gates Foundation to develop a community-oriented model of maternal and newborn health in rural Ethiopia and to position it for scale up. [3] Emory University implemented MaNHEP, in collaboration with John Snow Research and Training Inc., University Research Co. LLC, and Addis Ababa University. In 2014, Emory conducted a case study of the project focusing on recognition of and biomedical care seeking for maternal and newborn complications. The Ethiopia case study, was one of six country studies that included India, Indonesia, Nigeria, Tanzania and Uganda. All case studies were framed by the Delay Model. [4] In an earlier 2016 publication, we focused on findings pertaining to illness recognition and care seeking for maternal complications. [5] In this paper, we detail the main findings on illness recognition and care seeking for newborn complications and their implications for policy, programming and research.

Methods

Study site

As described in our recent publication focusing on illness recognition and care seeking for maternal complications [5], the study was conducted in the two most populous federal regions of Ethiopia, Oromia and Amhara (Fig. 1). [1] The districts were largely rural and included Degem, Kuyu and Warra Jarso in Oromia Region and North Achefer, South Achefer and Mecha in Amhara Region (estimated population 350,000). Each district has an urban center and around six health centers each of which oversee five or six health posts. From each district, one health center and two health posts were randomly selected. Cases of newborn complications occurring within the previous 6 months were identified and sampled from the catchment areas of these facilities, as described below. A case was defined as a mother, her newborn and the witnesses to the newborn's illness event.

Sampling and data collection

This section presents a summary of sampling and data collection procedures. For further details on sampling, the interview guide, reporting and maintainance of data

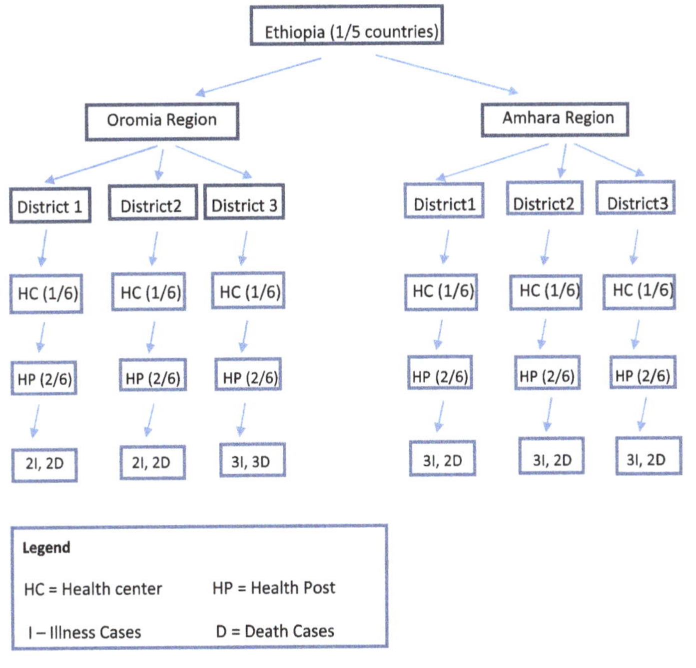

Fig. 1 Sample design

quality, see our previous publication on recognition and care seeking for maternal complications [5].

In the six districts, the study aimed to involve 30 cases: for each of the six districts, 3 mothers who perceived that their newborn became ill during the first month of life and was alive at 28 days of life, 2 mothers whose newborn became ill and died within 28 days of life and several witnesses to each event . Representation of diverse views and availability of cases were considerations in sampling. The inclusion criteria for these mothers were: female, age 18–49 years, gave birth in the previous 6 months, residence in the MaNHEP project area, perceived her newborn became ill within the first month of life and willing and able to participate. The final sample consisted of 16 cases in which the newborn survived to 28 days of life, and 13 cases in which the newborn died within 28 days of life, for a total sample size of 29 cases (Fig. 1).

After obtaining verbal informed consent using standard disclosure procedures, the study team used illness narrative interviews to collect data. The illness narrative is a qualitative rendering of an illness event by those who experienced the illness, along with those who were witnesses to the event. [6]

The narrative interviews were conducted with a primary caregiver, usually the mother of the newborn, and several witnesses to the illness event, who varied in number from one-to-three additional persons including her husband, mother-in-law, mother, sibling or neighbor. Although the interviews prioritized the primary caregiver who was usually the mother, other witnesses participated to a greater or lesser extent depending on personality and their role in the management of the illness episode. Thus, it turned out that the main or only respondent(s) in 13 of the 29 interviews was the mother; the mother and her husband in seven interviews; the mother and another person such as her mother-in-law or mother in five interviews; and persons other than the mother in four interviews.

Shortly after the interviews were conducted, "expanded field notes" on them were developed from memory, field notes, and audiotape recordings.

Analysis

. Coding procedures are detailed in our previous publication on illness recognition and care seeking for maternal complication. [5] A codebook, based on the illness narrative guide content and containing code definitions and inclusion and The analysis involved thematic content analysis using NVivo 10 based on the Delay Model [4]; re-coding of care-seeking pathways into: biomedical and non-biomedical or late biomedical categories; and univariate analysis to identify respondent characteristics and thematic code frequencies. Further details on these analyses are available in an earlier publication on care seeking for compications of pregnancy and child birth. [7] We also conducted a multiple correspondence analysis (MCA) to detect underlying structures in the illness recognition data. MCA is an exploratory qualitative data analysis technique. Perceived symptoms and causes (please refer below to the list of symptoms and causes) were treated as nominal variables with multiple levels, and the correlations among them were projected in a 2-dimensional visual "map." Proximity between different levels of these variables and between groups of individuals associated with the levels in the map were examined for clusters or patterns of symptoms and causes in relation to outcomes. A clustering of symptoms and causes suggests illness recognition on the part of respondents. Grouping individuals by an external outcome variable allow one to examine whether clusters of symptoms and causes are associated with differential outcomes-e.g. babies survived or did not survive the first 28 days of life. MCA was performed using the statistical software R [8].

Ethical approval

Before initiating the study, ethical review of and approval for the study was obtained from Emory University Institutional Review board and the Oromia and Amhara Regional State Health Bureaus.

Results

Sample characteristics

Of the 29 cases, a majority of mothers were between 19 and 29 years of age (55%) and had never attended school (62%). A majority of mothers (62%) also had given birth in a health facility. Mothers from Oromia attended more years of school than their Amhara counterparts (80% versus 43%). Of the cases, 13 cases involved newborns that had died. Of the newborns that had died, nearly all died within the first week of life (11 died day 1–3, 1 died between 4 and 7 days, and 1 died between 7 and 28 days). There were no notable differences in maternal age or education between the the group of newborns who died and those who survived. On the other hand, more babies born at home died than babies born in a health facility (eight out of the nine babies versus five of eighteen babies, respectively). The two babies who were born on the way to a health facility both survived.

Delay 1

Perceived symptoms and their severity

Mothers and witnesses to the illness event mentioned a number of symptoms in their newborns. In order of frequency, many mothers mentioned inability to breastfeed (72%), followed by vomiting (41%), fever (38%), coughing, sneezing and/or stuffy nose (38%), continuous crying and weak or difficult breathing (31% each) and cold body (24%). Symptoms mentioned by between 10 and 20% of mothers included swollen uvula, weak or no crying, weakness and diarrhea. Lastly, symptoms mentioned by less than 10% of mothers included inability to pass urine or stool, change in stool color and weight loss, as well as hiccups, frothing from the mouth, bleeding from the nose and mouth, moaning, rash, swollen umbilical cord, and swelling on the back of the head and neck.

Symptoms were often mentioned in clusters. For example, eight Amhara mothers and witnesses among the total of 29 mothers noticed that the baby was unable to breastfeed, vomited and/or had a fever, high temperature on the back of the neck, in addition to a red swollen uvula. Three mothers and witnesses observed that their baby had a cough, congested nose or difficult breathing in conjunction with inability to breastfeed, fever or vomiting. Others mentioned continuous crying, inability to breastfeed, vomiting and diarrhea, along with fever and increasing weakness.

> "He refused to suck my breast and when he did suck on it, he vomited soon afterwards. He cried a lot and he was sweating and had high fever. There was a sound inside his stomach when he was crying."(Mother, Oromia).

Of the 13 babies who died, several mothers and witnesses reported that their baby cried continuously after birth, was unable to breastfeed, lost weight and had a fever. Another mother noticed that her baby felt very cold and was silent until she died, whereas a father and his mother observed that their twin babies were coughing and had a congestion, difficulty breathing and were cold. Finally, one mother and the two grandmothers realized that their twin babies were born too soon, observing that they were very small and thin, weak and/or making moaning sounds.

Seventeen of the twenty-nine mothers and witnesses believed that their newborn's illness symptoms were serious; whereas in four cases, they thought the symptoms indicated the babies' condition was hopeless. One woman, whose newborn experienced two separate illness episodes, perceived the initial illness to be serious, but the second illness episode as not serious.

> "Yes, I was worried that the baby had fever and spent the whole night crying. I was worried that he may die. A baby cries and stops but my baby cried continuously. He also did not breastfeed and had vomiting and diarrhea." (Mother, Amhara).

> "When they [twins] came out from the womb, they were born with many problems. Even if the elder one was crying, they were coughing since birth and their body was as cold as iron. So I did not think they would start breastfeeding." (Grandmother, Oromia).

Some mothers and witnesses also reported changing perceptions of severity as symptoms presented. In three out of the 29 cases, they thought that the symptoms were not serious or that the baby would get better. Four families believed that the symptoms were not serious, but then serious when these symptoms persisted or other symptoms appeared.

> As one mother poignantly described, "I did not think that the baby was going to die. It was in the evening around nine that she was born and started to have difficulty breathing and sucking the breast. I was thinking that she may start sucking the breast next morning but she did not and her breathing problem persisted. Then she became weaker and weaker the following evening..." (Mother, Oromia).

Comparison of assessments of illness severity within cases of newborns who died versus cases of newborns who survived showed that, among the former,cases which were deemed to be hopeless were more frequent (4 of 13 cases versus 0 of 16 cases, respectively), cases which were deemed to be initially or ultimately not serious were more frequent (5 of 13 cases versus 2 of 16 cases, respectively), whereas cases which were judged to be serious were less frequent (4 of 13 cases versus 14 of 16 cases, respectively).

Perceived causes

Mothers and witnesses mentioned a number of causes for the observed symptoms. In order of frequency these included fallen uvula – a condition involving a red and swollen uvula and resulting in inability to breastfeed and fever (28%, Amhara only), prolonged labor and common cold (17% each), pregnancy workload and poor hygiene as well as supernatural causes such as God, evil eye or evil spirits (10% each). Causes mentioned in less than 10% of cases included maternal conditions such as bleeding, abdominal cramping, HIV, poor diet or malnutrition, eating bad food, physical sprain and maternal cough, as well as exposure to environmental and metaphysical elements resulting in a local illness known as *mitch* and the use of a scented soap for bathing, evil spirits or pre-term birth resulting in an illness known as *tilla*. Causes also included newborn conditions such as being in a bad position (e.g., breech), being malnourished (e.g., due to twins), being born too soon, having the umbilical cord around the neck as well as improper cord tying. The causes mentioned by mothers and caregivers in 90% of cases might be considered as "physical" or "biological."

Symptoms were sometimes thought to have multiple causes. For example, prolonged labor was associated with maternal twins or a baby that was in a bad position. In turn, prolonged labor was seen by some as a cause for inability to breast feed, continuous crying, difficult breathing or a cold body. A baby born too soon was associated with supernatural forces. Among some Amhara respondents, symptoms such as an inability to breastfeed, vomiting and fever were attributed to a swollen uvula which was, in turn, thought to be a result of natural processes, a heavy workload during pregnancy, bodily sprain or exposure to cold. Among Oromo respondents, these symptoms were thought to be caused by exposure to *mitch*, inadequate diet or poor hygiene. A cough, difficulty breathing and fever were often attributed to a common cold which was, in turn, thought to be a result of exposure to cold weather, a bad smell or lack of hygiene. As one father described,

> "I have found out that he had difficulty breathing, fever, coughing and vomiting. I thought the problem was a common cold due to the cold weather and the smell from the cattle we share our house with." (Father, Oromia).

Illness recognition

The MCA bi-plot map (Fig. 2) of the top 11 contributing variable levels for symptoms and causes reported by mothers and witnesses in each case shows that two MCA dimensions explained almost 40% (dimension 1 and 2 explains ~ 24 and 14%) of the variance in the data respectively. The cases are color-coded by two outcome groups: 1 = died within first 28 days, 2 = survived more than 28 days. One can see in the upper left quadrant of the map that symptoms of cough and congestion are correlated with causes common cold and poor hygiene, and that most of these newborns were among those that survived more than 28 days. Similarly, in the lower left quadrant one can see that symptoms of red swollen uvula and fever are associated the condition of fallen uvula, a folk category reported in Amhara only. In the lower right quadrant, symptoms of "weak or no cry," "difficulty breathing," "cold body," and the cause "born too soon" were clustered together, and most of the newborns in this quadrant died within the first 28 days. The cases falling into the two outcome categories (marked by green and brown triangles) appear separated and associated with different kinds of symptoms and causes, and the 95% confidence ellipses drawn around the

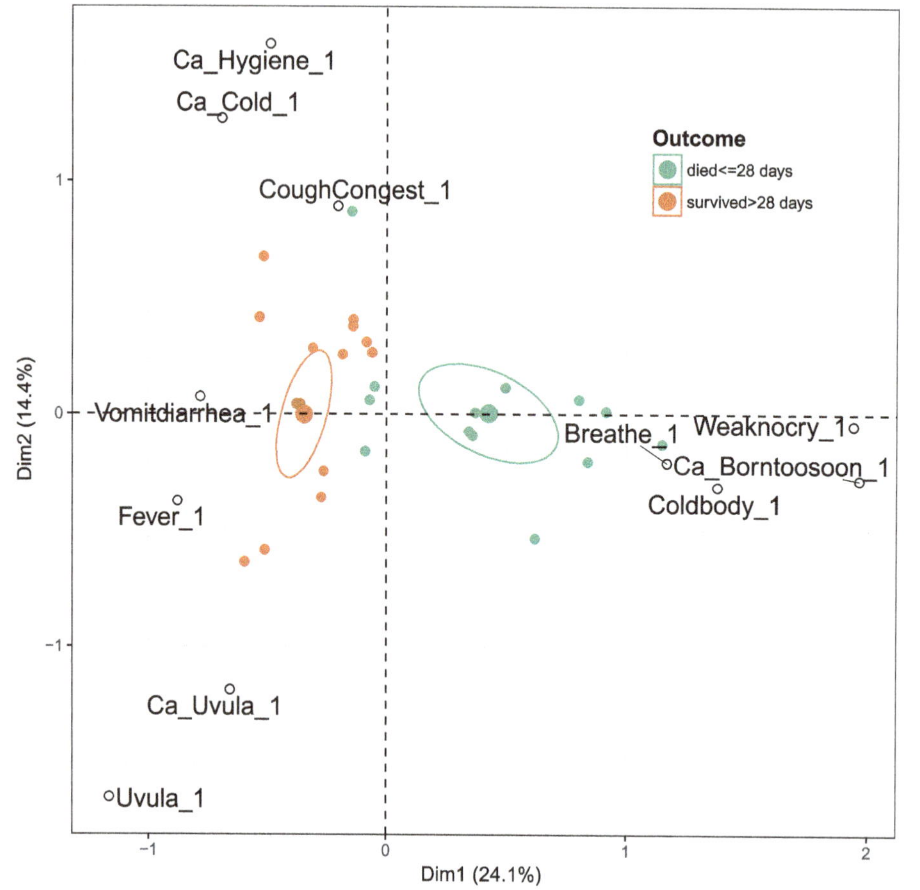

Fig. 2 Multiple correspondence analysis of perceived symptoms, causes and outcomes

mean point of the two groups of individuals do not overlap, indicating that the group means were significantly different. There is heterogeneity in symptoms and causes among the cases in which the newborns survived.

Decision-makers and time to make a decision to seek care

Decision-makers included parents of the newborn as well as other close members of the family such as their parents, a sister, sister-in-law, daughter or neighbor. Although the decision to seek biomedical care was often made in consultation with others, the final decision-makers were often the parents (8 out of 29 cases) or the mother herself (8 cases). Fathers were less often the sole decision maker (4 cases). As one woman commented:

> The baby spent the night crying a lot. It got even worse at night. I then decided that I would take the baby to the health center. Neighbors were complaining that I should not go to the health center before the baby was baptized. They said that an evil spirit would attack me. I ignored them and took the baby to the health center. (Amhara mother).

Of the 16 cases in which biomedical care was pursued, the time from illness recognition to the decision to seek care varied, from less than 12 h (six cases), 12–24 h (five cases), 25–72 h (two cases) togreater than 72 h (three cases, on days 5, 7 and 28).

Delay 2

Care seeking pathways

Mothers and families took different pathways to access care for their newborns. Of the 16 newborns who survived the illness event, twelve families (75%) sought biomedical care (Table 1). Two newborns first received care at a health center. Seven newborns were first treated at home or by a local healer and secondly received care at a hospital, health center, health post or by an HEW who was called-in to the home. One of these newborns was subsequently treated at home and at a health center as third and fourth steps of care. Three newborns received two treatments at home or by a local healer who was called-in before being taken to a health center. One of them was also subsequently treated by a local healer who was called-in as a first step of care. Of the four surviving newborns who did not receive biomedical care (25%), two received treatment at home and two were treated by a local healer who was called-in. One of the former was also subsequently treated by a local healer.

Of the 13 newborns who died, ten families (77%) did not seek biomedical care and were treated or cared for only at home (Table 2). Of the remaining three newborns, two received treatment at a health center and one at a hospital.

For analytical purposes, we chose to define care seeking at a health facility as a first or second step in response to newborn illness symptoms as 'timely

Table 1 Biomedical and non-biomedicalcare-seeking steps taken by families of 16 surviving newborns

First Step	Second Step	Third Step	Fourth Step
Biomedical care			
Health Center ($n = 2$)			
Home ($n = 5$)	Hospital/Health Center/Post ($n = 5$)	Home ($n = 1$)	Health Center ($n = 1$)
Home ($n = 1$)	Home ($n = 1$)	Health Center ($n = 1$)	
Home ($n = 2$)	Home Call-in ($n = 2$)	Health Center ($n = 1$)	Home Call-in ($n = 1$)
Home Call-in ($n = 1$)	Hospital ($n = 1$)	Health Center ($n = 1$)	
Home Call-in ($n = 1$)	Home ($n = 1$)	Health Center ($n = 1$)	
Non-Biomedical care			
Home ($n = 2$)	Home Call-in ($n = 1$)		
Home Call-in ($n = 2$)			

Table 2 Biomedical and non-biomedicalcare-seeking steps taken by families of 13 newborns who died

First Step	Second Step	Third Step	Fourth Step
Biomedical care			
Health Center			
(*n* = 2)			
Hospital			
(*n* = 1)			
Non-Biomedical care			
Home			
(*n* = 10)			

biomedical care seeking'. According to our definition, 12 of 29 families (41%) sought timely biomedical care in the neonatal period.

Timely biomedical care seeking was more frequent in the case of newborns who survived (8 of 16) compared to newborns who died (4 of 13). It was also associated with some characteristics of families. Timely biomedical care seeking was more frequent among younger mothers aged 19 to 29 years of age versus mothers older than 29 years of age (8 of 17 versus 3 of 10, respectively), mothers who delivered in a health facility as opposed to in a home or on the way to a health facility (10 of 18 versus 2 of 11, repectively), and, to a lesser extent, those who perceived the illness episode to be serious as compared to those who perceived it to be initially or ultimately not serious or hopeless (8 of 12 versus 10 of 17, respectively).

Symptoms and causes that appeared to have triggered biomedical care seeking were coughing, sneezing or stuffy nose associated with the common cold and poor maternal hygiene; and prolonged labor associated with maternal cramping and bleeding. Other symptoms included continuous crying, vomiting, malnutrition and improper cord tying. Symptoms that were as likely to trigger care seeking as not were difficulty breastfeeding and fever, both associated with a number of causes. Finally, symptoms and causes that were not associated with biomedical care seeking included swollen red uvula associated with the folk illness fallen uvula; and difficulty breathing, weak or no crying, and cold body associated with being born too soon or to supernatural causes. Few families relied on local traditional healers and birth attendants as a first or second step of care (6 of 29), in almost all cases for a fallen uvula.

Facilitators, delayers and barriers to care seeking

Respondents reported a number of factors that facilitated, delayed or prevented their use of health facility care. Facilitators included physical and financial accessibility of HEWs or health posts, as well as health education and advice from HEWs, health workers or neighbors. Factors that either delayed or prevented care seeking included postpartum restrictions on women's movement, perceived physical or spiritual vulnerability and weakness of post-natal women and newborns, hopelessness, the hope that the baby will get better, fear of travelling during the day time which may expose one to *mitch*, the evil eye or curious neighbors, or fears of poor treatment at the health facility. Other delaying factors were clinic hours, rain or night time hours, poor communications, distance, lack of transportation and financial constraints, e.g., one family that had to wait several weeks to receive a loan from their funeral association to cover medical costs.

Discussion

Summary of findings

In relation to Delay 1, the study findings suggest that the mothers and witnesses did recognize certain illness symptoms in their newborn. On the one hand, a number of symptoms were reported in clusters and were associated with particular causes such as being born too soon (premature), a common cold or lack of hygiene, or a fallen uvula. On the other hand, frequently mentioned symptoms such as difficulty breastfeeding and fever, important danger signs from a biomedical perspective, were associated with a variety of causes. Although most mothers and witnesses considered the symptoms they observed to be serious, some considered them not serious or only gradually came to believe they were serious, which led to a wait-and-see approach. As mentioned previously, more caretakers who considered their newborns' illnesses symptoms to be hopeless or not serious were among those whose newborns died.

Symptoms or causes perceived as serious, however, did not necessarily lead to care seeking, as evident in the 10 families who did not seek biomedical care or sought late care. It is especially concerning that symptoms such as difficulty breastfeeding, fever, difficulty breathing, weak or no crying, and a cold newborn body did not trigger care seeking in all cases. Although the newborn's parents were the main decision makers, others such as their parents, a sister, sister-in-law, daughter or neighbor were often involved. Their considerations about whether to seek care are consistent with the Delay Model [4] and include cultural norms such as perceived vulnerability and postpartum restrictions on the movement of mothers and newborns, advice from health workers, accessibility of services and perceived quality of care, as well as environmental conditions, economic and logistical issues.

In relation to Delay 2, in spite of the above considerations, 12 of 29 families sought timely bio-medical care, most often after an initial attempt at home-based care. Importantly, 38% of these families made the decision to seek care on the day that they recognized their newborn's illness. And few families relied on local traditional healers and birth attendants as a first or second step of care (10% each), primarily for the traditional illness, fallen uvula. Timely biomedical care seeking was more common among younger mothers, mothers who had delivered in a health facility, babies who survived the neonatal period, and to some extent among families who perceived the illness episode to be serious.

Researchers examining illness recognition and care seeking typically conduct descriptive studies using mixed methods and situated in a variety of settings, often in South Asia and sub-Saharan Africa. Some of these studies found that newborn caretaker recognition of newborn illness symptoms to be poor [9, 10] whereas other studies found that care takers did recognize such symptoms [11, 12]. Findings from our study conform with the latter including symptom clusters associated with the common cold, the folk illness fallen uvula, and preterm babies and those with difficulty breathing, which are associated with different causes and outcomes. Previous studies have shown that perceived causes of newborn illness range from the supernatural to naturalistic which influence whether traditional or modern treatment is utilized [12, 13, 14]. In this study, illness responses exhibited some association with specific types of mostly naturalistic causes. Conceptions and responses related to the fallen uvula illness in Amhara region resemble the local illnesses recognized in other countries which are seen to be best treated with traditional medicine [10, 15]. Illness symptoms that are considered serious have been found to be associated with care seeking in some studies whereas this association was weaker in a study conducted in Ghana and also in our study [10, 16].

Use of biomedical care ranging from 14 to 39% of illness episodes have been reported in various studies as compared to 40% in this study [11, 17, 18]. One of these studies conducted in Nepal reported that half of those who sought medical care did so after the first 48 h from the onset of illness as compared to 38% who sought such care in the first day after symptoms were recognized in our study [14]. The data we have presented on the characteristics of newborn care takers who seek such care are often not available in similar studies and contrast with the findings of one study on characteristics associated with care seeking for children under five [19]. We have also found that newborn survival is associated with facility delivery, the assessment that illness symptoms are serious and with the use of biomedical care.

Previous research has also explicitly identified factors which delay or prevent care seeking for newborn illnesses. Barriers such as aspects of local understanding of illness including symptom recognition, causation and severity, associated use of traditional treatments, wait-and-see attitudes, hopelessnes, negative experiences at health facilities, and lack of physical and financial access have been discussed in various studies [10, 14, 17, 20]. While finding that symptom recognition is not as much of a constraint on care seeking, this study has also identified all these barriers in addition to the role of postpartum restrictions on the movement and perceived vulnerability of women and newborns, reluctance to travel during the day time, limited clinic hours, and environmental factors. Furthermore, enablers such as the physical and financial accessibility of health posts and health counseling and education from health workers and acquaintances have been identified.

Strengths and challenges

The illness narrative method generated data on the actual experience and diverse perspectives of witnesses to the event. The illness event timeline and neutral probes used in the narrative interview stimulate recall and increase validity of the data. The replicability of the narrative interviews is unknown.

Conclusions

The findings of this study show that mothers and other witnesses generally recognize certain newborn illness symptoms and their seriousness. Several of them did initially or ultimately consider symptoms to be not serious or hopeless. Recognition of the seriousness of symptoms does not always lead to timely biomedical care seeking, although in our setting care seeking appears to occur more frequently among younger mothers, as well as those who gave birth in a health facility. The findings thus indicate an urgent need to focus health education and behavior change efforts on the seriousness as well as treatability of illness symptoms and identified local cultural factors that impede care seeking such as traditional postpartum restrictions on women's movement and associated beliefs about the vulnerability of mothers and newborns to harmful metaphysical elements if taken outside of the home, hopelessness and, in the case of Amhara region, the folk illness, fallen uvula. Families must come to understand timely biomedical care will improve the chances of their newborns' survival. Continued efforts to reduce known environmental, logistic and economic barriers to care seeking are also needed.

Abbreviations

FMoH: Federal Ministry of Health; HDA: Health Development Army; HEW: Health Extension Worker; MaNHEP: Maternal and Newborn Health in Ethiopia Partnership; RHB: Regional Health Bureau; URC: University Research Company, LLC; USAID: United States Agency for International Development

Acknowledgements
The authors would like to thank Allisyn Moran, Supria Madhavan, and Neal Brandes of USAID, and Danielle Charlet and Jim Sherry of URC for their vision, technical and financial support to the six country case study teams, including the Ethiopia team. We also thank Abebe Gebremariam Gobezayehu, Solomon Tesfaye, Aynalem H/Michael Frew and Lelisse Tadesse of Emory University Ethiopia and Mulusew Lijalem Belew of the Amhara Regional Health Bureau for their logistic contributions and support in sampling and case identification, as well as Abel Mekonnen, Yeshi Mulatu, Serawit Omer and Getahun Shiferaw of the Consultancy for Social Development for their role in conducting the illness narratives and data coding. Finally, we would like to express our gratitude to the women and families who participated in the illness narratives. While participation sometimes elicited painful memories, the information shared will help to improve our understanding and addressing of factors that facilitate and impede timely biomedical care seeking for others who, in the future, may be faced with complications of pregnancy and childbirth.

Funding
This study was made possible through funding by the United States Agency for International Development Translating Research into Action (TRAction) Project "Systematic Review of Illness Recognition and Appropriate Care Seeking for Maternal and Newborn Complications" through University Research Co., LLC. Both USAID and University Research Company, LLC, contributed to the overall six-country study design and protocol, development and standardization of the illness narrative guide and procedures, and organized data analysis and writing workshops to support six country teams. The views expressed in this manuscript are those of the authors.

Authors' contributions
YA contributed to the development and standardization of the illness narrative guide and procedures, training of interviewers, oversight of data collection and data quality, the analysis, interpretation and write-up of the data. SP contributed to the multiple correspondence analysis, its interpretation and write-up. LS contributed to the overall six-country study design and common protocol, its adaptation to the Ethiopia context, the development and standardization of the illness narrative guide and procedures, the analysis, interpretation and write-up of the data. All authors have read and approve of the final manuscript.

Ethics approval and consent to participate
This study was reviewed by and exempted from oversight by the Emory University Institutional Review Board and by the Amhara and Oromia Regional Health Bureau Ethical Review Committees. Informed verbal consent was obtained from all participants according to standard disclosure procedures. The verbal consent procedure was approved by the Institutional Review Board and the Health Bureau Ethical Review Committees.

Competing interests
The authors declare that they have no competing interests.

Author details
[1]Consultancy for Social Development, P.O. Box – 70196, Addis Ababa, Ethiopia. [2]Nell Hodgson Woodruff School of Nursing, Emory University, 1520 Clifton Road NE, 30322 Atlanta, Georgia. [3]Nell Hodgson Woodruff School of Nursing and Rollins School of Public Health, Emory University, 1520 Clifton Road NE, 30322 Atlanta, Georgia.

References
1. Central Statistical Agency (CSA) [Ethiopia] and ICF. Ethiopia Demographic and Health Survey 2016. Addis Ababa, Rockville: CSA and ICF; 2016.
2. Department of Evidence, Information and Research (WHO, Geneva) and Maternal Child Epidemiology Estimation (MCEE) 2017. MCEE-WHO methods and data sources for child causes of death 2000-2016. Global Health Estimates Technical Paper WHO/HMM/IER/GHE/2017.1.
3. Sibley LM, Tesfaye S, Desta BF, Frew AH, Kebede A, Mohammed H, Hepburn K, Ethier-Stover K, Dynes M, Barry D, Gobezayehu AG. Improving maternal and newborn health care delivery in rural Amhara and Oromiya regions of Ethiopia through the maternal and newborn health in Ethiopia partnership. J Midwif Womens Health. 2014;59(S1):6–20.
4. Thaddeus S, Maine D. Too far to walk: maternal mortality in context. SocSci Med. 1994;38(8):1091–110.
5. Sibley L, Amare Y. Illness recognition and care seeking for maternal complications of pregnancy and birth in rural Amhara and Oromia regional states of Ethiopia. BMC Pregnancy Childbirth. 2016;17:384.
6. Yount K, Gittelsohn J. Reports of health-seeking behavior from the integrated illness history and a standard child morbidity survey. J Mixed Method Res. 2008;2(1):23–62.
7. Sibley L, Amare Y, Tesfaye S, Belew ML, Shiffra K, Barry D. Appropriateness and timeliness of care-seeking for complications of pregnancy and childbirth in rural Ethiopia: a case study of the maternal and newborn health in Ethiopia partnership. J Health Popul Nutr. 2017;36(Suppl 1):50.
8. The Comprehensive R Archive Network https://cran.r-project.org/. Accessed 2018.
9. Choi Y, El Arifeen S, Mannan I, Rahman SM, Bari S, Darmstadt GL, Black RE, Baqui AH, Projahnmo Study Group. Can mothers recognize neonatal illness correctly? Comparison of maternal report and assessment by community health workers in rural Bangladesh. Tropical Med Int Health. 2010;15(6):743–53.
10. Hill Z, Kendall C, Arthur P, Kirkwood B, Adjei E. Recognizing childhood illnesses and their traditional explanations: Exploring options for care-seeking interventions in the context of the IMCI strategy in rural Ghana. Tropical Med Int Health. 2003;8: 668–76.
11. Awasthi S, Verma T, Agarwal M. Danger signs of neonatal illnesses: perceptions of caregivers and health workers in northern India. Bull World Health Organ. 2006;84:819–26.
12. Engmann C, Adongo P, Akawire Aborigo R, Gupta M, Logonia G, Affah G, Waiswa P, Hodgson A, Moyer CA. Infant illness spanning the antenatal to early neonatal continuum in rural northern Ghana: local perceptions, beliefs and practices. J Perinatol. 2013;33:476–81.
13. Amare Y, Degefie T, Mulligan B. Newborn care seeking practices in central and southern Ethiopia and implications for community-based programming. Ethiop J Health Dev. 2012;27(1):3–7.
14. Mesko N, Osrin D, Tamang S, Shrestha BP, Manandhar DS, Manandhar M, Standing H, Costello AM. Care for perinatal illness in rural Nepal: a descriptive study with cross-sectional and qualitative components. BMC Int Health Hum Rights. 2003;3(1):3.
15. Awasthi S, Srivastava NM, Pant S. Symptom-specific care-seeking behavior for sick neonates among urban poor in Lucknow, northern India. J Perinatol. 2008;28:S69–75.
16. Amarasiri de Silva MW, Wijekoon A, Hornik R, Martines J. Care seeking in Sri Lanka: one possible explanation for low childhood mortality. Soc Sci Med. 2001;53(10):1363–72.
17. Bazzano AN, Kirkwood BR, Tawiah-Agyemang C, Owusu-Agyei S, Adongo PB. Beyond symptom recognition: care-seeking for ill newborns in rural Ghana. Tropical Med Int Health. 2008;13(1):123–8.
18. Chowdhury H, Thompson S, Ali M, Alam N, Yunus M, Streatfield P. Care seeking for fatal illness episodes in neonates: a population-based study in rural Bangladesh. BMC Pediatr. 2011;11:88.
19. Sutrisna B, Kresno S, Utomo B, Sutrisna B, Reingold A, Harrison G. Care-seeking for fatal illnesses in young children in Indramayu, West Java, Indonesia. The Lancet. 1993;342(8874):787–9.
20. Mohan P, Iyengar SD, Agarwal K, Martines JC, Sen K. Care-seeking practices in rural Rajasthan: barriers and facilitating factors. J Perinatol. 2008;28(S2): S31–7.

The power of practice: simulation training improving the quality of neonatal resuscitation skills in Bihar, India

Brennan Vail[1*], Melissa C. Morgan[1,2,3], Hilary Spindler[3], Amelia Christmas[4], Susanna R. Cohen[5] and Dilys M. Walker[3,6,7]

Abstract

Background: Globally, neonatal mortality accounts for nearly half of under-five mortality, and intrapartum related events are a leading cause. Despite the rise in neonatal resuscitation (NR) training programs in low- and middle-income countries, their impact on the quality of NR skills amongst providers with limited formal medical education, particularly those working in rural primary health centers (PHCs), remains incompletely understood.

Methods: This study evaluates the impact of PRONTO International simulation training on the quality of NR skills in simulated resuscitations and live deliveries in rural PHCs throughout Bihar, India. Further, it explores barriers to performance of key NR skills. PRONTO training was conducted within CARE India's AMANAT intervention, a maternal and child health quality improvement project. Performance in simulations was evaluated using video-recorded assessment simulations at weeks 4 and 8 of training. Performance in live deliveries was evaluated in real time using a mobile-phone application. Barriers were explored through semi-structured interviews with simulation facilitators.

Results: In total, 1342 nurses participated in PRONTO training and 226 NR assessment simulations were matched by PHC and evaluated. From week 4 to 8 of training, proper neck extension, positive pressure ventilation (PPV) with chest rise, and assessment of heart rate increased by 14%, 19%, and 12% respectively (all $p \leq 0.01$). No difference was noted in stimulation, suction, proper PPV rate, or time to completion of key steps. In 252 live deliveries, identification of non-vigorous neonates, use of suction, and use of PPV increased by 21%, 25%, and 23% respectively (all $p < 0.01$) between weeks 1–3 and 4–8. Eighteen interviews revealed individual, logistical, and cultural barriers to key NR skills.

Conclusion: PRONTO simulation training had a positive impact on the quality of key skills in simulated and live resuscitations throughout Bihar. Nevertheless, there is need for ongoing improvement that will likely require both further clinical training and addressing barriers that go beyond the scope of such training. In settings where clinical outcome data is unreliable, data triangulation, the process of synthesizing multiple data sources to generate a better-informed evaluation, offers a powerful tool for guiding this process.

Keywords: Neonatal resuscitation, Bihar, India, Simulation Training, Barriers to Care

* Correspondence: brennan.vail@ucsf.edu
[1]Department of Pediatrics, University of California San Francisco, 550 16th Street, 4th Floor, Box 0110, San Francisco, CA 94158, USA
Full list of author information is available at the end of the article

Background

In 2016, 43% of deaths in children under age five globally occurred during the neonatal period [1]. In India, neonatal deaths accounted for 56% under-five deaths [1] and over half of these deaths occurred in only four states: Bihar, Uttar Pradesh, Madhya Pradesh, and Rajasthan [2]. Bihar is a state in eastern India with the highest rural birth rate in the country [3] and the highest multidimensional poverty index in all of South Asia [4]. Nearly one-third of neonatal deaths in Bihar are due to intrapartum related events [5], and yet providers are not adequately trained to perform basic neonatal resuscitation (NR) [6, 7]. Approximately 10% of neonates require tactile stimulation to transition at the time of birth and 3–6% require positive pressure ventilation (PPV) [8]. It is estimated that the effective provision of basic NR could save over 60,000 infants in India alone annually [9].

Although, there are many NR training programs in low- and middle-income countries (LMICs) [10], very few studies have evaluated the impact of such programs on the quality of clinical skills amongst providers with limited formal medical education in rural community settings. One small study evaluating the skills of community health workers in Bangladesh found improvement in initial resuscitation practices (drying, tactile stimulation), neck extension, and mouth-to-mouth ventilation with training, though no statistical analysis was provided [11]. More studies have focused on providers at referral hospitals [12–18]. Results from these studies are variable, with some demonstrating improvements in initial resuscitation [12, 15, 17, 18] and PPV skills [12–17], while others showed no change in initial resuscitation skills [14] or time to initiation of PPV [12, 15]. Several studies assessed skills at one time point and thus could not sufficiently determine the impact of training [19–23]. Others reported only a composite evaluation of skills [24–28], which is less relevant for NR, where outcomes depend on adequate performance of initial steps before proceeding to more complex ones.

This study offers a unique large-scale evaluation of an eight week, in-situ NR training program developed by PRONTO International [29] and implemented in rural primary health centers (PHCs) across Bihar with providers with limited formal medical education. PRONTO training was conducted within a larger maternal and child health quality improvement project called *Apatkaleen Matritva evam Navjat Tatparta* (AMANAT) [30–32]. The specific objectives of this study were 1) to evaluate the impact of PRONTO training on the quality of NR skills in simulated resuscitations; 2) to evaluate the impact of PRONTO training on performance in live deliveries requiring resuscitation of a non-vigorous infant; and 3) to explore obstacles to performance of specific evidence-based practices (EBP) in NR in Bihar.

Methods

Study design and setting

This study employed a mixed methods approach to evaluate the impact of PRONTO training on the quality of NR skills. Quantitative methods were used for the first two objectives and qualitative methods were used for the third objective. The portion of PRONTO simulation training evaluated in this manuscript was conducted at PHCs, where the majority of labor and delivery care in Bihar is provided. Each PHC serves a predominately rural population of ~ 190,000 individuals (number based on monitoring and evaluation data from CARE India [30]). PHCs provide largely preventative health care with limited curative services [33]. The vast majority of obstetric and neonatal care at PHCs is provided by nurses with an Auxiliary Nurse Midwife (ANM) or General Nursing and Midwifery (GNM) qualification, which require 2 and 3.5 years of training after completion of secondary school, respectively [34]. PHCs frequently face staffing shortages, often having only one nurse on duty in the labor room at any given time [33]. PHCs are not staffed with specialists, including pediatricians [33], and, in general, doctors are unavailable to assist in the labor room. Caesarian sections and instrumented deliveries are only performed at higher levels of care and thus require referral out of PHCs [33].

AMANAT and PRONTO interventions

AMANAT is multi-faceted quality improvement project, implemented by CARE India [30] in collaboration with the Government of Bihar, which seeks to improve maternal and child health outcomes in the state using a mentorship model of education [30–32]. AMANAT mentors are nurses with a Bachelor's degree in nursing recruited from across India. Mentees are ANMs and GNMs employed at PHCs.

PRONTO International training consists of in-situ simulations of a variety of neonatal and obstetric emergencies, which are supplemented by teamwork and communication activities, skills stations, and case-based learning [29]. Within AMANAT, PRONTO was responsible for training mentors to teach mentees emergency obstetric and neonatal care. Doctors were not included in the PRONTO training at PHCs as they were not part of the larger AMANAT program at PHCs and were infrequently involved in labor and delivery care in these facilities. Using a train-the-trainer model, PRONTO provided six days of training for mentors on simulation facilitation, team building, communication skills, and debriefing skills before mentoring began, and a four-day refresher training three months into the mentoring period. Over each 8-month phase, mentor pairs rotated between four PHCs, spending one week per month at each PHC conducting simulations. On average, seven NR simulations were conducted at each PHC over the 8 month training cycle.

In the PRONTO curriculum, normal spontaneous vaginal delivery (NSVD) simulations were introduced in week 2 and NR and postpartum hemorrhage (PPH) simulations were introduced in week 3 of training. Notably, bedside mentoring often began earlier, as mentors attended live deliveries during teaching hours with mentees to provide real-time instruction on any complications that arose. Formal assessment simulations were conducted for NSVD, PPH, and NR at weeks 4 and 8 of training. Pre-training assessments were not conducted, providing mentees time to adjust to simulation prior to being evaluated. NR simulations were conducted with the NeoNatalie™ [35] mannequin in situ in the labor rooms where mentees worked. All simulations were video-recorded to enable video-assisted debriefing as well as for programmatic evaluation.

Study population

ANMs/GNMs with labor room duties and interest in the mentoring program were selected for participation as mentees in AMANAT and PRONTO training. This analysis evaluates the clinical NR skills of mentees in both real and simulated deliveries in phases 2 and 3 of AMANAT mentoring conducted between September 2015 and July 2016. During this period, approximately 88% of mentees were ANMs and 12% were GNMs.

Interview participants were mentors who served as simulation facilitators. Twenty mentors, one from each phase 4 mentor pair, were selected for interviews in January 2017 based on the following criteria: 1) mentor was currently employed by AMANAT at the time of interview, and 2) mentor had worked in ≥2 phases of AMANAT (equivalent to 16 months in 8 different PHCs). Two interviewees were unable to participate due to illness and personal travel.

Study procedures

Mentee performance in simulated resuscitations

Evaluation of the quality of mentees' NR skills in simulated resuscitations was based on video-recorded assessment simulations from weeks 4 and 8 of training. At each PHC, mentees were selected by random lottery to participate in the NR assessment simulation for a given week. Assessments were announced but the lottery was conducted immediately prior to simulations. The simulated scenario began with a neonate found apneic while breastfeeding 15 min after birth, progressing to require suctioning, stimulation, and PPV. This simulation was chosen by mentors in place of a simulation beginning with a birth as it involved less set up and was thus easier to facilitate in high volume PHCs. Additionally, it allowed mentees to focus only on NR during the assessment rather than progressing from NSVD management to NR. Assessment videos were transferred to encrypted USB drives and transported to Patna, the capital of Bihar, where they were uploaded to an encrypted server and transferred to University of California San Francisco (UCSF). Videos were then coded by one of the lead investigators with pediatric clinical experience for pre-defined NR quality indicators selected by a team of clinical and simulation experts at UCSF and the University of Utah. The coder was blinded to time of assessment (week 4 vs. 8 of training). After the completion of coding, indicators least likely to be subject to bias due to simulation artifact were selected for inclusion in the analysis. Variable definitions are provided in Table 1.

Mentee performance in live resuscitations

Mentors attended births occurring in the PHCs during daytime working hours from Monday through Saturday. Mentors were asked to assess mentees' skills immediately after observed live deliveries using a smart phone application based on the OpenDataKit platform [36]. The application asked mentors to subjectively evaluate specific NR skills by indicating if the skill 'went well' or 'needed improvement.' This manuscript only evaluates mentees' performance during live deliveries in which the neonate was non-vigorous.

Table 1 Definition of key variables

Binary variables	
Stimulation	Clinically adequate stimulation performed prior to initiation of PPV
Suction	Suction performed prior to initiation of PPV
Neck extension	Neck extended in the proper sniffing position using towel roll or head tilt
PPV with chest rise	PPV with three consecutive breaths with visible chest rise
PPV rate 40–60 breaths/minute	PPV delivered at a rate of 40–60 breaths per minute
Heart rate assessed	Heart rate assessed at any point during the resuscitation
Time-based variables	
Mentee hands on neonate	Time elapsed between the mother calling for help and the nurse mentee placing hands on the neonate to begin the clinical evaluation
Neonate placed on warmer	Time elapsed between the mother calling for help and the neonate being placed on the warmer to begin the resuscitation
Initiation of PPV	Time elapsed between the mother calling for help and the initiation of PPV
PPV with chest rise	Time elapsed between the mother calling for help and the third consecutive breath of PPV with visible chest rise

PPV positive pressure ventilation

Barriers to evidence-based NR practices

Mentors were interviewed about the barriers to EBP in NR that they had observed mentees facing in PHCs. Study procedures for the qualitative portion of this manuscript have been described in detail in a separate manuscript [37]. In brief, a semi-structured interview guide was developed and piloted with a former AMANAT mentor. A portion of the interview guide asked mentors about each of the following skills before and after training: warming/drying/stimulating, measuring heart and respiratory rates, achieving chest rise during PPV, and performing the resuscitation with adequate urgency. The interview guide allowed the interviewer the flexibility to ask open-ended questions regarding barriers to these skills and to further explore emerging themes. One-on-one interviews were conducted in English by one of the lead investigators in a private room at PHCs. If the interview was conducted outside of business hours or private space was unavailable, the interview was conducted in a private location near the PHC. All interviewees were fluent in English. Interviews were observed by a local Hindi-speaking member of the PRONTO team in case minor phrase translations were required. Interview duration ranged from 45 to 75 min.

After 18 interviews, the interviewer concluded data saturation had been reached as no new barriers to care were being identified. However, this manuscript only presents barriers specifically linked by mentors to one of the skills evaluated in simulated or live resuscitations in an attempt to provide context for quantitative trends. Thus, this manuscript is not an exhaustive exploration of barriers to care, and other barriers that were not explicitly linked to a specific resuscitation skill are explored in a separate manuscript [37].

Analysis

All quantitative analyses were conducted using IBM SPSS Statistics 23 [38].

Mentee performance in simulated resuscitations

Assessment simulations from weeks 4 and 8 of training were paired by PHC. Simulation videos that were corrupt or could not be paired were discarded. Simulations where the mentor stepped in to assist mentees or where the clinical scenario deviated from the assessment scenario were also discarded. The percentage of simulations in which mentees correctly completed key NR tasks, meeting quality indicators, at weeks 4 and 8 of training was compared using McNemar's Test for paired proportions. The median time to mentee completion of key NR tasks at weeks 4 and 8 was compared using the Wilcoxon Signed Rank Test due to violation of the normality assumption of parametric methods.

Mentee performance in live resuscitations

The percentage of live deliveries in which mentors felt mentees adequately performed key NR skills was graphed by week of training. Additionally, the percentage of deliveries in which NR skills 'went well' in weeks 1–3 was compared to weeks 4–8 using the Pearson Chi-Squared Test. Week 3 was chosen as the cut-off because NR simulations were introduced into the PRONTO curriculum at that time. If the expected cell count assumption was violated, a Fisher's Exact Test was substituted.

Barriers to evidence-based NR practices

Audio-recorded interviews were transcribed and analyzed by the interviewer. Qualitative analysis was conducted using the thematic content approach [39, 40], which included 1) data familiarization, 2) identifying codes and then themes, 3) developing a coding scheme and applying it to the data, and 4) refining and organizing codes consistent with the Braun and Clarke approach to thematic analysis [41]. Two interviews (10%) were selected at random for double coding to ensure consistency in identification of key themes.

Results

Mentee performance in simulated resuscitations

A total of 1342 mentees at 160 PHCs participated in phases 2 and 3 of AMANAT/ PRONTO training. A randomly selected subset of these mentees was evaluated in 279 NR assessment simulations, which were video-recorded and coded for quality indicators. This analysis includes 226 (81%) assessment videos, or 113 PHC-matched week 4 and 8 video pairs.

From week 4 to 8 of training, there was a 13.5 percentage-point increase in proper neck extension ($p = 0.01$), a 19.0 percentage-point increase in PPV with visible chest rise ($p < 0.01$), and an 11.6 percentage-point increase in assessment of heart rate during resuscitations ($p < 0.01$). There was no statistically significant change between weeks 4 and 8 in adequate stimulation, suction, or delivery of PPV with the proper rate (Table 2). Additionally, there was no statistically significant change in median time to completion of key NR tasks (Table 3).

Mentee performance in live resuscitations

Mentee performance was evaluated in a total of 3195 live deliveries in phases 2 and 3. Amongst these, 252 (8%) were complicated by birth of a non-vigorous neonate. From early to later weeks of training, the percentage of deliveries in which mentees' identification of non-vigorous neonates, suctioning, and PPV 'went well' increased by 20.7, 25.4, and 22.7 percentage-points respectively (all $p < 0.01$). The percentage of deliveries in which mentors felt mentees performed adequate

Table 2 Percent of simulations in which mentees correctly performed key NR skills at weeks 4 and 8 of training ($N = 113$ matched pairs)

Key NR skill	N[a]	Week 4	Week 8	Percentage-point change[c]	*P*-value[d]
		n (%)[b]			
Stimulation	107	38 (35.5)	26 (24.3)	−11.2	0.08
Suction	111	69 (62.2)	78 (70.3)	8.1	0.25
Neck extension	104	78 (75.0)	92 (88.5)	13.5	0.01
PPV with chest rise	100	66 (66.0)	85 (85.0)	19.0	< 0.01
PPV rate 40–60 breaths/min	106	39 (36.8)	52 (49.1)	12.3	0.08
Heart rate assessed	112	97 (86.6)	110 (98.2)	11.6	< 0.01

NR Neonatal resuscitation, *PPV* Positive pressure ventilation
[a]N = total number of PHC-matched week 4 and 8 simulation pairs in which key NR skill could be evaluated
[b]n = number of week 4 and 8 simulations in which key NR skill was completed % = percent of week 4 and 8 simulations in which key NR skill was completed
[c]Percentage-point difference in completion of key NR skill from week 4 to 8 of training
[d]McNemar's Test of paired proportions

stimulation was high at baseline (94%) and did not change significantly (Table 4). The week-wise trend in these four variables is illustrated in Fig. 1.

Barriers to evidence-based NR practices

High level themes and illustrative quotations of barriers to 1) initial resuscitation, 2) measuring heart and respiratory rates, 3) achieving chest rise during PPV, and 4) performing the resuscitation with adequate urgency are summarized in Table 5.

Initial resuscitation

Prior to training, mentors explained mentees did not understand the clinical significance of the initial steps of resuscitation (warming, drying, stimulating, and suction) and did not know how to properly perform these steps. Rather, they performed traditional practices including holding the neonate upside down, over stimulating, and massaging the chest. Additionally, equipment issues, including the availability of clean, dry cloths precluded effective initial resuscitations.

After training, mentors felt that mentees knew how to perform warm/dry/stim in an evidence-based manner. However, mentors reported that mentees often forgot to perform these initial resuscitation steps in a perceived rush to begin ventilation. On the other hand, mentors felt mentees still did not understand the clinical indications for suctioning and were too quick to jump to this step. Supply issues remained a barrier to initial resuscitation after training. Mentors explained that equipment, including mucus extractors, was often unavailable or disorganized and thus inaccessible when urgently needed.

Measurement of heart and respiratory rates

Mentors explained that prior to training, mentees did not know how to measure vital signs, were inaccurate in their counting, or were unaware of normal parameters and their clinical significance for neonates. This was likely connected to the belief, prior to training, that the management of non-vigorous neonates was the responsibility of doctors. Mentors also explained that mentees' goal in resuscitations was simply to make the baby cry, so vital signs were frequently overlooked.

This goal remained true after training. Mentors reported that mentees frequently forgot to check vital signs because they were too focused on simply making the neonate cry. Nevertheless, mentors felt that mentees understood the significance of vital signs after training. However, they still could not measure them accurately, often because they did not have or could not read a clock.

Table 3 Time to mentee completion of key NR skills in simulation at weeks 4 and 8 of training ($N = 113$ matched pairs)

Time in seconds to key NR skill	N[a]	Week 4	Week 8	Difference in seconds[c]	*P*-value[d]
		Median (IQR)[b]			
Mentee hands on neonate	98	9 (6–17)	11 (7–22)	2	0.55
Neonate placed on warmer	105	35 (24–56)	38 (26–62)	3	0.95
Initiation of PPV	106	83 (48–111)	84 (66–114)	1	0.90
PPV with chest rise	58	116 (88–178)	137 (92–195)	21	0.76

NR Neonatal resuscitation, *PPV* Positive pressure ventilation, *IQR* Inter-quartile range
[a]N = total number of PHC-matched week 4 and 8 simulation pairs in which key NR skill could be evaluated
[b]Median time in seconds to completion of key NR skill (inter-quartile range)
[c]Difference in median number of seconds to completion of key NR skill from week 4 to 8 of training
[d]Wilcoxon Signed-Rank Test

Table 4 Percent of live deliveries in which mentees successfully completed key NR Skills in the early versus later weeks of training ($N = 252$)

Key NR skill	Weeks 1–3		Weeks 4–8		Percentage-point change[c]	*P*-value
	N[a]	*n* (%)[b]	N[a]	*n* (%)[b]		
Identification of non-vigorous infant	66	32 (48.5)	156	108 (69.2)	20.7	< 0.01[d]
Warm/dry/stimulate	65	60 (92.3)	144	139 (96.5)	4.2	0.29[e]
Suction	63	27 (42.9)	145	99 (68.3)	25.4	< 0.01[d]
PPV	48	12 (25.0)	109	52 (47.7)	22.7	< 0.01[d]

NR Neonatal resuscitation, *PPV* Positive pressure ventilation
[a]N = number of live deliveries in which performance of NR skill was required and recorded
[b]n = number of live deliveries in which NR skill was successfully completed; % = percent of live deliveries in which NR skill was successfully completed
[c]Difference in percent of live deliveries in which NR skill was completed from early to late weeks of training
[d]Pearson Chi-Squared Test
[e]Fisher's Exact Test

PPV with chest rise

Mentors explained that knowledge of all aspects of PPV, including clinical significance, mask selection, rate of delivery, and assessment of effectiveness was lacking before training. If ventilation was provided, it was often given mouth-to-mouth or by using a self-inflating bag on the mother's abdomen without knowledge of proper technique. Similar to the measurement of vital signs, mentors explained that some mentees believed that doctors were responsible for managing non-vigorous neonates prior to training, which meant they did not initiate ventilation themselves.

After training, mentors felt mentees had accepted the responsibility of providing PPV, but that they continued to have difficulty with mask seal, rhythm, and assessment of PPV effectiveness. Approximately two-thirds of mentors reported observing continued difficulty with neck extension after training, while one-third of mentors felt mentees had mastered this skill. Additionally, mentors reported mentees did not know when to stop PPV for reassessment because mentees did not have or could not read a clock. The availability of ventilation bags and different mask sizes, particularly preterm masks, was identified as a barrier after training-- likely persistent from before training but more frequently identified after PPV became an accepted duty of mentees. Finally, one mentor felt the traditional belief that oxygen was important in addressing respiratory distress was a barrier to performing PPV with self-inflating bags with no oxygen source after training.

Urgency

Mentors explained that mentees did not understand the concept of the golden minute or the significance of achieving effective ventilation within that timeframe prior to training. Additionally, they did not know how to accurately identify non-vigorous neonates requiring resuscitation. Further, mentors explained the traditional practice in Bihar was to patiently wait for neonates to cry, which commonly delayed resuscitations. Other

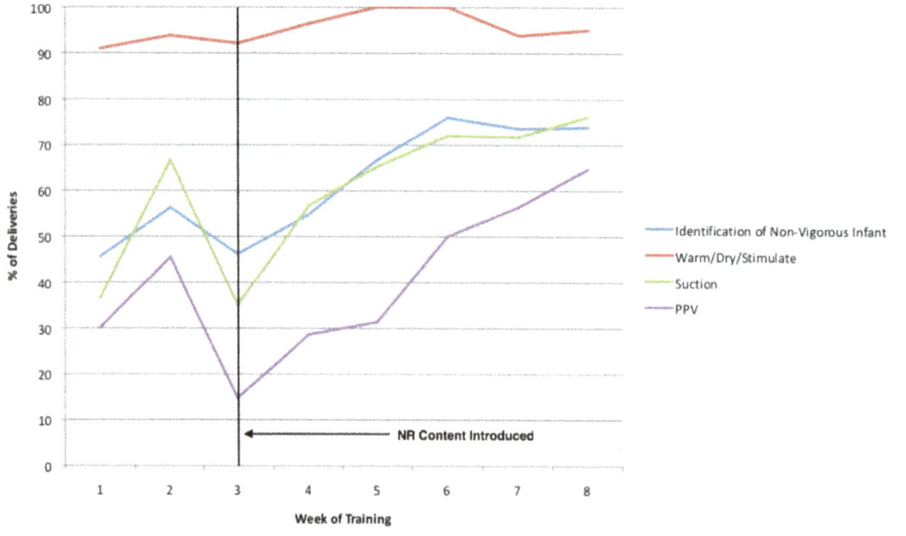

Fig. 1 Trend in the Percent of Live Deliveries in which Mentees Successfully Completed Key NR Skills by Week of Training

Table 5 Barriers to Evidence-Based Practices in Neonatal Resuscitation Before and After Training

Barrier	Before training	After training
Initial resuscitation		
Knowledge	"They were not knowing ok there is a need to stimulate... and they were not knowing ok why they need to dry the baby."	"So much suctioning is there… with the help of drying or stimulating the baby can be saved, but in spite of that they used to go for suctioning… like if baby didn't cry means ok get… sucker, get sucker."
Traditional Practices	"They'll hold the baby upside down, they will shake the baby here and there, they'll beat the baby… but… the proper stimulation they were not aware [that] they should rub the baby back or they should flick [the feet]."	
Equipment	"They used to dry the baby but… not with a clean or dry cloth."	"Baby was [asphyxiated with] thick meconium… suction, all the thing[s] [were] not available and we don't know where they are."
Focus on Later Management		"[Mentees] think that if the baby is not crying, they have to take [the baby] immediately to the warmer, so they forget the stimulation part."
Measurement of heart and respiratory rates		
Knowledge	"Actually before… [mentees] were not knowing ok heart rate and respiration[s] are two different things… then we started teaching them anatomy. Respiration- this is the work of lungs… and heart rate- this is the work of heart."	
Skill		"[Mentees] don't have timers to see or… just for name sake they see… or they don't see it properly… the counting goes here and there. They don't get it accurately."
Equipment		"Some sisters [are] having trouble while checking the heart rate because… watch is not available."
Focus on Later Management	"The goal is the baby should cry. [Mentees] don't see for the respiration rate or for the heart rate, they just see that the baby cries… keep on stimulating so that the baby cries."	"Until [mentees] see the baby [cry], they will give bag and mask, bag and mask. In between… check heart rate, respiratory rate, they were not doing."
Role of MD	"[Mentees] said… 'what's heart rate? How do we check that? That's doctor's thing, they do that with the stethoscope.'"	
PPV with chest rise		
Knowledge	"They were not knowing about the PPV. If any of the [mentees] knew, she was not knowing the correct rhythm… how much time you need to do, how you need to. She only knew ok we need to do."	
Skill	"[Mentees] just pump [the Ambu bag]… according to the baby['s] size they don't use the [correct] mask. Whatever mask they get, they will connect that and they will pump it."	"[Mask] seal is not good for most of the time… and the rhythm also. Some of the mentees, they forget the [ventilation] rhythm also."
Traditional Practices	"Before… in some facilities [mentees] were giving mouth to mouth ventilation… that time they didn't know how to use bag and mask ventilation."	"PPV they are doing but they have more belief in oxygen. If we will put the oxygen… baby will be crying they believe only."
Equipment		"In some PHC we don't have zero [size] mask… we have only one number mask, so it is not as effective, because in preterm baby we can't use the big one."
Role of MD	"Before training [mentees] were not doing [PPV]… they didn't know how to use bag and mask ventilation. They only know… we can't use, doctor has to do."	
Urgency		
Knowledge	"Actually they are not aware what is the effect [of delay]. Until we… know what is the effect, we will not take precaution."	"[Mentees] can't… understand when [the neonates] need resuscitation or not. Sometimes they identify very well but… sometime[s] they waiting for… crying… It's not proper timing."

Table 5 Barriers to Evidence-Based Practices in Neonatal Resuscitation Before and After Training *(Continued)*

Barrier	Before training	After training
Skill	"To cut the cord, to take the baby to the NBCC, and to start [the] resuscitation, it will take more than 5 min they were telling."	"It will take time, especially drying the baby, wiping it, stimulating it, clamping… the cords."
Traditional Practices	"Because their old practice is like... they… will wait, they'll tell, 'Baby will cry now, sister this is normal baby will cry now.'"	"They are thinking it might be crying… they are waiting for some time. But when we are there we are telling them not crying so go fast!"
Equipment		"Golden minute… [mentees] don't have articles for clamping or… they search for suctioning, for mucus extractor… availability is not there in the PHC, so they go outside to get."
Facility Layout		"NBCC is in another room… this is labor room, so next to labor room is NBCC, so that takes [mentees] more than a minute to take the baby from labor room to NBCC."
Maternal Management	"For one to two to three minutes [mentees] will wait… because [until] the placenta is removed, they will concentrate on that. Ok, the placenta is removed, after that they see, ok, baby is not crying. Then they will start with the Ambu."	
Human Resources		"Sometimes only one staff is there for delivery… she will be taking care of the mother and then baby is not crying..."

PPV Positive pressure ventilation, *PHC* Primary health center, *NBCC* Newborn care corner

delays were created by slow cord clamping and performance of the initial NR steps. Finally, mentors described mentees' focus on maternal management as a barrier to timely NR prior to training.

After training, mentors explained mentees were better at identifying non-vigorous neonates and knew about the golden minute; however, some mentors expressed concern some mentees still did not truly understand its clinical significance. Additionally, mentors explained mentees could not read a clock to facilitate timely resuscitations. Regarding skills, mentors explained mentees' inefficiencies in initial resuscitation and cord cutting continued to delay resuscitations after training. One mentor felt that mentees spent too much time trying to seal the mask. Overall, mentors felt more practice performing NR with proper timing was necessary. Other frequently mentioned barriers to urgency that were likely persistent from before training were the traditional practice of patiently waiting for the infant to cry, long distances between labor rooms and the newborn care corners (NBCCs), insufficient staffing, and issues with supply availability, functionality, and organization.

Discussion

PRONTO International's NR simulation training, implemented within the AMANAT quality improvement initiative, had a positive impact on key NR skills amongst ANM/GNM mentees working in rural PHCs across Bihar. Nevertheless, there is room for continued improvement in nearly all NR skills, likely due to the need for additional training as well as significant barriers that go beyond the scope of clinical skills training. For each of the key skills evaluated in this manuscript-- initial resuscitation, assessment of vital signs, performance of PPV, and urgency in resuscitations-- we present a triangulated discussion of simulation data, live delivery data, and barriers to care identified by mentors in qualitative interviews to facilitate a more nuanced understanding of the positive impacts of PRONTO training and areas for improvement.

Mentees' performance of the initial NR steps, including warming, drying, stimulating, and suctioning, was variable. This is consistent with previously published studies [12, 14]. In interviews, mentors suggested that knowledge of EBPs increased with training. However, there was no significant change in the percentage of simulated NR scenarios in which mentees provided clinically adequate stimulation prior to PPV from week 4 to 8 of training. In observed live deliveries, there was similarly no significant change in stimulation between the early and later weeks of training; although, the rate of stimulation was high at baseline. This knowledge-skill gap may be explained by mentors' observation that mentees frequently forgot initial NR steps in a perceived rush to start PPV. Moreover, the fact that the simulated scenario did not begin with a birth may have also contributed to mentees' relative failure to perform initial steps in simulation compared to live deliveries. Regarding suctioning, there was significant improvement in live deliveries, but not in simulated resuscitations. Despite this improvement in live deliveries, about a quarter of live-born neonates deemed to require suctioning did not receive it during week 8 of training, perhaps due to the supply issues highlighted by mentors.

Assessment of vital signs, including heart rate and respiratory rate, was evaluated only in simulated resuscitations. A significant improvement was observed from week 4 to 8 of training. Mentors explained that vital signs were often not assessed before training due to inadequate knowledge and a prevalent belief that NR was the doctor's responsibility. This suggests the observed change in simulation data, which did not include a true pre-training measurement, may underestimate the impact of training on this skill. Notably, while simulation data captured whether or not mentees checked heart rate, it did not assess the accuracy of heart rate measurements. Mentors explained in interviews that mentees have difficulty reading a clock, suggesting this may be an area for future improvement. This will likely require innovative solutions to help providers identify normal versus abnormal vital signs without the need to count precise rates.

Proper delivery of PPV is the chief focus of many NR trainings. A significant improvement in PPV skills was observed in both simulated and live resuscitations following PRONTO training. Previous studies have similarly reported improvement in PPV skills post-training [12–17]. During week 8, mentees achieved chest rise in 85 and 65% of simulated and live resuscitations, respectively. Other studies report comparable [12, 15] or lower rates of effective PPV [14, 16]. In interviews, mentors explained mentees continued to struggle with mask seal, rhythm, and real time assessment of PPV effectiveness. These observations are supported by the simulation data, which demonstrated no change in the use of the proper rate of PPV following training. Although interviewees disagreed about mentees' ability to perform proper neck extension, a significant improvement in this skill was observed in simulations from week 4 to 8. Mentors felt the persistent PPV knowledge-skill gap was due to insufficient practice as well as lack of availability of functional supplies in PHCs. The need for more practice with longer trainings is not an unfamiliar challenge amongst NR programs in LMICs [42] and the PRONTO training is unique in that it was conducted over 8 months. Nonetheless, given the departure PPV represents from traditional practices in Bihar, interviewees felt even this duration of training was insufficient.

Urgency is another key area for improvement. No significant change was observed in the time to completion of key NR tasks in simulations. In fact, the median time to effective chest rise trended upward non-significantly from week 4 to 8 of training. Other studies have similarly reported both increased and unchanged durations of time to PPV initiation [12, 15]. Nonetheless, mentors described a perceived rush to start ventilation after training that negatively impacted initial resuscitation measures. The discrepancy between the perceived urgency and true time to completion of key tasks may be related to barriers such as inability to read a clock, distance between labor rooms and NBCCs, and both supply and human resources shortages. Other barriers to urgency identified by interviewees included poor understanding of the true significance of the golden minute and continued performance of traditional clinical practices such as waiting indefinitely for the infant to cry. Timely identification of non-vigorous neonates in live deliveries improved significantly; however, mentees still failed to identify nearly a quarter of live-born neonates deemed non-vigorous by mentors at the end of training.

These results have informed the next iteration of the PRONTO curriculum, which will include greater emphasis on quick identification of non-vigorous neonates, beginning resuscitations with appropriate initial resuscitation measures, recognition of vital sign abnormalities without counting specific rates, and timely initiation of effective PPV. Nevertheless, this study has several limitations. Foremost, due to the unreliable birth registry system in Bihar, there are no reliable clinical outcome data on which to base the impact of this training program. For this reason, we used simulation data as a proxy.

The simulation data lack a true pre-training measurement, which may cause an underestimation of the true impact of training. Nonetheless, this was a conscious choice to allow mentees to adapt to simulation procedures prior to evaluation given their lack of familiarity with this method of learning [42]. The assessment simulation was also not changed between week 4 and 8. However, this is unlikely to have led to an overestimation of the impact of training given the aim of this study was to assess the quality of basic NR skills, which should follow an algorithm that is relatively independent of the clinical scenario in uncomplicated resuscitations. Additionally, simulation data represent the performance of only a subset of mentees who participated in the NR assessment simulations at week 4 and 8 of training. However, as the selection process was random, the impact of selection bias is likely minimal. Finally, this data is based on a single video assessor, which could have introduced interpretation bias. However, the potential for this bias was minimized by blinding the assessor to week of training and by choosing an assessor who was independent from training implementation.

The live birth data represent a convenience sample and could be biased, as data were collected by mentors who were not blind to week of training and who had somewhat limited clinical training themselves, as most were early in their nursing career. Further, live delivery data provide only a binary and subjective assessment of whether key NR steps went well or not. Nevertheless, these data provide the only assessment of performance in live deliveries, as medical record keeping is inconsistent. The investigators felt that a more rigorous assessment of resuscitations in real time would impact clinical care or preclude data collection given the high delivery volume at PHCs.

Qualitative interview data could be influenced by desire of mentors to please the interviewer as well as by any preconceptions mentors may have had about intrapartum or postnatal care in Bihar. We attempted to mitigate these potential biases by clearly stating during the consent process that interviews were not a performance evaluation and by selecting interviewees with at least 16 months of mentoring experience in PHCs. Finally, not all qualitative interview data regarding barriers to care is included in this manuscript. Rather, logistical, cultural, and structural barriers to immediate neonatal care and NR are more fully explored in a separate manuscript [37] and this manuscript only presents barriers explicitly linked by mentors to specific NR skills assessed in simulated and live resuscitations.

Conclusion

PRONTO simulation training conducted within the AMANAT intervention had a positive impact on knowledge and the use of evidence-based NR practices amongst numerous ANMs/GNMs working in rural PHCs throughout Bihar. Nevertheless there is a need for ongoing improvement, which will require addressing many barriers to care that extend beyond the scope of clinical skills training. Data triangulation, incorporating both quantitative and qualitative methodologies, offers a powerful tool for guiding this process in settings such as Bihar where clinical outcome data are unreliable, yet the need for improvement in neonatal care is great.

Abbreviations

ANM: Auxiliary nurse midwife; EBP: Evidence-based practices; GNM: General nursing and midwifery; IQR: Inter-quartile range; LMIC: Low- and middle-income countries; NBCC: Newborn care corner; NR: Neonatal resuscitation; NSVD: Normal spontaneous vaginal delivery; PHC: Primary health center; PPH: Postpartum hemorrhage; PPV: Positive pressure ventilation; UCSF: University of California San Francisco

Acknowledgements

The authors would like to thank the entire CARE India team for their support in facilitating PRONTO International simulation training as part of the AMANAT program throughout Bihar. We would also like to express our sincere appreciation for all phase 2-4 mentors for their commitment to teaching and their willingness to participate in qualitative interviews. Thank you also to the phase 2-4 participates for their commitment to the training and willingness to learn. Special thanks to Rebecka Thanaki, Renu Sharma, and Praicey Thomas for their help in arranging and facilitating qualitative interviews. Lastly, thank you to the entire PRONTO International team for their tireless work throughout implementation and evaluation of the training program.

Funding

This study was funded by the Bill and Melinda Gates Foundation. The funding body had no role in the design of the study; the collection, analysis, and interpretation of data; or in writing the manuscript.

Authors' contributions

BV designed data collection tools, coded all simulation videos, conducted all interviews, performed qualitative and quantitative data analysis, and drafted and revised the manuscript. MM provided clinical expertise and made substantial contributions to the design of data collection tools, data analysis, and manuscript revision. HS was also involved in study design and critical revision of the manuscript. AC was involved in PRONTO curriculum design, supervision of PRONTO training, provided expert local opinion for qualitative analysis, and critically revised the manuscript. SC was involved in PRONTO curriculum design, study design, and made significant contributions during manuscript revision. DW is the principal investigator for the evaluation of PRONTO in Bihar and made significant contributions to all aspects of study design and manuscript preparation. All authors have approved this manuscript for submission.

Competing interests

DW and SC are founding members of PRONTO International and sit on its board of directors. None of the other authors have any conflicts of interest to declare.

Author details

[1]Department of Pediatrics, University of California San Francisco, 550 16th Street, 4th Floor, Box 0110, San Francisco, CA 94158, USA. [2]Maternal, Adolescent, Reproductive, and Child Health Centre, London School of Hygiene and Tropical Medicine, Keppel Street, London WC1E 7HT, UK. [3]Institute for Global Health Sciences, University of California San Francisco, 550 16th Street, San Francisco, CA 94158, USA. [4]PRONTO International, State RMNCH+A Unit, C-16 Krishi Nagar, A.G. Colony, Patna, Bihar 80002, India. [5]College of Nursing, University of Utah, 10 South 2000 East, Salt Lake City, UT 84112, USA. [6]Department of Obstetrics and Gynecology and Reproductive Services, University of California San Francisco, 1001 Potrero Ave, San Francisco, CA 94110, USA. [7]PRONTO International, 1820 E. Thomas Street APT 16, Seattle, WA 98112, USA.

References

1. GBD 2016 Mortality Collaborators. Global, regional, and national under-5 mortality, adult mortality, age-specific mortality, and life expectancy, 1970–2016: a systematic analysis for the Global Burden of Disease Study 2016. Lancet. 2017;390:1084–150.
2. Ministry of Health & Family Welfare Government of India. INAP India Newborn Action Plan. 2014.

3. Registrar General of India. Sample registration system (SRS) statistical report 2013. New Delhi: 2013. Available from: http://www.censusindia.gov.in/vital_statistics/SRS_Reports_2013.html.
4. Oxford Poverty & Human Development Initiative. Multidimensional Poverty Index 2016 Highlights ~ South Asia. University of Oxford. 2016.
5. Dogra V, Khanna R, Jain A, Kumar AM, Shewade HD, Majumdar SS. Neonatal mortality in India's rural poor: findings of a household survey and verbal autopsy study in Rajasthan. Bihar and Odisha J Trop Pediatr. 2015;61(3):210–4.
6. Agrawal N, Kumar S, Balasubramaniam SM, Bhargava S, Sinha P, Bakshi B, et al. Effectiveness of virtual classroom training in improving the knowledge and key maternal neonatal health skills of general nurse midwifery students in Bihar, India: a pre- and post-intervention study. Nurse Educ Today. 2016;36:293–7.
7. Chauhan M, Sharma J, Negandhi P, Reddy S, Sethy G, Neogi SB. Assessment of newborn care corners in selected public health facilities in Bihar. Indian J Public Health. 2016;60(4):341–2.
8. Lee AC, Cousens S, Wall SN, Niermeyer S, Darmstadt GL, Carlo WA, et al. Neonatal resuscitation and immediate newborn assessment and stimulation for the prevention of neonatal deaths: a systematic review, meta-analysis and Delphi estimation of mortality effect. BMC Public Health. 2011;11(Suppl 3):S12.
9. Kamath-Rayne BD, Griffin JB, Moran K, Jones B, Downs A, McClure EM, et al. Resuscitation and obstetrical care to reduce Intrapartum-related neonatal deaths: a MANDATE study. Matern Child Health J. 2015;19(8):1853–63.
10. Reisman J, Arlington L, Jensen L, Louis H, Suarez-Rebling D, Nelson BD. Newborn Resuscitation Training in Resource-Limited Settings: A Systematic Literature Review. Pediatrics. 2016;138(2):e20154490.
11. Dynes M, Rahman A, Beck D, Moran A, Pervin J, Yunus M, et al. Home-based life saving skills in Matlab, Bangladesh: a process evaluation of a community-based maternal child health programme. Midwifery. 2011;27(1):15–22.
12. Ersdal HL, Vossius C, Bayo E, Mduma E, Perlman J, Lippert A, et al. A one-day "helping babies breathe" course improves simulated performance but not clinical management of neonates. Resuscitation. 2013;84(10):1422–7.
13. Couper ID, Thurley JD, Hugo JF. The neonatal resuscitation training project in rural South Africa. Rural Remote Health. 2005;5(4):459.
14. Makene CL, Plotkin M, Currie S, Bishanga D, Ugwi P, Louis H, et al. Improvements in newborn care and newborn resuscitation following a quality improvement program at scale: results from a before and after study in Tanzania. BMC Pregnancy Childbirth. 2014;14:381.
15. Seto TL, Tabangin ME, Josyula S, Taylor KK, Vasquez JC, Kamath-Rayne BD. Educational outcomes of helping babies breathe training at a community hospital in Honduras. Perspect Med Educ. 2015;4(5):225–32.
16. Singhal N, Lockyer J, Fidler H, Keenan W, Little G, Bucher S, et al. Helping babies breathe: global neonatal resuscitation program development and formative educational evaluation. Resuscitation. 2012;83(1):90–6.
17. Carlo WA, Wright LL, Chomba E, McClure EM, Carlo ME, Bann CM, et al. Educational impact of the neonatal resuscitation program in low-risk delivery centers in a developing country. J Pediatr. 2009;154(4):504–8.e5.
18. Kamath-Rayne BD, Josyula S, Rule ARL, Vasquez JC. Improvements in the delivery of resuscitation and newborn care after helping babies breathe training. J Perinatol. 2017;37(10):1153–60.
19. Goudar SS, Somannavar MS, Clark R, Lockyer JM, Revankar AP, Fidler HM, et al. Stillbirth and newborn mortality in India after helping babies breathe training. Pediatrics. 2013;131(2):e344–52.
20. Hoban R, Bucher S, Neuman I, Chen M, Tesfaye N, Spector JM. 'Helping babies breathe' training in sub-Saharan Africa: educational impact and learner impressions. J Trop Pediatr. 2013;59(3):180–6.
21. Jeffery HE, Kocova M, Tozija F, Gjorgiev D, Pop-Lazarova M, Foster K, et al. The impact of evidence-based education on a perinatal capacity-building initiative in Macedonia. Med Educ. 2004;38(4):435–47.
22. Musafili A, EssÈn B, Baribwira C, Rukundo A, Persson L. Evaluating helping babies breathe: training for healthcare workers at hospitals in Rwanda. Acta Paediatr. 2013;102(1):e34–8.
23. Reisman J, Martineau N, Kairuki A, Mponzi V, Meda AR, Isangula KG, et al. Validation of a novel tool for assessing newborn resuscitation skills among birth attendants trained by the helping babies breathe program. Int J Gynaecol Obstet. 2015;131(2):196–200.
24. Bookman L, Engmann C, Srofenyoh E, Enweronu-Laryea C, Owen M, Randolph G, et al. Educational impact of a hospital-based neonatal resuscitation program in Ghana. Resuscitation. 2010;81(9):1180–2.
25. Hosokawa S. Impact of neonatal resuscitation training workshop in Mongolia. Int Med J. 2011;18(2):133–6.
26. McClure EM, Carlo WA, Wright LL, Chomba E, Uxa F, Lincetto O, et al. Evaluation of the educational impact of the WHO essential newborn care course in Zambia. Acta Paediatr. 2007;96(8):1135–8.
27. Opiyo N, Were F, Govedi F, Fegan G, Wasunna A, English M. Effect of newborn resuscitation training on health worker practices in Pumwani hospital Kenya. PLoS One. 2008;3(2):e1599.
28. Woods J, Gagliardi L, Nara S, Phally S, Varang O, Viphou N, et al. An innovative approach to in-service training of maternal health staff in Cambodian hospitals. Int J Gynaecol Obstet. 2015;129(2):178–83.
29. PRONTO International. Available from: http://prontointernational.org [Accessed 20 Feb 2016].
30. CARE India. Available from: https://www.careindia.org [Accessed 20 Feb 2016].
31. Das A, Nawal D, Singh MK, Karthick M, Pahwa P, Shah MB, Mahapatra T. Evaluation of the mobile nurse training (MNT) intervention – a step towards improvement in intrapartum practices in Bihar. India BMC Pregnancy and Childbirth. 2017;17(1):266.
32. Das A, Nawal D, Singh MK, Karthick M, Pahwa P, Shah MB, Mahapatra T, Chaudhuri I. Impact of a nursing skill-improvement intervention on newborn-specific delivery practices: an experience from Bihar. India Birth. 2016;43(4):328–35.
33. Sharma, BP. Rural health statistics. Government of India Ministry of Health and Family Welfare Statistics Division 2015.
34. Indian Nursing Council. Types of Nursing Programs. Available from: http://www.indiannursingcouncil.org/nursing-programs.asp?show=prog-type [Accessed 2 June 2017].
35. Laerdal Medical. NeoNatalie. Available from: https://www.laerdal.com/us/products/simulationtraining/obstetrics-pediatrics/neonatalie/. Accessed 22 Aug 2018.
36. OpenDataKit. Available from: https://opendatakit.org [Accessed 12 May 2017].
37. Vail B, Morgan MC, Dyer J, Chrismas A, Cohen SR, Joshi M, Gore A, Mahapatra T, Walker DM. Logistical, cultural, and structural barriers to immediate neonatal care and neonatal resuscitation in Bihar, India. BMC pregnancy and childbirth. 2017. Under review.
38. IBM Corp. Released 2013. IBM SPSS statistics for Macintosh, version 23.0. Armonk: IBM Corp.
39. Green J, Thorogood N. Qualitative methods for Health Research. 3rd ed. London: SAGE; 2014.
40. Pope C, Mays N. Qualitative research in health care. 2nd ed. London: BMJ Books; 2000.
41. Braun V, Clarke V. Using thematic analysis in psychology. Qual Res Psychol. 2006;3:77–101.
42. Rule ARL, Tabangin M, Cheruiyot D, Mueri P, Kamath-Rayne BD. The call and the challenge of pediatric resuscitation and simulation research in low-resource settings. Simul Healthc. 2017;12(6):402–6.

Mosaic Tetrasomy of 9p24.3q21.11 postnatally identified in an infant born with multiple congenital malformations

Irene Plaza Pinto[1,2*], Lysa Bernardes Minasi[2,3], Raphael Steckelberg[4,5], Claudio Carlos da Silva[1,2,3,6,7] and Aparecido Divino da Cruz[1,2,3,6]

Abstract

Background: Supernumerary Marker Chromosomes consist in structurally abnormal chromosomes, considered as an extra chromosome in which around 70% occur as a de novo event and about 30% of the cases are mosaic. Tetrasomy 9p is a rare chromosomal abnormality described as the presence of a supernumerary isochromosome 9p. Clinical features of tetrasomy 9p include a variety of physical and developmental abnormalities.

Case presentation: Herein, we reported a postnatal case of a newborn who died in early infancy with multiple congenital malformations due to a mosaic de novo tetrasomy 9p detected by Chromosomal Microarray Analysis. Conventional cytogenetics analysis of the proband was 47,XY,+mar[45]/46,XY[5]. The parental karyotypes presented no visible numerical or structural alterations. Microarray Analysis of the proband revealed that the marker chromosome corresponded to a mosaic de novo gain at 9p24.3q21.11.

Conclusions: Chromosomal Microarray Analysis was helpful to identify the origin of the supernumerary marker chromosome and it was a powerful tool to carry out genetic diagnostic, guiding the medical diagnosis. Furthermore, the CMA allowed observing at the first time in Central Brazil the tetrasomy 9p and partial tetrasomy 9q in mosaic, encompassing a large duplicated region with several morbid genes, in an infant with multiple congenital malformations.

Keywords: SMC, Chromosome 9, Congenital disorders, Genetics, CMA

Background

Supernumerary Marker Chromosomes (SMC) are structurally abnormal chromosomes whose origin cannot to be adequately established by G banding karyotyping [1, 2]. In general, SMC are seen as an extra chromosome in metaphase spreads with an incidence rate of 0.43/1000 in postnatal cases and about 1/1000 in prenatal testing. Approximately 70% of SMC occur de novo and about 30% of the cases are mosaic [3, 4].

Tetrasomy 9p is a rare chromosomal abnormality described as the presence of a supernumerary isochromosome 9p, initially found as a SMC. Further investigation of the SMC commonly shows involvement of the entire 9p, or the entire 9p with part of the heterochromatic region of 9q, or yet the entire 9p with heterochromatic region of 9q, and part of the euchromatic material of 9q [5, 6]. Moreover, around 30% of known cases of tetrasomy 9p exhibits chromosome mosaicism. Both constitutive and mosaic SMC of chromosome 9 comprises a clinically noticeable syndrome [3, 7, 8].

Clinical phenotype of tetrasomy 9p includes a variety of physical and developmental abnormalities. Commonly,

* Correspondence: iplazapinto@gmail.com
[1]Biotechnology and Biodiversity PhD Program, Federal University of Goias, Rede Centro Oeste de Pós-Graduação de Pesquisa e Inovação, Rua 235, n. 40, Setor Leste Universitário, Goiânia, GO 74605-050, Brazil
[2]Replicon Research Group, Department of Biology, Pontifical Catholic University of Goias, Rua 235, n. 40, Setor Leste Universitário, Goiânia, GO 74605-050, Brazil
Full list of author information is available at the end of the article

patients have distinctive facial appearances with hypertelorism, cleft lip or palate, ear anomalies, and micrognathia [3, 9]. In addition, recurrent clinical features include developmental delay, central nervous system anomaly, limb defects, postnatal growth failure, congenital heart disease, renal anomalies, and short neck with excess nuchal skin [8].

Herein, we report a postnatal case of a newborn who had multiple congenital malformations due to a mosaic de novo tetrasomy of 9p and partial tetrasomy of 9q detected by Chromosomal Microarray Analysis (CMA).

Case presentation

The proband was a preterm newborn boy, the first child of non-consanguineous parents, born at 31 weeks gestation to a 44-year old father and a 43-year old mother by cesarean section. At birth, the child weighed 1,480 g, measured 44 cm in crown-to-heel length, and exhibited multiple congenital anomalies. The newborn was transferred to the Intensive Care Units (ICU) immediately after birth. His general health condition deteriorated progressively, leading to his death at 105th days after birth. The newborn had brain malformation, including ventriculomegaly and corpus callosum dysgenesis, cleft lip and palate, retrognathism, hypertelorism, clenched hands with overlapping fingers, and hypotonia. Additionally, he revealed mild heart septal hypertrophy, ambiguous genitalia, enlarged kidneys without corticomedullary differentiation, and gallbladder with tiny cystic formations (Fig. 1). His mother had three miscarriages from previous marriages and one miscarriage with her current husband. The remaining of his family history was otherwise unremarkable.

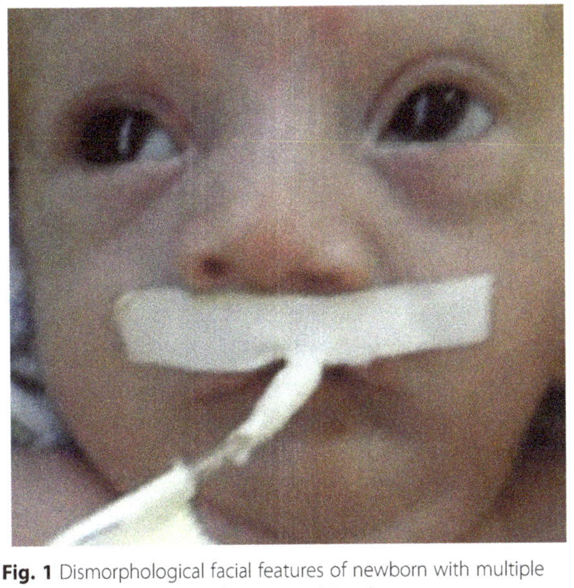

Fig. 1 Dismorphological facial features of newborn with multiple congenital malformations from Central Brazil

Both parents signed a written informed consent and the mother signed as the legal representative for the child. Peripheral blood was obtained to isolate genomic DNA for CMA using Qiagen QIAamp® DNA Mini kit (Hilden, Germany). Karyotyping was performed in a private laboratory through conventional cell culture, harvesting, and GTG banding with a > 550 bands resolution following standard procedures [10]. Chromosome analyses were done using Zeiss Axio Scope (Jena, Germany) and the software IKAROS® (Metasystems Corporation, Altlussheim, Germany). All laboratory procedures were carried out following international standardized protocols and consensual criteria of quality.

The CMA was carried out on proband and his biological parents using the GeneChip® CytoScanHD™ (Affymetrix, Santa Clara, USA) following the manufacturer's recommendations without modifications. Chromosomal analyses were done using the Chromosome Analysis Suite (ChAS®) software (Affymetrix, Santa Clara, USA) and the CNVs found in the patient were analyzed in comparison with public databases, including Database of Genomic Variants (DGV), Database of Chromosomal Imbalance and Phenotype in Humans using Ensemble Resources (DECIPHER), and CytoScanHD™ Array Database. Furthermore, CNVs were classified according to their nature, based on [11, 12].

The proband showed a male karyotype with a large submetacentric SMC in 90% of the analyzed metaphases after counting 50 metaphase spreads. His karyotype was 47,XY,+mar[45]/46,XY[5], suggesting 10% mosaicism. The parental karyotypes and CMA results had no visible numerical or structural alterations. The proband's CMA revealed the marker chromosome corresponded to a de novo 70.77 Mb gain at arr[GRCh37] 9p24.3q21.11 (203,861_70,974,662)× 4[0.3] dn with 30% mosaicism, encompassing 286 genes, including 152 OMIM morbid genes (Fig. 2).

Discussion and conclusions

Chromosomal alterations associated with a spectrum of multiple congenital anomalies are most frequently numerical and are identified in 0.3–1% of newborns [13, 14]. Partial tetrasomy 9 is not yet a well recognizable clinical syndrome due to the limited number of postnatal cases described to date. Moreover, patients with partial tetrasomy 9 have variable phenotypes depending on the size and position of the duplicated region and the degree of mosaicism [6–8, 15].

Here we reported a case of a boy who died postneonataly in early infancy whose karyotype indicated an additional SMC which origin could not be determined by GTG-banding. Microarray analysis showed 47,XY,+mar[45]/46,XY[5].arr [GRCh37] 9p24.3q21.11(203,861_70,974,662)× 4[0.3] dn. Copy Number Variations (CNVs) within the region of gain

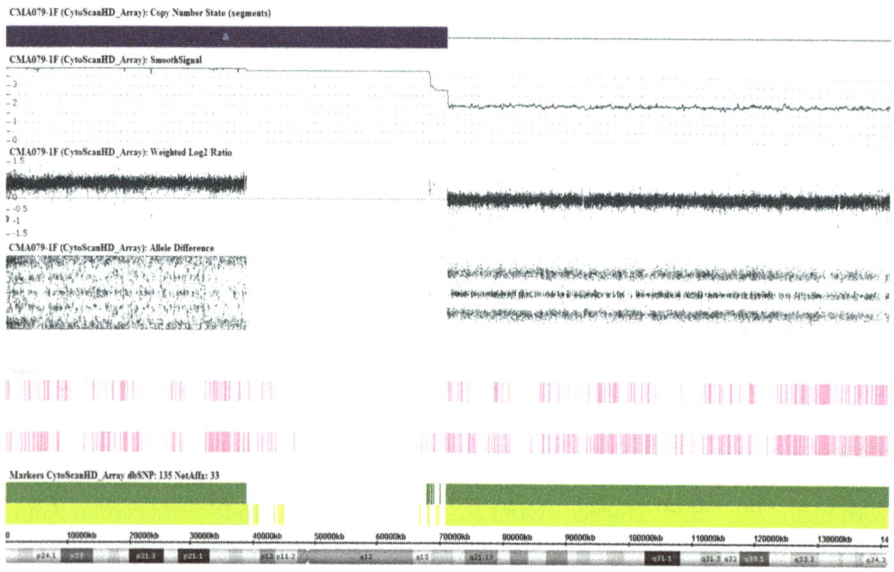

Fig. 2 ChAS® (Affymetrix, USA) interface indicating the results of Chromosomal Microarray Analysis showing the derivative chromosome 9 responsible for tetrasomy 9p extended distally to 9q21.11

indicated tetrasomy, revealing full tetrasomy 9p and partial tetrasomy 9q, including the proximal euchromatic region of the long arm in a mosaic state. Parental CMA were uneventful.

According to [4], about of 40% of all SMCs are derived from non-acrocentric autosomes and the risk of an abnormal phenotype is approximately 28%. Mosaic tetrasomy of 9p most commonly arises as a de novo chromosomal rearrangement resulting from an early sporadic error in embryonic development. Thus, the risk of recurrence is relatively low and this has important implications in genetic counseling for the family [16]. Furthermore, it is important to emphasize the mother history of miscarriage because either a cryptic translocation or some aberrant chromosomal constitution restricted to the mother's gonads, most likely as a gonadal mosaicism, could be responsible for her failure to conceive health offspring. However, the family refused to undergo genetic counseling and refused any additional genetic testing.

Tetrasomy 9p is a rare disorder firstly described by [17]. Up to now, at least 34 postnatal cases have been previously reported in medical literature, varying greatly in chromosomal range and phenotype severity. Although the affected population is small, males seemed to be slightly more affected than females [5]. The clinical severity of tetrasomy 9p varies from neonatal death to mild developmental delay and minor anomalies [9, 18, 19]. Furthermore, when the tetrasomic segment extend to 9q22-9q32 it is common to observe intrauterine growth retardation, skeletal anomalies, cleft lip/palate, and heart defects [15].

According to some authors, three different types of supernumerary isochromosome 9p have been described so far. There are tetrasomies containing exclusively the entire 9p, some includes the entire 9p and a small proportion of the heterochromatic region of 9q, and yet some harbors the entire 9p and a large portion of 9q extending to 9q21, including both heterochromatic and euchromatic regions of 9q [3, 5, 6]. The tetrasomy was categorized as the third type of SMC involving chromosome 9, with breakpoints at 9q21.11 and isochromosome 9p, justifying the severity of symptoms in the studied proband.

There is a positive correlation between degree of mosaicism and the severity of the phenotype in infants having tetrasomy 9p. However, the breakpoint of 9q extended distally to 9q21.11, which encompasses a large duplicated region with several OMIM morbid genes. This finding supports the claim the nature of the involved genes was more crucial than the level of mosaicism in defining phenotype's severity in our proband.

The CMA was helpful to identify the origin of the SMC in the proband born to parents with normal karyotypes. In addition, it was an effective method to identify the tetrasomy 9p and partial tetrasomy 9q in mosaic in an infant with multiple congenital malformations for the first time in Central Brazil. Rare and complex phenotypes must always be investigated to define subsets and allow the phenotype/genotype correlation. Furthermore, it was recommended to the family to undergo a non-directive genetic counseling to help understanding the familial implications of genetic contribution to disease and the chance of recurrence.

Abbreviations

ChAS: Chromosome Analysis Suite; CMA: Chromosomal Microarray Analysis; CNVs: Copy Number Variations; DECIPHER: Database of Chromosomal Imbalance and Phenotype in Humans using Ensemble Resources; DGV: Database of Genomic Variants; ICU: Intensive Care Units; OMIM: Online Mendenlian Inheritance in Man; SMC: Supernumerary Marker Chromosomes; SNP: Single Nucleotide Polymorphism

Acknowledgments

The authors wish to thank Dr. Rinaldo W. Pereira and the Rede ExeGenes for supporting the betterment of genetic diagnosis in Central Brazil. We are also grateful for Mr. Sean M. Quail's contribution for proofreading the manuscript and assistance with the English language. This work was sponsored by a grant from CNPq (Edital 031/564465/2010-10) and FAPEG (2011.6002.19.1847.1134-03). IPP holds a scholarship from CAPES/UFG.

Authors' contributions

IPP, LBM, RS, CCS and ADC have made substantial contributions to conception and design the experiment. RS was the patient's attending physician. IPP performed CMA experiments. IPP, LBM, CCS, and ADC analyzed the data. IPP, ADC and LBM wrote the paper. All authors read and approved the final manuscript.

Competing interests

The authors declare that they have no competing interests.

Author details

[1]Biotechnology and Biodiversity PhD Program, Federal University of Goias, Rede Centro Oeste de Pós-Graduação de Pesquisa e Inovação, Rua 235, n. 40, Setor Leste Universitário, Goiânia, GO 74605-050, Brazil. [2]Replicon Research Group, Department of Biology, Pontifical Catholic University of Goias, Rua 235, n. 40, Setor Leste Universitário, Goiânia, GO 74605-050, Brazil. [3]Genetics Master's Program, Pontifical Catholic University of Goias, Rua 235, n. 40, Setor Leste Universitário, Goiânia, GO 74605-050, Brazil. [4]Maternity Hospital Amparo, Av T-12 n° 280 Setor Bueno, Goiânia, GO, Brazil. [5]Dr Henrique Santillo Rehabilitation and Readjustment Center, Av. Ver. José Monteiro, 1655, Setor Negrão de Lima, Goiânia, GO, Brazil. [6]Human Cytogenetics and Molecular Genetics Laboratory, Secretary of Goias State for Public Health, Goiânia, GO, Brazil. [7]State University of Goias, Eseffego, Goiânia, Goiás, Brazil.

References

1. Liehr T, Cirkovic S, Lalic T, et al. Complex small supernumerary marker chromosomes - an update. Mol Cytogenet. 2013;31(6):46–51.
2. Liehr T. Small supernumerary marker chromosomes. 2017. http://ssmc-tl.com/sSMC.html. Accessed 08 Feb 2017.
3. Jafari-Ghahfarokhi H, Moradi-Chaleshtori M, Liehr T, Hashemzadeh-Chaleshtori M, Teimori H, Ghasemi-Dehkordi P. Small supernumerary marker chromosomes and their correlation with specific syndromes. Adv Biomed Res. 2015;27(4):140–6.
4. Jang W, Chae H, Kim J, et al. Identification of small marker chromosomes using microarray comparative genomic hybridization and multicolor fluorescent in situ hybridization. Mol Cytogenet. 2016;8(9):61–70.
5. El Khattabi L, Jaillard S, Andrieux J, et al. Clinical and molecular delineation of Tetrasomy 9p syndrome: report of 12 new cases and literature review. Am J Med Genet A. 2015;167(6):1252–61.
6. Chen CP, Wang LK, Chern SR, et al. Mosaic tetrasomy 9p at amniocentesis: prenatal diagnosis, molecular cytogenetic characterization, and literature review. Taiwan J Obstet Gynecol. 2014;53(1):79–85.
7. Düzcan F, Ergin H, Aytan M, Tepeli E, Özdemir Ö, Basaran S. Non-mosaic Tetrasomy 9p in an infant with multiple congenital anomalies. Gynecol Obstet Reprod Med. 2007;13(2):114–6.
8. Ogino W, Takeshima Y, Nishiyama A, Yagi M, Oka N, Matsuo M. Mosaic tetrasomy 9p case with the phenotype mimicking Klinefelter syndrome and hyporesponse of gonadotropin-stimulated testosterone production. Kobe J Med Sci. 2007;53(4):143–50.
9. Di Bartolo DL, El Naggar M, Owen R, et al. Characterization of a complex rearrangement involving duplication and deletion of 9p in an infant with craniofacial dysmorphism and cardiac anomalies. Mol Cytogenet. 2012;5(1):31–6.
10. Verma RS, Babu A. Human chromosomes: Principles and Techiniques. 2nd ed. New York: MacGraw-Hill; 1995.
11. Miller DT, Adam MP, Aradhya S, et al. Consensus statement: chromosomal microarray is a first-tier clinical diagnostic test for individuals with developmental disabilities or congenital anomalies. Am J Hum Genet. 2010;86(5):749–64.
12. Battaglia A, Doccini V, Bernardini L, et al. Confirmation of chromosomal microarray as a first-tier clinical diagnostic test for individuals with developmental delay, intellectual disability, autism spectrum disorders and dysmorphic features. Eur J Paediatr Neurol. 2013;17(6):589–99.
13. Starke H, Nietzel A, Weise A, et al. Small supernumerary marker chromosomes (SMCs): genotype-phenotype correlation and classification. Hum Genet. 2003;114(1):51–67.
14. Pratte-Santos R, Ribeiro KH, Santos TA, Cintra TS. Analysis of chromosomal abnormalities by CGH-array in patients with dysmorphic and intellectual disability with normal karyotype. Einstein (Sao Paulo). 2016;14(1):30–4.
15. Zhou YC, Zhang C, Zhai JS, et al. A patient with unusual features and a 69.5 Mb duplication from a de novo extra der (9): a case report. Mol Med Rep. 2015;12(1):155–8.
16. Campbell IM, Shaw CA, Stankiewicz P, Lupski JR. Somatic mosaicism: implications for disease and transmission genetics. Trends Genet. 2015;31(7):382–92.
17. Ghymers D, Hermann B, Distèche C, Frederic J. Partial tetrasomy of number 9 chromosome, and mosaicism in a child with multiple malformations (author's transl). Humangenetik. 1973;20(3):273–82.
18. Frémond ML, Gitiaux C, Bonnet D, et al. Mosaic Tetrasomy 9p: a Mendelian condition associated with pediatric-onset overlap myositis. Pediatrics. 2015;136(2):e544–7.
19. Oh M, Cho IJ, Shin S, Lee ST, Choi JR. Isolated 9p duplication with der(Y)t(Y; 9)(q12;p13.2) in a male patient with cardiac defect and mental retardation confirmed by chromosomal microarray. Ann Lab Med. 2016;36(2):191–3.

Association between ambient air pollutants and preterm birth in Ningbo, China

Wen-Yuan Liu[1†], Zhe-Bin Yu[2,3†], Hai-Yan Qiu[1†], Jian-Bing Wang[2,3†], Xue-Yu Chen[2] and Kun Chen[2,3*]

Abstract

Background: Exposure to air pollutants has been related to preterm birth, but little evidence can be available for $PM_{2.5}$, O_3 and CO in China. This study aimed to investigate the short-term effect of exposure to air pollutants on risk preterm birth during 2014–2016 in Ningbo, China.

Methods: We conducted a time-series study to evaluate the associations between daily preterm birth and major air pollutants (including $PM_{2.5}$, PM_{10}, SO_2, NO_2, O_3 and CO) in Ningbo during 2014–2016. A General Additive Model extend Poisson regression was used to evaluate the relationship between preterm birth and air pollution with adjustment for time-trend, meteorological factors and day of the week (DOW). We also conducted a subgroup analysis by season and age.

Results: In this study, a total of 37,389 birth occurred between 2014 and 2016 from the Electronic Medical Records System of Ningbo Women and Children's Hospital, of which 5428 were verified as preterm birth. The single pollutant model suggested that lag effect of $PM_{2.5}$, PM_{10}, NO_2 reached a peak at day 3 before delivery and day 6 for SO_2, and no relationships were observed for O_3 and preterm birth. Excess risks (95% confidence intervals) for an increase of IQR of air pollutant concentrations were 4.84 (95% CI: 1.77, 8.00) for $PM_{2.5}$, 3.56 (95% CI: 0.07, 7.17) for PM_{10}, 3.65 (95% CI: 0.86, 6.51) for SO_2, 6.49 (95% CI: 1.86, 11.34) for NO_2, – 0.90 (95% CI: -4.76, 3.11) for O_3, and 3.36 (95% CI: 0.50, 6.30) for CO. Sensitivity analyses by exclusion of maternal age < 18 or > 35 years did not materially alter our results.

Conclusions: This study indicates that short-term exposure to air pollutants (including $PM_{2.5}$, PM_{10}, SO_2, NO_2) are positively associated with risk of preterm birth in Ningbo, China.

Keywords: Preterm birth, Air pollution, Time-series analysis, $PM_{2.5}$, PM_{10}, SO_2

Background

Preterm birth, defined as less than 37 weeks of gestations, is the second largest direct cause of child deaths among children less than 5 years [1]. There are 15 million premature birth annually worldwide and China contributed 1.1 million (rank 2nd worldwide) according to international survey data [2]. Preterm birth account for 75% of perinatal mortality and more than half the long-term morbidity [3]. Moreover, the survived preterm babies are at increased risk of neuro-developmental impairments, respiratory and gastrointestinal complications [3]. The etiology of preterm birth remains unclear yet many risk factors have been explored.

There is increasing evidence that exposure to ambient air pollutants is associated with preterm birth [4–9]. A systematic review has reported positive associations between air pollutants and risk of adverse birth outcomes including preterm birth [5]. And a recent meta-analysis of 23 studies has also showed that a significantly increased risk of preterm birth with interquartile range increase in particulate matter exposure during pregnancy

* Correspondence: ck@zju.edu.cn
†Wen-Yuan Liu, Zhe-Bin Yu, Hai-Yan Qiu and Jian-Bing Wang contributed equally to this work.
[2]Department of Epidemiology and Biostatistics, School of Public Health, Zhejiang University, Hangzhou 310058, China
[3]Research Center for Air Pollution and Health, Zhejiang University, Hangzhou 310058, China
Full list of author information is available at the end of the article

[10]. It should be noted that findings of exposure to air pollution and preterm birth from Western countries may not be applicable to the Chinese populations due to higher air pollution levels, genetic and physiological differences. However, a recent systematic review, included all studies in China, showed the effect of air pollution on preterm birth was inconsistent [11].

In this study, we used birth data during 2014–2016 in Ningbo, Zhejiang Province, China, and conducted a time-series study to investigate the association between exposure to ambient air pollutants and risk of preterm birth.

Methods

Study population

This study was conducted in Ningbo, which located in the southeast of China and composed of six districts and has a metropolitan area population of 7.8 million. We obtained anonymous births information from the Electronic Medical Records System (EMRS) in Ningbo Women and Children's Hospital (the largest women's hospital in Ningbo) from 2014 January 1st to 2016 December 31st. A total of 40,968 birth records were included in the EMRS. Duplicated records ($n = 2305$), non-live birth records ($n = 230$), twin pregnancy and multiple pregnancies ($n = 1274$) and birth records with extreme gestational age (< 20 weeks) ($n = 160$) were excluded from this study. Finally, a total of 37,389 eligible births were included in our study.

Preterm birth

Preterm birth was defined as a singleton live-birth delivery before 37 completed weeks of gestation(< 259 days) [1]. Gestational age was calculated based on the date of women's last menstrual period (LMP). For women who had no LMP date, gestational age was substituted by a clinical estimate. A total of 5428 preterm births were finally included for the current analysis. The number of preterm births was calculated for each day from 2014 January 1st to 2016 December 31st. The study was reviewed and approved by Committee of ethics, Ningbo Women and Children's Hospital.

Air pollution and meteorological exposure

Daily meteorological data including mean temperature (degree Celsius) and relative humidity(percent) were collected from the Ningbo Meteorological Bureau. Daily values for temperature and relative humidity were calculated by averaging 24 hourly monitoring data.

Daily mean concentrations of air pollutants, including particulate matter (aerodynamic diameter less than or equal to 2.5 μm ($PM_{2.5}$) and 10 μm (PM_{10})), sulfur dioxide (SO_2), nitrogen dioxide (NO_2), Ozone (O_3) and carbon monoxide (CO) during 2014 to 2016, were collected from the Environmental Monitoring Center of Ningbo City (http://www.nbemc.net/aqi/home/index.aspx). The daily concentrations of each pollutant were averaged from the available monitored results of eight stations which were monitored by the China National Quality Control. The eight stations were "Shi Jian Ce Zhong Xin", "Tai Gu Xiao Xue", "San Jiang Zhong Xue", "Wan Li Xue Yuan", "Huan Bao Da Lou", "Long Sai Yi Yuan", "Qian HuShui Chang" and "Wan Li Guo Ji". The distribution of these 8 monitor stations in Ningbo was shown in Additional file 1: Figure S1. Air pollutants were measured in the unit of micrograms per cubic meter(μg/m^3) except milligrams per cubic meter (mg/m^3) for CO.

Statistical analysis

Distribution of daily number of preterm births follows the Poisson distribution due to its small probabilities. Thus, we used a Generalized Additive Model (GAM) extended Poisson regression [12] to explore the potential effect of air pollution on premature birth. This method has been widely used in air pollution time-series studies [13–22] because of its non-parametric flexibility.

We firstly built a basic model based on the daily number of preterm births without air pollution variables. To control for non-linear trend between preterm birth and time or weather conditions, we added time-dependent variables including calendar time, temperature and relative humidity via natural spline functions. Degree of freedom (df) for natural spline functions were adopted by generalized cross-validation (GCV) scores [12]. Day of the week was also included as a dummy variable in the basic models. Then, each air pollutant was added into a single-pollutant model separately. The number of gestations at risk of preterm birth was used as an offset. In brief, we fitted the following model to evaluate the effect of air pollutants on preterm birth:

$$\begin{aligned}\mathrm{Log}[E(Y_t)] = \alpha + \beta Z_t &+ S\ (\text{time},\ df)\\ &+ S\ (\text{temperature},\ df)\\ &+ S\ (\text{relative humidity},\ df)\\ &+ DOW_t(\text{day of the week}) + \text{Offset}_t\end{aligned}$$

In this formula, t represents the day of the observation; Y_t represents daily number of preterm births, $E(Y_t)$ stands for the expected values for the number of premature births on day t. α is residual, β is the regression coefficient, and Z_t is the average concentration of air pollutants on the observed day or over several days. S (time, df) is the calendar time smoothing spline function, S (temperature, df) is the daily temperature smoothing spline function, S (relative humidity, df) is the daily relative humidity smoothing spline function, and DOW_t is a dummy variable with Monday as a reference. The corresponding degree of freedom for time, temperature and relative humidity in the spline function were 7, 7 and4 in the final model.

We investigated the acute effect on the risk of preterm birth by adding the concentration of each pollutant into the model for a 1-day exposure window with lag-time from 1 to 6 days before birth. Cumulative effect was also calculated by including the lag moving average (Avg1-Avg6) into the model. Relative risks (RRs) and 95% confident intervals (CIs) were calculated by the regression coefficient β of air pollutants. And we reported excess risks (ERs) and 95% CIs that represented a percent increase in daily preterm birth risk per IQR increase in air pollutant concentrations. ER was calculated as follows: $ER = (RR - 1) \times 100\%$. We also examine the exposure-response curve by using a natural spline function for certain pollutants in the GAM model. Goodness of fit of the model was assessed by using Akaike Information Criterion (AIC). The best df for each air pollutant was indicated by the lowest AIC value in the GAM model.

Sensitivity analysis by exclusion of maternal age < 18 or > 35 years in preterm birth records was conducted to evaluate the robustness of our results, because women aged < 18 or > 35 years had a higher possibility to develop a preterm birth [23]. And we further divided the study period into cold period (November to April) and warm period (May to October). Models were fitted separately in two periods to check if any difference in the effect of air pollutants on preterm birth during warm and cold periods. 95% confidence interval for the difference in effect estimates between two strata (a potential effect modifier) was calculated as follows:

$$\left(Q1\text{-}Q2 \pm 1.96\sqrt{SE1 + SE2}\right)$$

Where Q1 and Q2 are the adjusted estimates from two strata (e.g. cold and warm period), and SE1, SE2 are the corresponding standard errors [24].

Continuous variables with normal distribution were presented as mean ± standard deviation (SD), and non-normal variables were reported as median ± interquartile range (IQR). Spearman's correlation coefficient was used for the correlations between ambient air pollutants and meteorological factors. $P < 0.05$ was considered statistically significant. All statistical analyses were conducted by using R 3.3.1.

Results

Descriptive results of exposure and outcomes

The descriptive results of air pollution and meteorological data are shown in Table 1. The mean daily concentrations of $PM_{2.5}$, PM_{10}, SO_2, NO_2, O_3 and CO during 2014 to 2016 were 43.73 μg/m³, 69.69 μg/m³, 16.56 μg/m³, 40.50 μg/m³, 64.33 μg/m³, 1.06 mg/m³, respectively. Concentrations of air pollutants were higher in the cold period than those in the warm period except for O_3. Daily mean ambient temperature and relative humidity were 17.4 °C and 76.8%.

A total of 5428 preterm births were identified among the total valid births of 37,159. Overall prevalence of preterm birth was 14.61%. The number of births in women with the maternal age < 18 or > 35 years was 3452, among which 714 births were diagnosed as preterm birth (20.68%). And the corresponding prevalence of preterm birth during cold and warm periods was 14.63% and 14.58%, respectively.

Correlation between ambient air pollutants and meteorological factors

Table 2 shows the Spearman's correlation analysis of air pollution and meteorological measures. $PM_{2.5}$ was

Table 1 Air pollution and meteorological data in Ningbo, China (2014–2016)

	Mean ± SD			Minimum	P_{25}	P_{50}	P_{75}	IQR	Maximum
	ALL year	Cold Period[a]	Warm Period						
Air pollutants									
SO_2 (μg/m³)	16.56 ± 9.05	18.91 ± 10.25	14.25 ± 6.97	5.90	10.53	13.70	19.09	8.56	74.08
NO_2 (μg/m³)	40.50 ± 16.88	49.85 ± 15.99	31.28 ± 11.94	5.59	28.00	37.38	51.34	23.34	115.00
PM_{10} (μg/m³)	69.69 ± 38.37	87.03 ± 41.75	52.60 ± 24.85	10.18	42.90	60.20	85.31	42.41	287.10
$PM_{2.5}$ (μg/m³)	43.73 ± 26.26	55.64 ± 29.38	31.99 ± 15.55	4.24	25.50	37.38	54.11	28.62	196.93
O_3 (μg/m³)	64.33 ± 29.71	53.46 ± 25.07	75.05 ± 30.05	8.17	42.99	61.96	83.02	40.03	244.30
CO (mg/m³)	1.06 ± 0.35	1.13 ± 0.39	0.99 ± 0.28	0.04	0.88	1.00	1.19	0.31	2.92
Meteorology									
Temperature (°C)	17.42 ± 8.10	10.64 ± 5.17	24.10 ± 3.76	−4.47	10.23	18.69	23.94	13.71	32.25
Relative Humidity (%)	76.8 ± 11.80	74.29 ± 13.38	79.19 ± 9.33	32.96	69.82	77.81	85.47	15.65	97.60

$PM_{2.5}$: particulate matter less than 2.5 μm in aerodynamic diameter, *PM_{10}*: particulate matter less than 10 μm in aerodynamic diameter, *SO_2*: sulfur dioxide, *NO_2*: nitrogen dioxide, *O_3*: Ozone, *CO*: carbon monoxide

[a]Cold period was from November to April, and warm period was from May to October

Table 2 Correlation between air pollutants and meteorological factors in Ningbo, China

	SO_2	NO_2	PM_{10}	$PM_{2.5}$	CO	O_3	Temperature	Relative humidity
SO_2	1.00							
NO_2	0.59	1.00						
PM_{10}	0.69	0.74	1.00					
$PM_{2.5}$	0.66	0.74	0.95	1.00				
CO	0.22	0.45	0.43	0.47	1.00			
O_3	−0.13	−0.46	−0.13	−0.17	− 0.29	1.00		
Temperature	−0.39	− 0.62	− 0.52	−0.50	− 0.20	0.37	1.00	
Relative humidity	−0.39	−0.04	− 0.36	−0.24	0.08	−0.33	0.21	1.00

$PM_{2.5}$: particulate matter less than 2.5 μm in aerodynamic diameter, *PM_{10}*: particulate matter less than 10 μm in aerodynamic diameter, *SO_2*: sulfur dioxide, *NO_2*: nitrogen dioxide, *O_3*: Ozone, *CO*: carbon monoxide
All correlations were statistically significant ($P < 0.01$)

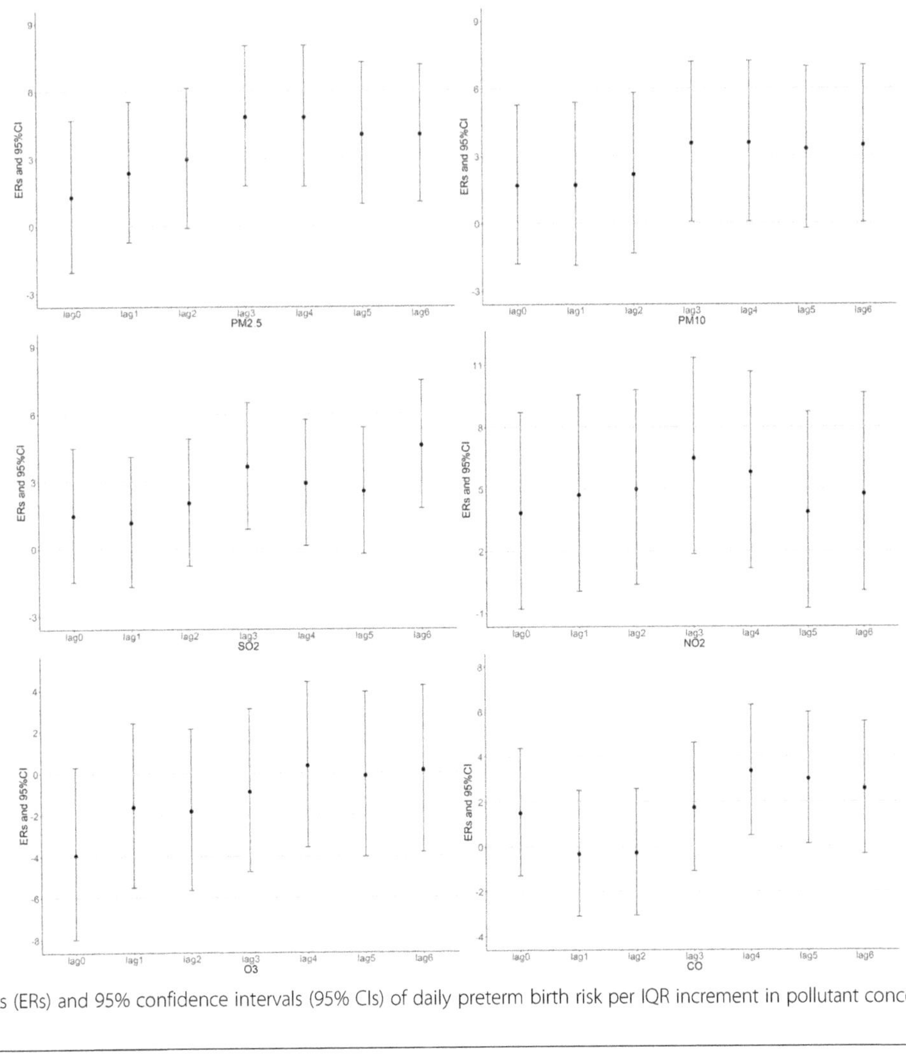

Fig. 1 Excess Risks (ERs) and 95% confidence intervals (95% CIs) of daily preterm birth risk per IQR increment in pollutant concentrations at different lag days

positively associated with SO_2, NO_2, PM_{10} and CO, but negatively associated with O_3. The strong correlation was observed for $PM_{2.5}$ and NO_2 (Spearman's Rho = 0.74, $P < 0.01$). And two weather variables were negatively related to SO_2, NO_2, $PM_{2.5}$, PM_{10} and CO, but positively related to Ozone.

Short-term effects for preterm birth

Fig 1 shows the association between air pollutants and daily preterm births at lag0–6 days. The largest ERs were observed at Lag3 for $PM_{2.5}$, PM_{10} and NO_2, Lag6 for SO_2 and Lag 4 for CO. No significant associations were observed for Ozone and preterm births. The associations between cumulative concentrations and preterm births at different lag days (Avg1-Avg6) are shown in the Additional file 2: Table S1. Figure 2 shows the dose-response curve between certain air pollutants and risk of preterm births by using a natural spline function for air pollutants in GAM models. Nonlinear association was observed for PM_{10}, SO_2 and preterm births.

Table 3 and Additional file 3: Table S2 show the excess risks and 95% CIs for short-term exposure to air pollutants and daily preterm birth stratified by maternal age and season. The associations between $PM_{2.5}$, PM_{10}, SO_2, NO_2 and preterm birth tended to be attenuated after we restricted the analysis in women with the maternal age of 18–35 years, but the associations still remained significant. In season-specific analyses, the adverse effect of $PM_{2.5}$, SO_2 and NO_2 on preterm birth were stronger in cold period and attenuated in warm period as compared with the whole year. Similar results were observed for the effect of four air pollutants ($PM_{2.5}$, PM_{10}, SO_2 and NO_2) in cold and warm periods when maternal age was restricted from 18 to 35 years. No significant associations were observed for Ozone. No significant interaction effect was observed for season and maternal age on the association of short-term exposure to air pollution and preterm birth (Additional file 4: Table S3).

Table 4 provides ERs and 95% CIs from two-pollutant models. The effect of air pollutants on daily preterm

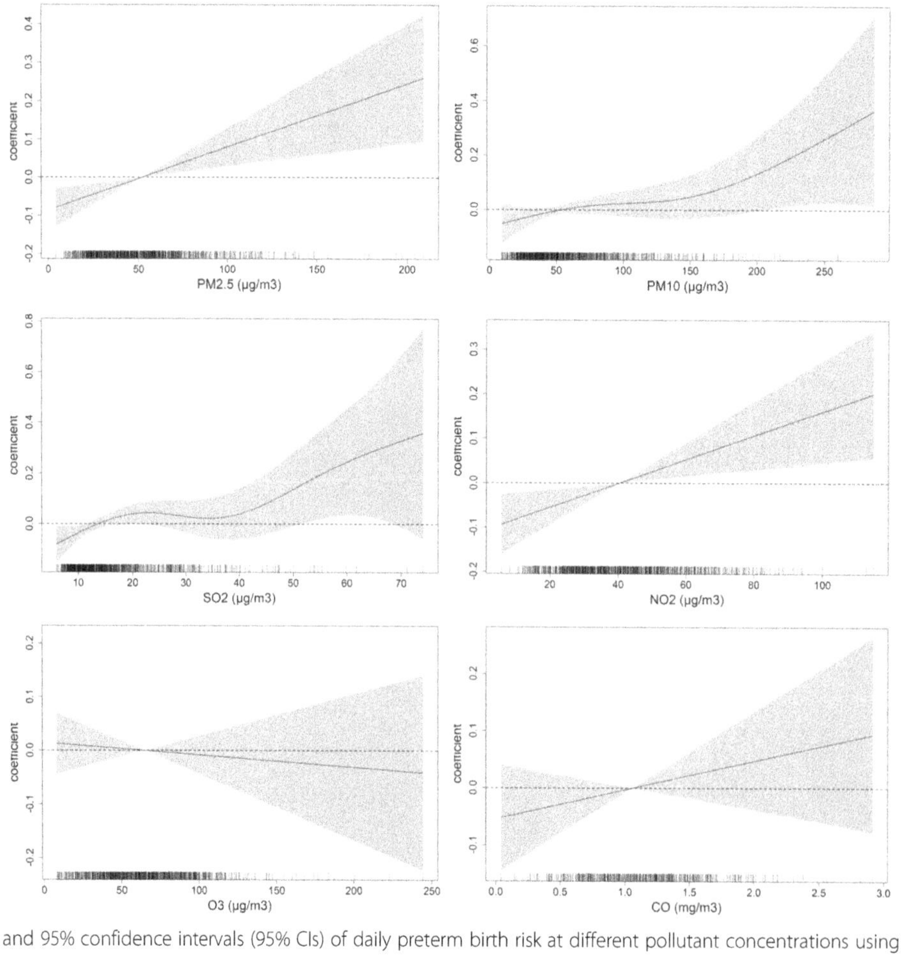

Fig. 2 Coefficients and 95% confidence intervals (95% CIs) of daily preterm birth risk at different pollutant concentrations using natural spline functions

Table 3 Excess risks (ERs) and 95% confidence intervals of preterm birth per IQR increment in air pollutant concentrations in warm and cold periods in Ningbo, China

	All births			Gestational women age between 18 and 35			Gestational women under 18 or above 35		
	Annual	Cold period	Warm period	Annual	Cold period	Warm period	Annual	Cold period	Warm period
$PM_{2.5}$ [b]	4.84 (1.77,8.00)[c]	4.92 (1.47,8.50)[c]	4.06 (− 2.55,11.12)	4.53 (1.09,8.09)[c]	4.65 (0.71,8.74)[c]	3.17 (− 4.23,11.15)	9.40 (0.74,18.80)[c]	12.24 (2.40,23.04)[c]	− 1.93 (− 18.95,18.67)
PM_{10} [b]	3.56 (0.07,7.17)[c]	5.11 (1.04,9.35)[c]	1.87 (−5.26,9.53)	4.88 (0.88,9.03)[c]	6.74 (2.12,11.58)[c]	2.64 (− 5.42,11.39)	13.22 (2.55,25.00)[c]	16.73 (4.50,30.40)[c]	0.65 (−19.38,25.66)
SO_2 [b]	3.65 (0.86,6.51)[c]	4.93 (1.64,8.33)[c]	1.44 (− 3.70,6.85)	6.56 (3.39,9.82)[c]	7.04 (3.29,10.92)[c]	5.53 (−0.32,11.71)	8.46 (0.21,17.40)[c]	10.95 (1.37,21.45)[c]	2.79 (− 12.58,20.87)
NO_2 [b]	6.49 (1.86,11.34)[c]	9.25(3.45,15.38)[c]	3.12(−5.08,12.02)	6.66(1.42,12.17)[c]	10.32(3.69,17.37)[c]	2.7(−6.26,12.51)	14.20 (1.18,28.90)[c]	7.40(−7.79,25.09)	−2.94(− 23.32,22.87)
O_3 [b]	− 0.90 (− 4.76,3.11)	−6.35 (− 12.78,0.55)	3.23 (− 1.81,8.53)	− 2.76 (− 7.1,1.79)	− 3.86 (− 10.69,3.49)	1.55 (− 3.91,7.32)	−4.11 (− 14.14,7.10)	−8.96 (− 24.85,10.28)	−1.23 (− 14.53,14.15)
CO [b]	3.36 (0.50,6.30)[c]	5.16 (1.33,9.13)[c]	1.89 (−2.71,6.71)	0.37 (−2.84,3.70)	2.29 (− 1.16,5.87)	0.40 (− 4.60,5.66)	7.82 (0.85,15.28)[c]	10.44 (1.71,19.92)[c]	4.14 (−7.37,17.08)

$PM_{2.5}$: particulate matter less than 2.5 μm in aerodynamic diameter, *PM_{10}*: particulate matter less than 10 μm in aerodynamic diameter, *SO_2*: sulfur dioxide, *NO_2*: nitrogen dioxide, *O_3*: Ozone, *CO*: carbon monoxide

[a] ERs were calculated per IQR increment for each air pollutant

[b] Lag day (lag 3 for $PM_{2.5}$, PM_{10}, NO_2, SO_2, O_3, lag4 for CO) were used

[c] $P<0.05$

Table 4 Excess risks (ERs) and 95% confidence intervals (CIs) of daily preterm birth in two-pollutant models

	Two-pollutant models[a]	ERs and 95% CIs
$PM_{2.5}$	–	4.84 (1.77, 8.00)
	NO_2	3.44 (−0.47, 7.50)
	SO_2	3.70 (−0.02, 7.52)
PM_{10}	–	3.56 (0.07, 7.17)
	NO_2	0.42 (−4.13,5.20)
	SO_2	1.15 (−3.21, 5.69)
SO_2	–	3.65 (0.86, 6.51)
	$PM_{2.5}$	1.69 (−1.55, 5.08)
	PM_{10}	3.09 (−0.41, 6.72)
	NO_2	2.18 (−1.07,5.52)
NO_2	–	6.49 (1.86, 11.34)
	$PM_{2.5}$	3.09 (−3.61, 9.11)
	PM_{10}	6.11 (−0.03,12.62)
	SO_2	4.55 (−0.80, 10.18)

$PM_{2.5}$: particulate matter less than 2.5 μm in aerodynamic diameter, *PM_{10}*: particulate matter less than 10 μm in aerodynamic diameter, *SO_2*: sulfur dioxide, *NO_2*: nitrogen dioxide
[a]Lag day 3 for $PM_{2.5}$, PM_{10}, NO_2, SO_2 were used

birth became nonsignificant after controlling for other air pollutants in the two-pollutant models.

Discussion

In this study, we performed an ecological time-series study to examine the short-term effect of air pollutants on preterm birth during 2014–2016 in Ningbo. We found that $PM_{2.5}$, PM_{10}, SO_2 and NO_2 were significantly associated with increased risk of preterm birth during 1-week preceding delivery. Single pollutant analysis using General Additive Model indicated that the effect of $PM_{2.5}$, PM_{10}, and NO_2 reached a peak value at lag day 3 and SO_2 at lag day 6. The corresponding ERs for an increased concentration of IQR were 4.84 (95% CI: 1.77, 8.00) for $PM_{2.5}$, 3.56 (95% CI: 0.07, 7.17) for PM_{10}, 3.65 (95% CI: 0.86, 6.51) for SO_2, and 6.49 (95% CI: 1.86, 11.34) for NO_2, respectively.

The observed effect of particulate matter ($PM_{2.5}$, PM_{10}) were consistent with several previous studies [13, 25–29]. A ten- year time-series study conducted in Rome [30] has detected a significant effect of PM_{10} on preterm-birth risk. An updated meta-analysis 10 of 23 studies has showed an increased risk with an IQR increase in PM_{10} exposure during pregnancy (pooled OR = 1.03, 95% CI:1.01–1.05). Limited studies in China can be available to evaluate the effect of PM exposure on preterm birth. A birth cohort conducted in Lanzhou, China between 2010 and 2012 [26] also found that exposure to high levels of ambient PM_{10} could increase the risk of preterm birth, and another prospective birth cohort in China confirmed the adverse effect on preterm birth risk of $PM_{2.5}$ exposure [23]. Our study also indicated significant associations for $PM_{2.5}$, PM_{10} exposure and preterm birth, but the RRs were relatively lower. The discrepancies could be explained by the different design, population and particulate matter level.

Our study found significant associations between maternal exposure to SO_2, NO_2 and preterm birth 1 week proceeding delivery. SO_2 was consistently associated with preterm birth according to a systematic review of 25 studies conducted in China [11]. Previous time-series studies conducted in China and Atlanta, USA also observed that increased NO_2 concentration was associated with preterm birth risk [13, 27]. The effects of O_3 and CO were less well-studied because the monitoring network of these air pollutants by Chinese government started from 2013. In our study, we found no significant effect of CO and O_3 on preterm birth, even after stratified by maternal age and season. However, a previous study reported an increase of 5% in risk of preterm birth per 100 $\mu g/m^3$ increase in CO concentrations in the second trimester of pregnancy [23, 31]. Further studies are needed to confirm the effect of carbon monoxide and the critical windows of exposure to these air pollutants.

In our study, the effect of air pollutants on preterm birth risk tended to be stronger in cold period than that in warm period, although this difference was not statistically significant. Previous studies have also showed that the effect of air pollutants on preterm birth varied in different seasons [32]. This seasonal discrepancy may be explained by a higher level of air pollutants in cold period as Table 1 shows. Furthermore, residents may reduce time to go outdoors due to high temperature and frequent rain during warm seasons [17] thus the chance of exposure to ambient air pollution is relatively lower as compared with cold seasons.

The association between short-term exposure to certain air pollutants and risk of preterm birth may suggest that air pollution can motivate the biologic mechanism of labor and thus leading to preterm birth. Potential mechanisms for this association could be explained by inflammation, endocrine disruption, hemodynamic responses, oxidative stress and endothelial dysfunction [33]. When air pollutants are inhaled into the body, oxidative stress and intrauterine inflammation may induce preeclampsia [34] and preterm premature rupture of membranes [35], which could contribute a significant part of the causes of preterm birth.

Our study had several important strengths. Firstly, we used time-series Generalized Additive Model extended Poisson regression to adjust for the confounding effects of long-time trends, meteorological factors and season. In addition, our study provided evidence for the effect of previously less well-studied air pollutants (O_3 and CO).

Our study also had several limitations. Average data from fixed monitoring locations were used to represent air pollution exposure, which could affect our results. And ecological study design could underestimate the effect of air pollution when monitoring data was used to represent individual exposure level [36]. It should also be noted that our analyses were not adjusted for infant gender, maternal smoking status and education level due to lack of these individual risk factors. Future studies with individual risk factors especially time varying factors (such as maternal smoking exposure) are needed to confirm our findings. Besides, early obstetric ultrasound was used to estimate the gestational age instead of LMP for a small portion of women who forgot their last menstrual period. There are also other hospitals can be selected in the region, but medical records in other hospitals cannot be available in the current study. We believe that these issues would not affect our results. Finally, we cannot identify the independent effect of each pollutant due to high correlations between pollutants.

Conclusions

In summary, this study examined the association between concentrations of air pollutants ($PM_{2.5}$, PM_{10}, SO_2, NO_2, O_3 and CO) and risk of preterm birth in Ningbo. Our results suggested that short-term exposure to four pollutants ($PM_{2.5}$, PM_{10}, SO_2 and NO_2) were associated with preterm birth risk in Ningbo. These findings might have important implications in preventing preterm birth while further studies are still needed.

Additional files

Additional file 1: Figure S1. Location of air quality monitor stations in Ningbo city.

Additional file 2: Table S1. Association between cumulative air pollution concentrations and risk of preterm birth.

Additional file 3: Table S2. Excess risks (ERs) and 95% confidence intervals of preterm birth per IQR increment in air pollutant concentrations stratified by season and maternal age in Ningbo, China.

Additional file 4: Table S3. Difference of estimates and 95% confidence intervals (95% CIs) of air pollutants on risk of preterm birth between subgroups.

Funding

This study was supported by the Air Pollution and Health Research Center, Zhejiang University (NO.519600-I21502), Health and Family Planning Commission of Zhejiang Province (NO.2014KYB356 and NO.2014KYA273), Science and Technology bureau of Ningbo (NO.2014B82003), Key laboratory of maternal-fetal medicine, Ningbo Women and Children's Hospital (NO.2010A22011). The sponsors had no role in the design and conduct of the study; in the collection, management, analysis, and interpretation of the data; or in the preparation, review, or approval of the manuscript.

Availability of data and materials

The study did not contain confidential patient data. No further data will be shared because all the data supporting the findings is contained within the manuscript.

Authors' contributions

WYL collected the data and drafted the manuscript. ZBY performed the statistical analysis. HYQ assisted in data management and analyses. XYC assisted in manuscript editing. JBW and KC contributed in the study design and manuscript editing. All authors read and approved the final manuscript.

Competing interests

The authors declare that they have no competing interests.

Author details

[1]Key laboratory of maternal-fetal medicine, Ningbo Women and Children's Hospital, Ningbo 315012, China. [2]Department of Epidemiology and Biostatistics, School of Public Health, Zhejiang University, Hangzhou 310058, China. [3]Research Center for Air Pollution and Health, Zhejiang University, Hangzhou 310058, China.

References

1. Goldenberg RL, Culhane JF, Iams JD, Romero R. Epidemiology and causes of preterm birth. LANCET. 2008;371(9606):75–84.
2. Blencowe H, Cousens S, Oestergaard MZ, Chou D, Moller AB, Narwal R, Adler A, Vera GC, Rohde S, Say L, et al. National, regional, and worldwide estimates of preterm birth rates in the year 2010 with time trends since 1990 for selected countries: a systematic analysis and implications. LANCET. 2012;379(9832):2162–72.
3. Muglia LJ, Katz M. The enigma of spontaneous preterm birth. N Engl J Med. 2010;362(6):529–35.
4. Polichetti G, Capone D, Grigoropoulos K, Tarantino G, Nunziata A, Gentile A. Effects of ambient air pollution on birth outcomes: an overview. Crit Rev Environ Sci Technol. 2013;43(12):1223–45.
5. Stieb DM, Chen L, Eshoul M, Judek S. Ambient air pollution, birth weight and preterm birth: a systematic review and meta-analysis. Environ Res. 2012;117:100–11.
6. Shah PS, Balkhair T, KSGD P. Air pollution and birth outcomes: a systematic review. Environ Int. 2011;37(2):498–516.
7. Sun X, Luo X, Zhao C, Chung NR, Lim CE, Zhang B, Liu T. The association between fine particulate matter exposure during pregnancy and preterm birth: a meta-analysis. BMC Pregnancy Childbirth. 2015;15:300.
8. Liu C, Sun J, Liu Y, Liang H, Wang M, Wang C, Shi T. Different exposure levels of fine particulate matter and preterm birth: a meta-analysis based on cohort studies. Environ Sci Pollut Res Int. 2017.
9. Khader Y, Abdelrahman M, Abdo N, Awad S, Al-Sharif M, Elbetieha A, Malkawi M. Exposure to Air Pollution and Pregnancy Outcomes in the East Mediterranean Region: a Systematic Review. Int J Pediatrics-Mashhad. 2016;4(1):1255–71.
10. Li X, Huang S, Jiao A, Yang X, Yun J, Wang Y, Xue X, Chu Y, Liu F, Liu Y, et al. Association between ambient fine particulate matter and preterm birth or term low birth weight: an updated systematic review and meta-analysis. Environ Pollut. 2017;227:596–605.
11. Jacobs M, Zhang G, Chen S, Mullins B, Bell M, Jin L, Guo Y, Huxley R, Pereira G. The association between ambient air pollution and selected adverse pregnancy outcomes in China: a systematic review. Sci Total Environ. 2017;579:1179–92.
12. Hastie T, Tibshirani R. Generalized additive models for medical research. Stat Methods Med Res. 1995;4(3):187–96.

13. Darrow LA, Klein M, Flanders WD, Waller LA, Correa A, Marcus M, Mulholland JA, Russell AG, Tolbert PE. Ambient air pollution and preterm birth a time-series analysis. Epidemiology. 2009;20(5):689–98.
14. Yang Y, Li R, Li W, Wang M, Cao Y, Wu Z, Xu Q. The association between ambient air pollution and daily mortality in Beijing after the 2008 olympics: a time series study. PLoS One. 2013;8(10):e76759.
15. Fell DB, Buckeridge DL, Platt RW, Kaufman JS, Basso O, Wilson K. Circulating influenza virus and adverse pregnancy outcomes: a time-series study. Am J Epidemiol. 2016;184(3):163–75.
16. Schwartz J, Dockery DW, Neas LM. Is daily mortality associated specifically with fine particles? J Air Waste Manag Assoc. 1996;46(10):927–39.
17. Zheng PW, Wang JB, Zhang ZY, Shen P, Chai PF, Li D, Jin MJ, Tang ML, Lu HC, Lin HB, et al. Air pollution and hospital visits for acute upper and lower respiratory infections among children in Ningbo, China: A time-series analysis. Environ Sci Pollut Res Int. 2017;24(23):18860-69.
18. Souza JB, Reisen VA, Santos JM, Franco GC. Principal components and generalized linear modeling in the correlation between hospital admissions and air pollution. Rev Saude Publica. 2014;48(3):451–8.
19. Zhao A, Chen R, Kuang X, Kan H. Ambient air pollution and daily outpatient visits for cardiac arrhythmia in Shanghai, China. J Epidemiol. 2014;24(4):321–6.
20. Tam WW, Wong TW, Ng L, Wong SY, Kung KK, Wong AH. Association between air pollution and general outpatient clinic consultations for upper respiratory tract infections in Hong Kong. PLoS One. 2014;9(1):e86913.
21. Zhang F, Wang W, Lv J, Krafft T, Xu J. Time-series studies on air pollution and daily outpatient visits for allergic rhinitis in Beijing, China. Sci Total Environ. 2011;409(13):2486–92.
22. Rudez G, Janssen NA, Kilinc E, Leebeek FW, Gerlofs-Nijland ME, Spronk HM, Ten CH, Cassee FR, de Maat MP. Effects of ambient air pollution on hemostasis and inflammation. Environ Health Perspect. 2009;117(6):995–1001.
23. Qian Z, Liang S, Yang S, Trevathan E, Huang Z, Yang R, Wang J, Hu K, Zhang Y, Vaughn M, et al. Ambient air pollution and preterm birth: a prospective birth cohort study in Wuhan, China. Int J Hyg Environ Health. 2016;219(2):195–203.
24. Zeka A, Zanobetti A, Schwartz J. Individual-level modifiers of the effects of particulate matter on daily mortality. Am J Epidemiol. 2006;163(9):849–59.
25. Arroyo V, Diaz J, Ortiz C, Carmona R, Saez M, Linares C. Short term effect of air pollution, noise and heat waves on preterm births in Madrid (Spain). Environ Res. 2016;145:162–8.
26. Zhao N, Qiu J, Zhang Y, He X, Zhou M, Li M, Xu X, Cui H, Lv L, Lin X, et al. Ambient air pollutant PM10 and risk of preterm birth in Lanzhou, China. Environ Int. 2015;76:71–7.
27. Zhao Q, Liang Z, Tao S, Zhu J, Du Y. Effects of air pollution on neonatal prematurity in Guangzhou of China: a time-series study. Environ Health. 2011;10.
28. Sagiv SK, Mendola P, Loomis D, Herring AH, Neas LM, Savitz DA, Poole C. A time-series analysis of air pollution and preterm birth in Pennsylvania, 1997-2001. Environ Health Perspect. 2005;113(5):602–6.
29. Fleischer NL, Merialdi M, van Donkelaar A, Vadillo-Ortega F, Martin RV, Betran AP, Souza JP: Outdoor air pollution, preterm birth, and low birth weight: analysis of the world health organization global survey on maternal and perinatal health. Environ Health Perspect 2014, 122(4):425–430.
30. Effect of ambient temperature and air pollutants on the risk of preterm birth, Rome 2001–2010.
31. Rudra CB, Williams MA, Sheppard L, Koenig JQ, Schiff MA. Ambient carbon monoxide and fine particulate matter in relation to preeclampsia and preterm delivery in western Washington state. Environ Health Perspect. 2011;119(6):886–92.
32. He JR, Liu Y, Xia XY, Ma WJ, Lin HL, Kan HD, Lu JH, Feng Q, Mo WJ, Wang P, et al. Ambient temperature and the risk of preterm birth in Guangzhou, China (2001-2011). Environ Health Perspect. 2016;124(7):1100–6.
33. Suh YJ, Ha EH, Park H, Kim YJ, Kim H, Hong YC. GSTM1 polymorphism along with PM10 exposure contributes to the risk of preterm delivery. Mutat Res. 2008;656(1–2):62–7.
34. Wu J, Ren C, Delfino RJ, Chung J, Wilhelm M, Ritz B. Association between local traffic-generated air pollution and preeclampsia and preterm delivery in the south coast air basin of California. Environ Health Perspect. 2009;117(11):1773–9.
35. Aagaard-Tillery KM, Nuthalapaty FS, Ramsey PS, Ramin KD. Preterm premature rupture of membranes: perspectives surrounding controversies in management. Am J Perinatol. 2005;22(6):287–97.
36. Zeger SL, Thomas D, Dominici F, Samet JM, Schwartz J, Dockery D, Cohen A. Exposure measurement error in time-series studies of air pollution: concepts and consequences. Environ Health Perspect. 2000;108(5):419–26.

17

Agreement test of transcutaneous bilirubin and bilistick with serum bilirubin in preterm infants receiving phototherapy

Rinawati Rohsiswatmo[1,2], Hanifah Oswari[1], Radhian Amandito[2], Hikari Ambara Sjakti[1], Endang Windiastuti[1], Rosalina Dewi Roeslani[1] and Indrayady Barchia[1*]

Abstract

Background: This study compares the minimally invasive Bilistick and a noninvasive method with standard Total Serum Bilirubin (TSB) measurement in preterm newborns receiving phototherapy. We assess the agreement of Transcutaneous Bilirubinometer (TcB) and Bilistick bilirubin measurements with standard TSB measurement in preterm infants receiving phototherapy.

Methods: Bilirubin was measured by using TcB and Bilistick in 94 preterm infants in RSCM Jakarta Neonatal Ward from October 2016 to March 2017, with gestational ages of < 35 weeks, before phototherapy and after 24 and 48 h of phototherapy.

Results: There was significant correlation before, at 24 and 48 h of phototherapy between TSB and either TcB ($r = 0.874$; $r = 0.889$; $r = 0.878$ respectively; $p < 0.0001$), or Bilistick ($r = 0.868$; $r = 0.877$; $r = 0.918$ respectively; $p < 0.0001$). The mean difference and limits of agreement before, at 24 and 48 h of phototherapy between TcB and TSB were 0.81 ± 1.51 mg/dL (− 2.14 to 3.77 mg/dL); 0.43 ± 1.57 mg/dL (− 2.66 to 3.51 mg/dL); 0.41 ± 1.58 mg/dL (− 2.69 to 3.50 mg/dL), respectively. For Bilistick they were − 1.50 ± 1.47 mg/dL (− 4.38 to 1.38 mg/dL); − 1.43 ± 1.47 mg/dL (− 4.32 to 1.46 mg/dL); − 1,15 ± 1.31 mg/dL (− 3,72 to 1,42 mg/dL), respectively.

Conclusions: Both methods are reliable for measuring TSB before, during, and after phototherapy in preterm infants. TcB tends to overestimate while Bilistick underestimates TSB.

Keywords: Indonesia, Bilistick, Transcutaneous bilirubin, Phototherapy, Preterm infants

Background

Hyperbilirubinemia is one of the most common problems arising in the neonatal period. Hyperbilirubinemia in neonates often develops in the first week of life, ranging in frequency from 60% in term and 80% in preterm infants [1–3]. Phototherapy is still the primary treatment to prevent further complications for newborns with hyperbilirubinemia, especially for premature infants who have a higher risk of bilirubin encephalopathy [4]. During the course of phototherapy, it is necessary to monitor the bilirubin levels periodically until phototherapy is completed in order to prevent overtreatment. However, regular blood taking can cause problems such as anemia and increased risk of infection in newborns with hyperbilirubinemia. The risk increases especially in preterm infants with lower blood volume and altered immune status. Serum bilirubin measurement is a gold standard for measuring total serum bilirubin (TSB) levels for both detection and evaluation during phototherapy. However, this measurement is an invasive procedure that poses a higher risk of infection, pain, and requires a rather large amount of blood [5–7]. Currently, there are several alternatives for measurement of bilirubin levels. In this study, we will be focusing on the Bilistick System. Compared to TSB, which requires large volumes of blood, the Bilistick System requires only 25 μL of capillary blood. With regards to its cost, the Bilistick System is considerably cheaper than the non-invasive transcutaneous

* Correspondence: indrayady@yahoo.com
[1]Department of Child Health, Faculty of Medicine, Universitas Indonesia – Cipto Mangunkusumo Hospital, Jl Pangeran Diponegoro No. 71, Salemba, Kenari, Senen, Jakarta Pusat, DKI Jakarta 10430, Indonesia
Full list of author information is available at the end of the article

bilirubinometer (TcB); €1300 for transcutaneous bilirubin (JM 103) compared to €600 for Bilistick device (2016 Version) and €1.5 for each test strip and transfer pipette.

Several studies on transcutaneous and Bilistick bilirubin measurements have been conducted to assess the validity of both devices. The correlation between TcB and TSB results in previous studies was strong ($r = 0.835$; $p < 0.0001$), but this study did not measure bilirubin levels during phototherapy [8]. A previous meta-analysis study comparing the measurement of TcB and TSB levels during phototherapy obtained $r = 0.64$ (95% CI 0.43–0.77) on the measurement of transcutaneous bilirubin in the sternal region, but this study was performed on near-term and term infants [9].

Studies comparing Bilistick and serum bilirubin showed a strong correlation ($r = 0.961$ and $r = 0.914$; $P < 0.0001$) but they did not include infants receiving phototherapy [10]. A study comparing bilirubin measurement using transcutaneous bilirubin and Bilistick has been recently reported, with a similar limit of agreement of the Bilistick System (– 5.8 to 3.3 mg/dL) and JM-103 system (– 5.4 to 6.0 mg/dL) versus the clinical laboratory; however, this study only involved term infants and not those being treated by phototherapy [11].

To our knowledge, no previous study has been conducted comparing the measurement of TcB and Bilistick with total serum bilirubin during phototherapy in preterm infants. The aim of this study was to assess the agreement of TcB and Bilistick bilirubin measurements in hyperbilirubinemic preterm infants before and during phototherapy in the hope of determining the best alternative method for measurement of bilirubin levels to reduce the risk of anemia and infections in preterm infants. This is especially important for places with limited laboratory facilities that require measurement systems that are accurate, easy to use, inexpensive, and provide fast results.

Methods

Study population

This study was conducted in the Neonatology Division of the Department of Child Health Faculty of Medicine, Universitas Indonesia – Cipto Mangunkusumo Hospital (RSCM) Jakarta. The inclusion criteria were: hyperbilirubinemic preterm infants age ≤ 14 weeks, gestational age < 35 weeks old who are receiving phototherapy in the Neonatology Division of RSCM Jakarta and with signed parental consent for inclusion in the study. Exclusion criteria were: preterm infants with a prior history of phototherapy or previous exchange transfusion and all preterm infants with defects at the site of measurement. Decision to initiate phototherapy was based on the Indonesian Pediatric Society (IDAI) guidelines for preterm infants with hyperbilirubinemia [12]. Bilirubin measurement was conducted only for the first 48 h of phototherapy after which the neonate received standard therapy including continued phototherapy if indicated.

Laboratory investigations

For each participating hyperbilirubinemic newborn, a thorough explanation of the research was given to the parents and parental consent to participate in the study was obtained. Identification of the patient included: name, age, gender, parent's name and relationship with parents, gestational age, and history of phototherapy. Ballard score was calculated, then the weight was measured using baby scales (20 kg with 0.1 kg precision) (Seca, Germany), and body length and head circumference were measured using an infantometer and measuring tape (100 cm length with 0.1 cm precision) (Seca, Germany). For each infant, bilirubin was measured using TcB, Bilistick and total serum bilirubin lab measurement. The TcB measurement was performed 3 times in a row with Dragger JM 103 in the midsternum area, and the average of the 3 measurements was obtained. All measurements were made by a trained nurse or physician. For the Bilistick measurement, 25uL of capillary blood was collected by a nurse, and then applied to a test strip and inserted in the Bilistick reader. The TSB concentration is determined by reflectance spectroscopy within 3 min of loading.

The TSB measurement was performed by taking 0.6 ml of venous blood, putting it into a vacuum tube, and sending it to Cipto Mangunkusumo Hospital Clinical pathology laboratory in Jakarta, where they employed the chemical oxidation method utilizing vanadate as the oxidizing agent using the ADVIA Chemistry Total Bilirubin 2 device (Siemens, Germany).

Statistical analysis

Categorical data are presented in the form of frequency distribution, proportion, and percentage, while continuous-scale data are presented as mean and standard deviation or median and range. The correlation between the gold standard measurement and the tool under test was calculated using Pearson correlation (normal distribution) and Spearman correlation (abnormal distribution). Bland-Altman test was used to calculate the agreement of the mean difference between the gold standard measurement and the tested tool. The mean difference is expressed as mean ± SD, while the limit of agreement is calculated based on the mean ± 1.96

Table 1 Characteristics of subjects ($n = 94$)

Characteristics	
Gender	
Male	53 (56.4%)
Female	41 (43.6%)
Age (days) Mean ± SD (range)	2.94 ± 1.66 (1 to 10)
Gestational age (weeks) Mean ± SD (range)	31.27 ± 2.32 (26 to 34)
Weight (g) Mean ± SD (range)	1466.73 ± 442.24 (700 to 2450)

Table 2 Profile of bilirubin levels

Measurement	Bilirubin level
Before phototherapy	
Total serum bilirubin (mg/dL) Mean ± SD (range)	10.18 ± 2.91 (4.43 to 19.70)
Transcutaneous (mg/dL) Mean ± SD (range)	10.99 ± 3.07 (4.70 to 19.60)
Bilistick (mg/dL) Mean ± SD (range)	8.68 ± 2.78 (4.20 to 14.80)
24 h of phototherapy	
Total serum bilirubin (mg/dL) Mean ± SD (range)	9.75 ± 3.04 (3.25 to 18.20)
Transcutaneous (mg/dL) Mean ± SD (range)	10.18 ± 3.44 (1.90 to 19.70)
Bilistick (mg/dL) Mean ± SD (range)	8.33 ± 2.86 (3.20 to 17.90)
48 h of phototherapy	
Total serum bilirubin (mg/dL) Median ± SD (range)	8 (0.58 to 21.26)
Transcutaneous (mg/dL) Median ± SD (range)	7.9 (1.70 to 22.30)
Bilistick (mg/dL) Median ± SD (range)	6.85 (1.20 to 17.20)

SD. Statistical Package for the Social Sciences (SPSS) version 18.0 for Windows was used for all statistical analyses. This research was approved by the Medical Research Ethics Committee of the Faculty of Medicine, University of Indonesia and the licensing of research sites from Cipto Mangunkusumo Hospital.

Results

During the study period, there were 120 preterm infants less than 35 weeks of gestation who suffered hyperbilirubinemia and 96 of them (80%) had indications for phototherapy. Of these 96 infants, 2 infants were not treated with phototherapy due to clinical deterioration and eventual death. The remaining 94 infants were enrolled in the study.

The characteristics of 94 participants included in the study are reported in Table 1. There were 53 (56.4%) males and 41 (43.6%) females. The mean age of the subjects at the time of hyperbilirubinemia diagnosis was 2.9 days with a range of 1 to 10 days. The mean of gestational age of subjects was 31.3 weeks with a range of 26 to 34 weeks while mean weight of subjects was 1466.73 g with a range of 700 to 2450 g.

Profiles of total serum bilirubin, transcutaneous bilirubin, and Bilistick levels before phototherapy, and after 24 h and 48 h of phototherapy are reported in Table 2.

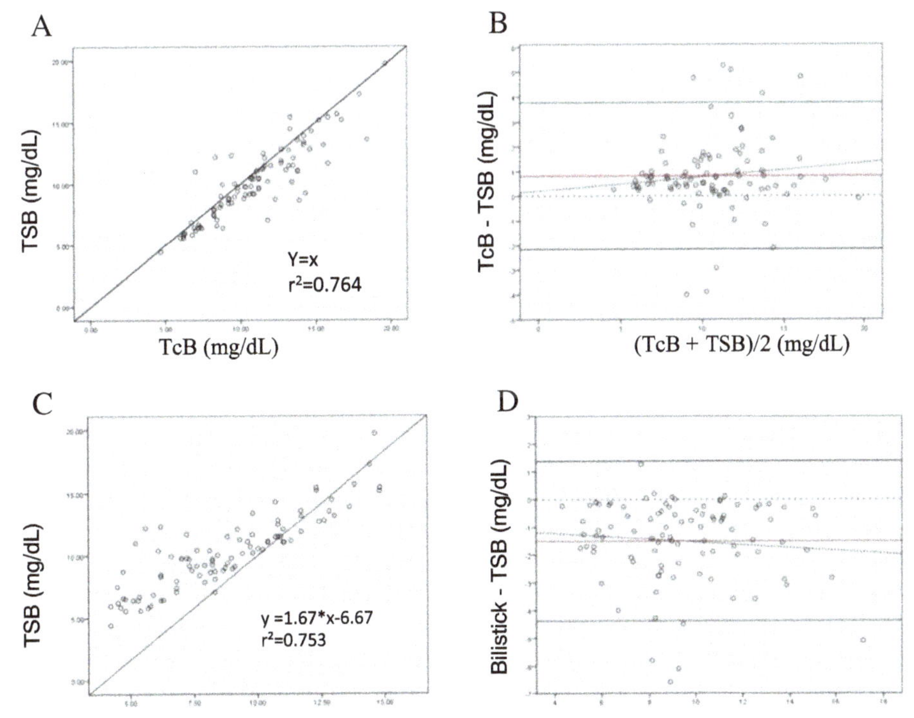

Fig. 1 Scatter and Bland Altman plot between TcB and TSB (**a** and **b**), Bilistick and TSB (**c** and **d**) before phototherapy, Y equation = linear equation obtained from linear regression analysis. Y = estimated TSB, X = Bilirubin level of the device being tested (red line) = average difference (black line) = agreement limit (dotted diagonal) = tendency of average difference (dotted line) = 0 point, standard to observe distance with red line

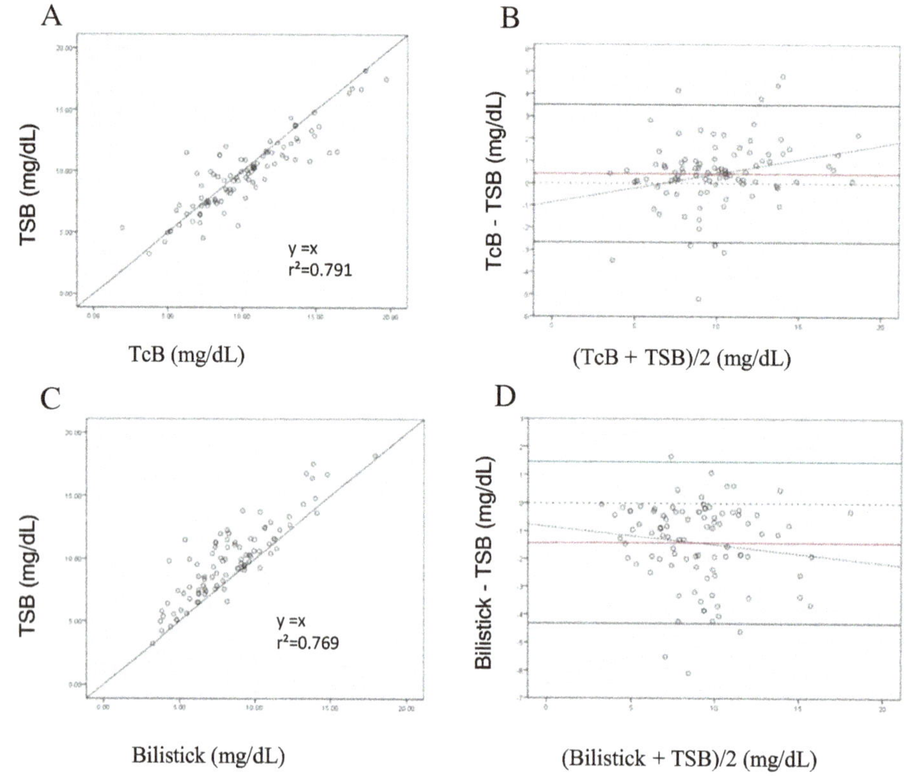

Fig. 2 Scatter and Bland Altman plots between TcB and TSB (**a** and **b**), Bilistick and TSB (**c** and **d**) at 24 h of phototherapy. Y equation = linear equation obtained from linear regression analysis. Y = estimated TSB, X = Bilirubin level of the device being tested (red line) = average difference (black line) = agreement limit (dashed line) = tendency of average difference (dotted line) = 0 point, standard to observe distance with red line

Kolmogorov-Smirnov and Shapiro-Wilk test were used to test the normality of data, from which we obtained a normal distribution with $p > 0.05$ for bilirubin measurement data before phototherapy and after 24 h of phototherapy. While for measurement of 48-h bilirubin phototherapy, we obtained an abnormal distribution with a value of $p < 0.05$.

The Pearson correlation test of total serum bilirubin level and transcutaneous bilirubin before phototherapy showed a significant positive correlation between total serum bilirubin and transcutaneous bilirubin (Fig. 1a) ($r^2 = 0{,}764$, $p < 0.0001$).

Transcutaneous bilirubin levels tended to overestimate total serum bilirubin before phototherapy with a mean difference of 0.81 mg/dL (SD 1.51) with a 95% CI of 0.50 to 1.12 and the limits of agreement were − 2.14 and 3.77 mg/dL. The Bland-Altman plot shows that the higher the bilirubin level, the wider the difference between the 2 methods (Fig. 1b).

As shown in Fig. 1c there was a significant and positive correlation between total serum bilirubin and Bilistick bilirubin measurement before phototherapy ($r^2 = 0.753$, $p < 0.0001$).

Bilistick tended to underestimate total serum bilirubin before phototherapy measurement with a mean difference of − 1.50 mg/dL (SD 1.47) with a 95% CI of − 1.80 to − 1.20 with the limits of agreement of − 4.38 and 1.38 mg/dL. The Bland-Altman plot shows the higher the bilirubin level, the wider the difference between Bilistick and total serum bilirubin measurement (Fig. 1d).

After 24 h of phototherapy, we found a significant positive correlation between total serum bilirubin and transcutaneous bilirubin ($r^2 = 0.791$, $p < 0.0001$ (Fig. 2a). TcB overestimates total serum bilirubin with a mean difference of 0.43 mg/dL (SD 1.57) with 95% CI of 0.10 to 0.75 and limits of agreement of − 2.66 and 3.51 mg/dL (Fig. 2b). There was a positive and significant correlation between total serum bilirubin and Bilistick bilirubin ($r^2 = 0.769$, $p < 0.0001$) (Fig. 2c). Bilistick underestimates total serum bilirubin with a mean difference − 1.43 mg/dL (SD 1.47) with 95% CI -1.73 to − 1.13 and the limits of agreement were − 4.32 and 1.46 mg/dL. The Bland-Altman plot shows the higher the bilirubin level, the wider the difference between Bilistick and total serum bilirubin measurement (Fig. 2d).

The same pattern was observed after 48 h of phototherapy. A significant and positive correlation was present between total serum bilirubin and transcutaneous bilirubin ($r^2 = 0.771$, $p < 0.0001$) (Fig. 3a); TcB overestimates total serum bilirubin with a mean difference of 0.41 mg/dL (SD 1.58) with 95% CI 0.08 to 0.73 and the limits of agreement were − 2.69 and 3.50 mg/dL. The Bland-Altman plot shows that the higher the bilirubin level the wider the difference between transcutaneous bilirubin level and total

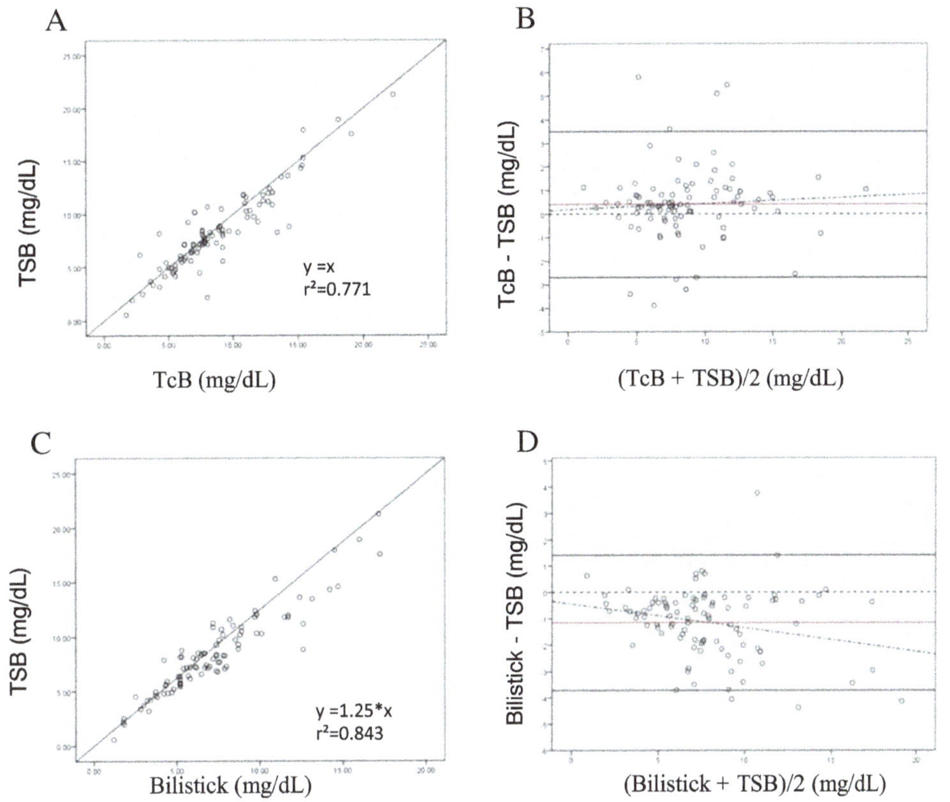

Fig. 3 Scatter and Bland Altman plot between TcB and TSB (**a** and **b**), Bilistick and TSB (**c** and **d**) at 48 h of phototherapy. Y equation = linear equation obtained from linear regression analysis. Y = estimated TSB, X = Bilirubin level of the device being tested (▬) = average difference (▬) = agreement limit (⋰) = tendency of average difference (▪▪▪▪▪▪) = 0 point, standard to observe distance with red line

serum bilirubin (Fig. 3b). A significant and positive correlation was also found between total serum bilirubin and Bilistick ($r^2 = 0.843$, $p < 0.0001$) (Fig. 3c). Bilistick bilirubin tends to underestimate total serum bilirubin with a mean difference of − 1.15 mg/dL (SD 1.31) with 95% CI -1.42 to − 0.88 and the limits of agreement were − 3.72 and 1.42 mg/dL. The Bland-Altman plot shows, the higher the bilirubin level, the wider the difference between Bilistick bilirubin level and total serum bilirubin (Fig. 3d).

Discussion

This study assessed the correlation and agreement of TcB and Bilistick bilirubin measurement with TSB before and during phototherapy in preterm infants of gestational age less than 35 weeks. There was a very strong and significant positive correlation between TcB and Bilistick bilirubin measurement with TSB before and after 24 or 48 h of phototherapy. The results we obtained were similar to the meta-analysis of TcB measurement in preterm infants [9]. Prior to phototherapy, JM 103 had a strong correlation of $r = 0.87$ (95% CI of 0.82–0.91), and an even stronger correlation with preterm infants of less than 32 weeks ($r = 0.89$ (95% CI of 0.82–0.93)) [13]. Other studies obtained even stronger correlations in preterm infants with a gestational age of less than 28 weeks ($r = 0.92$ and $r = 0.94$, [14, 15]). The result of correlation on 24-h phototherapy TcB measurement in our study was superior to previous studies in near term and term infants [9]. We assume this difference is due to our participants being premature infants with gestational ages of less than 35 weeks, as their thinner skin thickness may improve light absorption and reflection from the subcutaneous tissue to the appliance. The accuracy of Bilistick was also comparable with previous studies in term infants who did not receive phototherapy, suggesting that Bilistick may be reliably used in preterm infants before and after phototherapy [10, 11, 13–16].

Measurement of TcB before phototherapy and after 24 and 48 h of phototherapy tended to overestimate by 0.81, 0.43, and 0.41 mg/dL compared with TSB. These results did not greatly differ from previous studies [11, 13, 17, 18]. TcB measurement before phototherapy and after 24 h and 48 h of phototherapy overestimated bilirubin level with a mean difference of less than 1 mg/dL and showed very strong positive correlation. This led to the conclusion that TcB bilirubin measurement was reliable in preterm infants both before and during phototherapy. Why the TcB measurement tended to overestimate serum bilirubin is not clear, but we hypothesized that it is related to an increased blood flow in the skin, which is inversely proportional to weight gain and gestational age. This is revealed in our study of preterm infants with gestational ages of less than 35 weeks who have high blood flow and low skin thickness. Phototherapy increases blood flow in the skin by increasing the body temperature. An increase in body temperature of 0.5–1 °C leads to an increase of 3 times the blood flow in the skin [19]. In addition, some TcB devices while usable up to a bilirubin level of 20 mg/dL, the reliability of the result is questionable at levels above 15 mg/dL.

Bilistick measurement before phototherapy, and after 24 h and 48 h of phototherapy tended to underestimate by 1.5, 1.43, and 1.15 mg/dL compared with TSB. Bilistick measurement appears to be lower with a mean difference of less than 1.5 mg/dL. This result is similar with what was reported in term infants who did not receive phototherapy [11]. Since this is the first study performed in preterms using the Bilistick system, additional data needs to be collected to verify that this small underestimation is correct.

Based on the tendency of both methods to overestimate or underestimate, the Indonesian guideline for phototherapy or exchange transfusion might require some changes in cases where doctors decide to use the Bilistick alone. This underestimation would have led to 11 neonates not receiving phototherapy when phototherapy would have been indicated by traditional serum bilirubin measurements in our population.

Limitation

We did not use the newest version of Bilistick because it was not available during our time of study [11]. The population of our study includes mostly patients of Sumatran and Javanese descent, in whom skin tones do not contrast greatly enough between light and dark skin tone for transcutaneous bilirubin results to show any of the discrepancies reported in Caucasian and African-American races [20–22]. We also did not have enough samples to statistically analyze the difference between extreme premature and premature babies.

Conclusions

Both TcB and Bilistick show equal reliability and can be used as an alternative measurement methods for monitoring bilirubin levels in term and preterm newborns, as well as before and after phototherapy. However, TcB tends to overestimate TSB while Bilistick underestimates TSB.

Abbreviations

CI: Confidence Interval; RSCM: Cipto Mangunkusumo Hospital; SD: Standard deviation; SPSS: Statistical package for the social sciences; TcB: Transcutaneous bilirubin; TSB: Total serum bilirubin

Acknowledgements

We would like to thank the nursing staff, physicians, and laboratory analysts at our neonatal ward and NICU for their helpful cooperation in this study, as well as Claudio Tiribelli for providing us the Bilistick system. We would also kindly thank Thomas Mayers for his valuable help in proofreading our manuscript.

Authors' contributions

This work was carried out in collaboration between all authors. Authors IB, EW, and RR designed the study and interpreted the data. Authors IB, HO, and RA anchored the lab study, gathered the initial data, performed preliminary data analysis and managed the literature searches. Author IB and RDR produced the initial draft and IB, HAS, and RA wrote the manuscript. All authors read and approved the final manuscript.

Competing interests

The authors declare that they have no competing interests.

Author details

[1]Department of Child Health, Faculty of Medicine, Universitas Indonesia – Cipto Mangunkusumo Hospital, Jl Pangeran Diponegoro No. 71, Salemba, Kenari, Senen, Jakarta Pusat, DKI Jakarta 10430, Indonesia. [2]Neonatal Intensive Care Unit, Pondok Indah General Hospital, Jl Metro Duta Kav UE, Pondok Indah, Pondok Pinang, Kebayoran Lama, Jakarta Selatan, DKI Jakarta 12310, Indonesia.

References

1. Kliegman RM, Behrman RE, Jenson HB, Stanton BM. Nelson textbook of pediatrics e-book: Elsevier. Health Sciences; 2007.
2. Martin RJ, Fanaroff AA, Walsh MC. Fanaroff and Martin's neonatal-perinatal medicine E-book: diseases of the fetus and infant. Elsevier Health Sciences; 2010.
3. Slim G, Naous A, Naja Z, Naja AS, Rajab M. Effect of Instituting a Hospital Pre-discharge Bilirubin Screening on Subsequent Significant Hyperbilirubinemia in Term and Near Term Newborn. 2015.
4. Arnolda G, Nwe H, Trevisanuto D, et al. Risk factors for acute bilirubin encephalopathy on admission to two Myanmar national paediatric hospitals. Matern Health Neonatol Perinatol. 2015;1(1):22.
5. Grabenhenrich J, Grabenhenrich L, Bührer C, Berns M. Transcutaneous bilirubin after phototherapy in term and preterm infants. Pediatrics. 2014; 134(5):e1324–9.
6. Szabo P, Wolf M, Bucher HU, Fauchere J-C, Haensse D, Arlettaz R. Detection of hyperbilirubinaemia in jaundiced full-term neonates by eye or by bilirubinometer? Eur J Pediatr. 2004;163(12):722–7.
7. Uwurukundo J, Baribwira C, Basinga P, Niyibizi P, Mutigima E. Assessing the accuracy of the jm-102 transcutaneous bilirubin measurement in dark skin jaundiced neonates: case of University Teaching Hospital, Rwanda. Rwanda Med J. 2013;69(2):39–44.
8. Chang Y-H, Hsieh W-S, Chou H-C, Chen C-Y, Wu J-Y, Tsao P-N. The effectiveness of a noninvasive transcutaneous bilirubin meter in reducing the need for blood sampling in Taiwanese neonates. Clinical Neonatology. 2006;13(2):60–3.
9. Nagar G, Vandermeer B, Campbell S, Kumar M. Effect of phototherapy on the reliability of transcutaneous bilirubin devices in term and near-term infants: a systematic review and meta-analysis. Neonatology. 2016;109(3):203–12.

10. Zabetta CC, Iskander I, Greco C, et al. Bilistick: a low-cost point-of-care system to measure total plasma bilirubin. Neonatology. 2013;103(3):177–81.
11. Greco C, Iskander I, Akmal D, et al. Comparison between Bilistick system and transcutaneous bilirubin in assessing total bilirubin serum concentration in jaundiced newborns. J Perinatol. 2017;37(9):1028.
12. Kosim MS, Yunanto A, Dewi R, Sarosa GI, Usman A. Buku ajar neonatologi. Jakarta: IDI; 2008.
13. Nagar G, Vandermeer B, Campbell S, Kumar M. Reliability of transcutaneous bilirubin devices in preterm infants: a systematic review. Pediatrics. 2013;132(5):871–81.
14. Ahmed M, Mostafa S, Fisher G, Reynolds T. Comparison between transcutaneous bilirubinometry and total serum bilirubin measurements in preterm infants< 35 weeks gestation. Ann Clin Biochem. 2010;47(1):72–7.
15. Schmidt E, Wheeler C, Jackson G, Engle W. Evaluation of transcutaneous bilirubinometry in preterm neonates. J Perinatol. 2009;29(8):564.
16. Greco C, Arnolda G, Boo N-Y, et al. Neonatal jaundice in low-and middle-income countries: lessons and future directions from the 2015 don ostrow Trieste yellow retreat. Neonatology. 2016;110(3):172–80.
17. Campbell DM, Danayan KC, McGovern V, Cheema S, Stade B, Sgro M. Transcutaneous bilirubin measurement at the time of hospital discharge in a multiethnic newborn population. Paediatr Child Health. 2011;16(3):141–5.
18. Olusanya BO, Imosemi DO, Emokpae AA. Differences between transcutaneous and serum bilirubin measurements in black African neonates. Pediatrics. 2016;138:e20160907.
19. Wu PY, Wong W, Guerra G, et al. Peripheral blood flow in the neonate. 1. Changes in total, skin, and muscle blood flow with gestational and postnatal age. Pediatr Res. 1980;14(12):1374.
20. Taylor JA, Burgos AE, Flaherman V, et al. Discrepancies between transcutaneous and serum bilirubin measurements. Pediatrics. 2015;135(2):224–31.
21. Bhutta ZA, Yusuf K. Transcutaneous bilirubinometry in Pakistani newborns: a preliminary report. J Pakistan Med Assoc. 1991;41:155–6.
22. Wainer S, Rabi Y, Parmar SM, Allegro D, Lyon M. Impact of skin tone on the performance of a transcutaneous jaundice meter. Acta Paediatr. 2009;98(12):1909–15.

Growth during the first year in infants affected by neonatal abstinence syndrome

Tammy E. Corr[1*], Eric W. Schaefer[2] and Ian M. Paul[1,2]

Abstract

Background: Infants with neonatal abstinence syndrome (NAS) initially experience neurologic excitability, poor feeding, and/or hyperphagia in the setting of increased metabolic demand. Because the longitudinal effects of these early symptoms and behaviors on weight trends are unknown, we sought to contrast weight gain patterns through age 1 year for infants diagnosed with NAS with matched controls.

Methods: Retrospective cohort of 70 singletons with a gestational age of ≥37 weeks and an ICD-9 or ICD-10 diagnosis of NAS made ≤7 days after birth with institutional follow-up matched to patients without NAS. Infants were matched on gestational age (±2 weeks), birth weight (±20 g), sex (exact), and insurance type (exact). Quantile regression methods were used to estimate 10th, 25th, 50th, 75th and 90th percentiles of weight over time.

Results: The mean gestational age for an infant with NAS was 38.8 weeks (standard deviation [SD], 1.3). The mean birth weight was 3.141 kg (SD, 0.510). NAS patients had a median of 24 weights recorded between birth and 400 days (inter-quartile range [IQR], 16–32 weights). Patients without NAS had a median of 12 weights recorded (IQR, 10–16). Growth curves were similar over the first 400 days of life. Patients with NAS had non-significantly higher and lower estimated weights for the 90th and 10th percentiles, respectively.

Conclusion: Infants with a diagnosis of NAS grew similarly to controls during their first year. Given the frequently-encountered NAS symptoms of hyperphagia and irritability, future studies may evaluate whether early differences in caregiver feeding exist and whether they have longer-term impacts on growth.

Keywords: Neonatal abstinence syndrome, Neonatal opioid withdrawal syndrome, Infant growth, Infant nutrition, Pediatric obesity, Behavioral feeding, Comfort feeding, Parenting practices

Background

Neonatal abstinence syndrome (NAS) is a growing public health problem both nationally and globally [1–4]. Infants affected by neonatal abstinence syndrome display a number of symptoms and behaviors related to neurologic excitability including increased tone, tremors, hyperthermia, tachypnea, excessive crying, and increased time in an awake state [5]. Additionally, these infants often exhibit poor feeding with an uncoordinated suck as well as symptoms of gastrointestinal dysfunction such as regurgitation and emesis and loose or watery stools [5]. This constellation of neurologic and gastrointestinal symptoms may result in caloric intake that is inadequate and fails to meet the increased metabolic demands of the symptomatic infant resulting in hyperphagia [6].

Studies focused on caloric intake and growth of infants affected by NAS in the immediate neonatal period are inconsistent and sparse [6–9]. While some studies suggest weight loss in the neonatal period is greater in drug-exposed infants [7, 9], other studies report infants seem to compensate for this hypermetabolic state by increased intake [6], while still others propose that this hyperphagia can lead to excessive weight gain [8]. Even less is known about the feeding patterns and subsequent growth of these affected infants as they age [10].

Infants affected by NAS are symptomatically irritable and difficult to soothe. These characteristics along with early hyperphagia may lead to the development of aberrant feeding behaviors by caregivers with a tendency towards feeding to comfort. While infants have an innate

* Correspondence: tcorr@pennstatehealth.psu.edu
[1]Penn State College of Medicine, Department of Pediatrics, P.O. Box 850, 500 University Drive, Hershey, PA 17033-0850, USA
Full list of author information is available at the end of the article

ability to control their caloric intake [11, 12], parental feeding practices can alter eating behavior and affect subsequent weight gain and growth [13]. Therefore, we sought to estimate the weight patterns through age 1 year for infants affected by NAS compared with matched controls without NAS. We hypothesized that infants affected by NAS would have larger weight gains than those of matched controls and a tendency towards obesity.

Methods

Design

In this retrospective cohort study, electronic medical records (EMR) of all newborns ($N = 13{,}718$) hospitalized at the Penn State Milton S. Hershey Medical Center (HMC; Hershey, PA) between July 2008 and March 2016 were queried. HMC is a tertiary care center with a level IV neonatal intensive care unit (NICU) and an active maternal-fetal medicine (MFM) program. Data extracted from the EMR included birth weight, type of delivery (vaginal or Cesarean), sex, gestational age, singleton versus multiple birth, NICU stay, insurance status (public, private, self-pay), receipt of drugs (morphine, phenobarbital, clonidine) during birth hospitalization, total number of inpatient and outpatient visits within 13 months after birth, and weights and lengths entered in the EMR during inpatient or outpatient visits. Where data were missing from searchable fields of NAS patients, they were manually extracted from the clinical chart. For all transferred newborns with a diagnosis of NAS ($N = 127$), pre-transferal data were obtained by physically reviewing outside records.

Participants

Analysis was restricted to newborns of singleton birth with a gestational age ≥ 37 weeks and a diagnosis of NAS made ≤7 days after birth who had ≥3 weights recorded after discharge with ≥1 weight recorded between 100 and 400 days to ensure adequate follow up. NAS cases were identified using the ICD-9 diagnosis code 779.5 (drug withdrawal syndrome in a newborn) and the ICD-10 code P96.1 (neonatal withdrawal symptoms from maternal use of drugs of addiction). Each NAS patient was matched to 1 patient without NAS on gestational age (±2 weeks), birth weight (±25 g), sex, and insurance (private vs. public, exact match) using a greedy matching algorithm [14]. While the acceptable range for matching on gestational age was wide, the majority were exact matches, and only 1 match had a 2-week difference. Eligible matches were well singletons with no NICU stay, a gestational age of ≥37 weeks with record of birthweight who had ≥3 weights recorded after discharge with ≥1 weight recorded between 100 and 400 days. A total of 2900 patients without NAS met these inclusion criteria. For matching, self-pay was combined with Medicaid and missing insurance status was imputed as private.

Data analysis

We used a quantile regression model appropriate for longitudinal data to estimate 10th, 25th, 50th (median), 75th, and 90th percentiles of weight (measured in kg) as a function of time after birth. The penalized fixed-effects model in the R package "Regression Quantiles for Panel Data (rqpd)" was used to estimate the percentile curves [15]. The model includes separate intercepts for each patient to account for the correlation among repeated weights measured for a patient. Regularization was used to estimate the intercepts with the amount of regularization controlled by a tuning parameter (λ). Separate models were fitted for patients treated with NAS and their matched controls so that λ could be specified differently in each model and adjusted accordingly for the smaller number of weights recorded for matched controls. The parameter λ was set equal to 50 for NAS patients and to 20 for matched controls.

To estimate non-linear percentile curves, we used restricted cubic splines [16] with knots at each quartile of weight and a knot at 2 days after birth. The knot at 2 days was used to model the early and expected loss of weight in the first days after birth. All weights recorded from birth to 400 days after birth were used. Three obvious errors in recorded weights were deleted (e.g. a value of 0 kg). Final percentile curves were only shown to 390 days (approximately 13 months after birth). Non-parametric bootstrapping with 1000 bootstrap samples was used to test for differences between NAS patients and matched controls for each percentile curve. In these bootstrap samples, matched pairs were randomly selected, and all weights from selected patients were used in respective models fits in each bootstrap sample.

We conducted 2 subgroup analyses. First, we compared percentile curves of patients who did and did not receive pharmacologic therapy for NAS. Second, we compared patients with NAS who received pharmacologic therapy to their matched controls. The same methods were used as above with the following changes: λ was set to 20 and only 4 total knots were used (instead of 5) for patients with NAS who did not receive pharmacologic therapy due to the smaller number of weights recorded for this subgroup.

Results

Among the 234 neonates with a diagnosis of NAS and documented inpatient stay at our center, 70 (30%) met all inclusion criteria and were included in

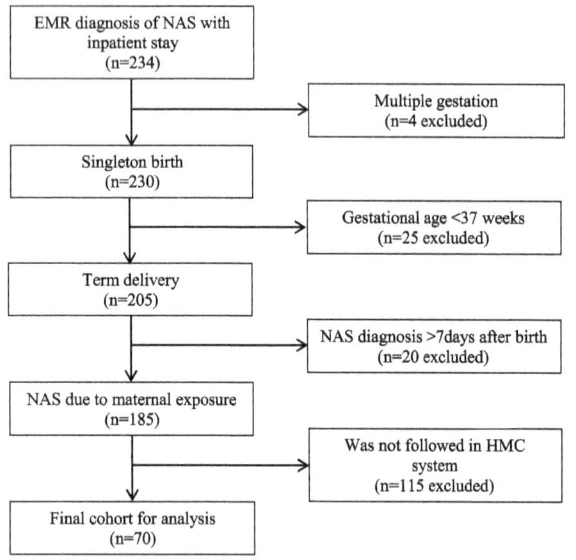

Fig. 1 Flow diagram of patients retained for analysis

the final analysis (Fig. 1). Thirty-seven percent of the NAS population was early term, 50% term, and 13% post term. NAS patients were primarily insured by Medicaid (81%). Similar to controls, about one third of NAS infants were born via C-section, and the majority (89%) were inborn. Nearly 75% of NAS patients had a NICU admission. Median lengths of stay were 11.1 days for patients with NAS and 2.2 days for controls (Table 1).

Fifty (71%) of the NAS patients were < 1 day old at the time of NAS diagnosis. An additional 14% were diagnosed on the day following birth, and the remaining 14% of patients were diagnosed between ages 2–5 days. Thirty-six (51%) of NAS patients did not receive pharmacologic treatment. Among NAS patients who required pharmacologic therapy, nearly all (97%) received treatment with morphine with 4 patients (12%) requiring the addition of a second agent (phenobarbital or clonidine) to manage their symptoms. One patient received treatment with phenobarbital alone.

Table 1 Demographic and birth characteristic of infants with NAS[a] and matched controls

Variable	NAS (*n* = 70)	Matched Controls (*n* = 70)	
Sex[b]			
Male	30 (43%)	30 (42.9%)	
Female	40 (57%)	40 (57.1%)	
Gestational age (weeks)[b]			
37	13 (19%)	13 (19%)	
38	13 (19%)	12 (17%)	
39	25 (36%)	28 (40%)	
40	10 (14%)	10 (14%)	
41	9 (13%)	7 (10%)	
Birth weight (kg)[b]			
Median	3.030	3.033	
(Interquartile range)	2.746–3.465	2.750–3.465	
Insurance[b]			
Private	13 (19%)	13 (19%)	
Medicaid/self-pay	57 (81%)	57 (81%)	
			P-value
Transferred from outside hospital	8 (11%)	0 (0%)	0.003
Type of delivery			0.990
Vaginal	48 (69%)	47 (67%)	
Cesarean	22 (31%)	23 (33%)	
NICU[c] stay	52 (74.3%)	0 (0%)	N/A[d]
Total length of stay (days)			< 0.001
Median (Interquartile range)	11.1 (5.3–22.3)	2.2 (1.9–2.6)	

NAS[a], Neonatal Abstinence Syndrome; [b]matched characteristic; *NICU*[c], Neonatal Intensive Care Unit; *N/A*[d], not applicable as controls were required to have no NICU stay; thus, the groups are different by definition

Patients with NAS had a total of 2072 weights recorded between birth and 400 days of age (median = 24, inter-quartile range 16–32) compared to 974 weights recorded (median = 12, inter-quartile range 10–16) during the same time period for matched controls. The majority (61%) of the weights for patients with NAS were recorded during the initial birth hospitalization with a median of 12 weights recorded during the birth hospitalization and a median of 9 weights recorded between newborn discharge and 400 days. In contrast, for matched controls, the median number of weights recorded during the birth hospitalization was 3, and a median of 10 weights were recorded between newborn discharge and 400 days.

Figure 2 displays individual growth trajectories of patients with NAS and their matched counterparts, while Fig. 3 shows the estimated percentile curves of weight as a function of time after birth for NAS patients and matched controls. Percentile estimates were generally similar between groups, although the 10th and 90th percentiles were wider for NAS patients. However, no differences were statistically significant between groups for any percentile.

In a subgroup analysis, Fig. 4 shows the percentile curves of patients with a diagnosis of NAS who received pharmacologic therapy ($N = 34$) and those who did not ($N = 36$). Differences between groups were non-significant for each percentile. In a separate subgroup analysis, Fig. 5 shows percentile curves of patients with NAS requiring pharmacologic therapy and matched controls. Differences were again non-significant.

Discussion

This retrospective, pilot analysis of data from a single center failed to reveal significant growth differences between birth and 1 year among those infants diagnosed with NAS when compared with matched controls. Further subgroup analysis of those NAS infants pharmacologically treated compared to matched controls did not demonstrate growth differences. These results conflict with our a priori hypotheses, which reflected known feeding difficulties and hyperphagia among infants with NAS.

Pediatric growth is a complex, multifactorial process influenced by genes, nutritional intake, the environment, overall health, and socioeconomic status (SES). In the newborn period, the NAS population is unique in its nutritional needs. The hypermetabolic state resulting from symptoms of withdrawal in combination with poor feeding places this patient population at risk for excessive weight loss in the neonatal period [7, 9]. While the neonate may compensate for this hypermetabolic state by increased intake [6], there is some evidence that these eating habits may lead to undue weight gain [8]. Our study failed to support either of these patterns of growth.

Instead, consistent with a previous investigation by Vance et al. [10], we found similar weight gain trends between infants affected by NAS and their matched counterparts. This likeness existed when comparing all infants with a diagnosis of NAS to matched controls and when comparing controls only to NAS patients with more severe disease who were treated with pharmacologic therapy. Reasons for this lack of difference may be due to our small sample size of just 70 patients. Indeed, there appears to be a trend, albeit non-significant, towards NAS patients having higher estimated weight values for the 90th percentile and smaller estimated values for the 10th percentile.

It is reasonable to presume differences may exist in the growth of this population for a number of reasons. Similar to previous study findings [3, 17], NAS patients cared for at our center were predominantly insured by Medicaid, a proxy for lower socioeconomic status [18]. There is an abundance of data that suggest children

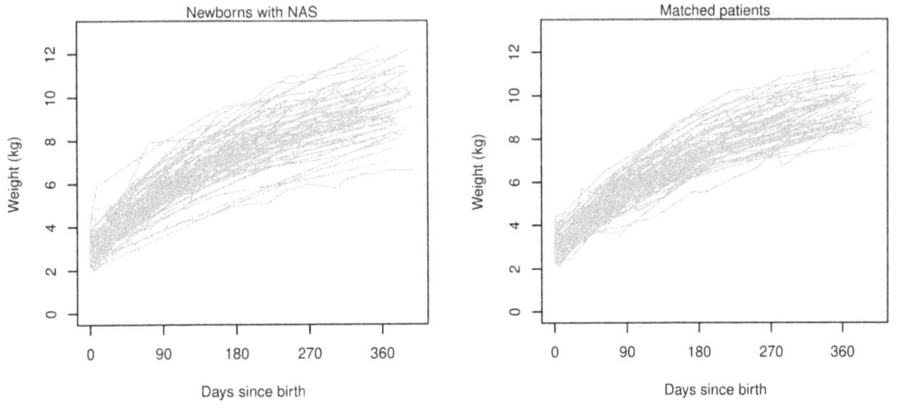

Fig. 2 Individual growth trajectories of weight for patients with neonatal abstinence syndrome (left) and matched comparison patients (right) show similar growth patterns

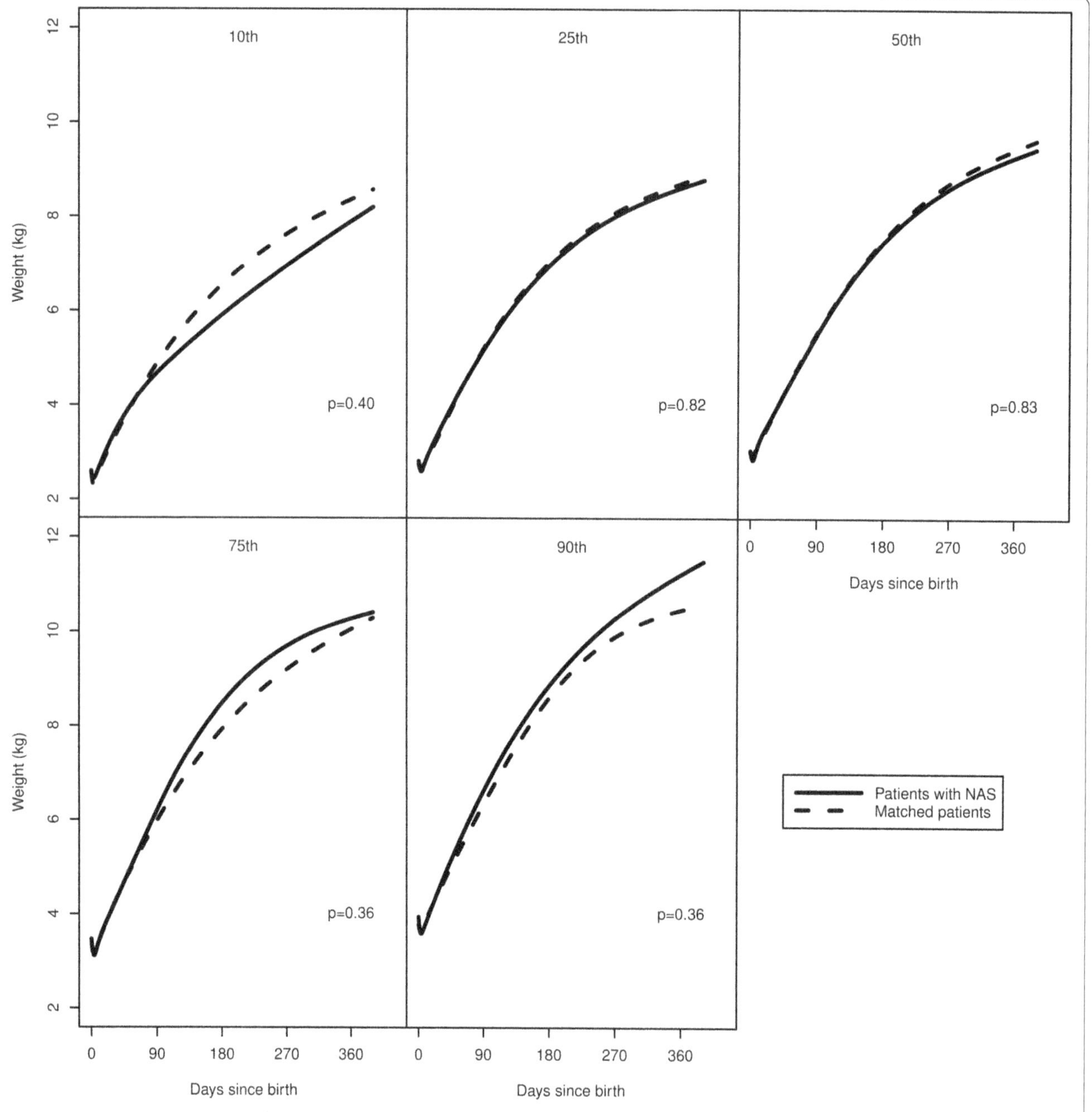

Fig. 3 Estimated percentile curves for patients with neonatal abstinence syndrome (NAS) and their matched comparison patients show similar growth patterns between patients with and without NAS

affected by poverty are at risk for abnormal weight gain. Wright et al. revealed that children of deprivation were 2.2 times more likely than children with adequate resources to have failure to thrive [19], and more recent data from developing countries suggest children from low-income households are at risk for both undernutrition and overnutrition [20, 21]. In developed countries such as the United States, there are numerous studies that indicate there is an inverse relationship between weight and SES [22–24].

However, the burden of NAS is experienced by members of all socioeconomic statuses, and deprivation alone is not the only reason to suspect variance in growth. There is compelling evidence to suggest early feeding behaviors affect childhood eating habits and weight [25, 26]. Hyperphagia and significant irritability are characteristic symptoms in newborns affected by NAS. In an effort to soothe these agitated infants, caregivers may feed to comfort under the incorrect assumption the infant is crying

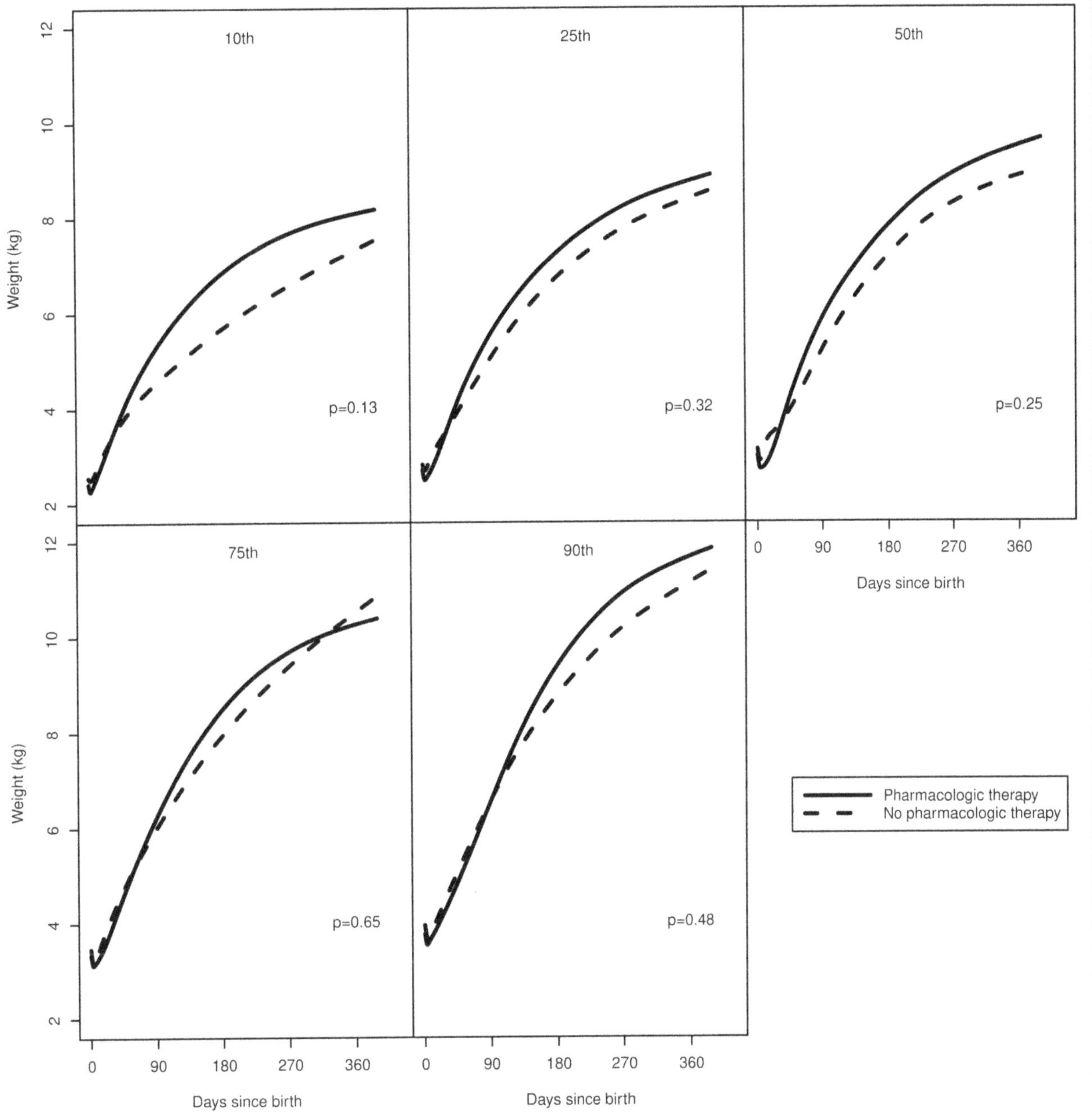

Fig. 4 Estimated percentile curves for patients with neonatal abstinence syndrome (NAS) stratified by pharmacologic therapy reveals no difference in growth between infants receiving pharmacologic treatment and those who do not

secondary to hunger. While infants have an innate ability to control their caloric intake [11, 12], parental feeding practices can alter eating behavior and affect subsequent weight gain and growth [13]. Therefore, it is reasonable to suspect that this population is at risk for development of abnormal feeding behaviors with a consequent tendency towards obesity. It is also equally plausible to presume this behavior is modifiable as recently demonstrated in the INSIGHT trial with infants not affected by NAS [27].

There are a number of limitations to our study. Our data are retrospective and gathered from a single center with a fairly homogenous population. Many patients ultimately received their post-discharge care outside the HMC system, and the resulting sample size is small and may conceal actual differences that exist in growth of this vulnerable population. Additionally, utilizing a hospital database for research depends on correct ICD coding. Failing to assign the relevant diagnostic code for an infant who displays symptoms of NAS may lead to

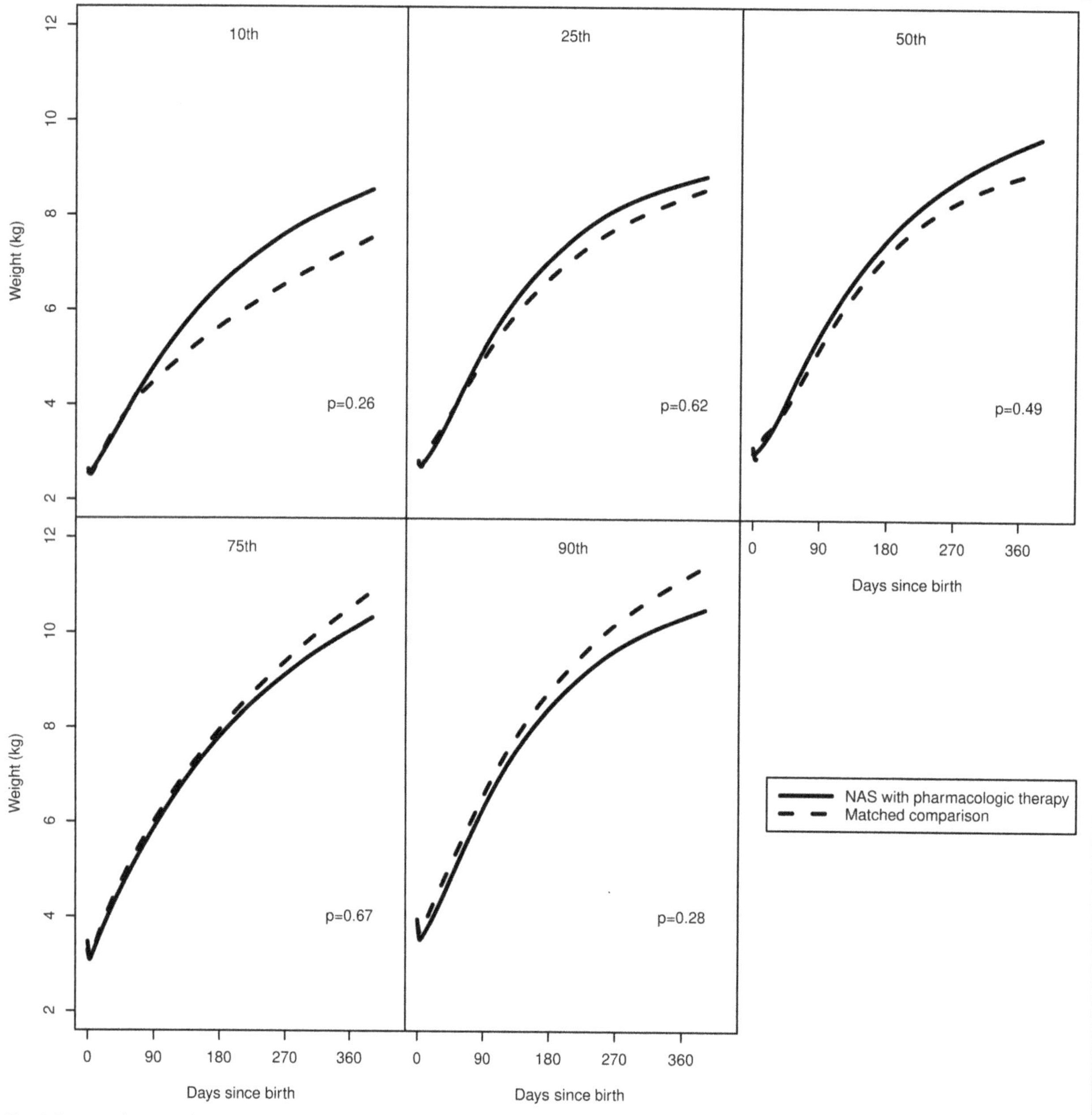

Fig. 5 Estimated percentile curves for patients with neonatal abstinence syndrome (NAS) who received pharmacologic therapy and matched comparison patients demonstrate no significant difference in growth over the first year

a falsely-low appreciation of the true extent of this syndrome at our institution. Conversely, inappropriately assigning a diagnosis of NAS to an infant being observed for NAS may lead to improper selection of the desired study population. Indeed, in our dataset, over half of the patients with a diagnosis of NAS did not receive pharmacologic management, suggesting that their symptoms were mild or they were inaccurately assigned such a diagnosis. Future research using a larger database with access to long-term follow-up data may clarify whether differences in growth exist between patients affected by NAS and their non-affected counterparts.

Conclusion

Infants with a diagnosis of NAS grew similarly to matched controls in this small, retrospective sample from a single center. Future studies may evaluate whether early differences in caregiver feeding exist, and if so, whether they have longer-term impacts on growth of these infants.

Abbreviations

EMR: Electronic medical records; HMC: Hershey Medical Center; IQR: Inter-quartile range; MFM: Maternal fetal medicine; NAS: Neonatal abstinence syndrome; NICU: Neonatal intensive care unit; SD: Standard deviation; SES: Socioeconomic status

Acknowledgements

The authors would like to acknowledge Jessica Beiler of the Penn State Health Pediatric Clinical Research Office for her assistance in data collection.

Funding

The first author received funding through the Penn State Children's Hospital, Children's Miracle Network to support the work completed in this study. They played no role in the design of the study or collection, analysis, and interpretation of data.

Authors' contributions

TC contributed to the conception and design of the study, interpretation of data, drafting the manuscript and approving the final version. ES contributed to the design of the study; acquisition, analysis, and interpretation of the data; drafting of the manuscript; and approving of the final version. IP contributed to the conception and design of the study, interpretation of data, editing of the manuscript, and approving of the final version of the manuscript.

Competing interests

The authors declare that they have no competing interests.

Author details

[1]Penn State College of Medicine, Department of Pediatrics, P.O. Box 850, 500 University Drive, Hershey, PA 17033-0850, USA. [2]Penn State College of Medicine, Department of Public Health Sciences, Hershey, PA, USA.

References

1. Patrick SW, Davis MM, Lehmann CU, Cooper WO. Increasing incidence and geographic distribution of neonatal abstinence syndrome: United States 2009 to 2012. J Perinatol. 2015;35(8):650–5.
2. Tolia VN, Patrick SW, Bennett MM, Murthy K, Sousa J, Smith PB, et al. Increasing incidence of the neonatal abstinence syndrome in U.S. neonatal ICUs. NEJM. 2015;372(22):2118–26.
3. Corr TE, Hollenbeak CS. The economic burden of neonatal abstinence syndrome in the United States. Addiction. 2017;112:1590–9.
4. Kocherlakota P. Neonatal abstinence syndrome. Pediatrics. 2014;134(2): e547–61.
5. Hudak ML, Tan RC. Neonatal drug withdrawal. Pediatrics. 2012;129(2): e540–e60.
6. Martinez A, Kastner B, Taeusch HW. Hyperphagia in neonates withdrawing from methadone. Arch Dis Child Fetal Neonatal Ed. 1999;80(3):F178–82.
7. Weinberger SM, Kandall SR, Doberczak TM, Thornton JC, Bernstein J. Early weight-change patterns in neonatal abstinence. Am J Dis Child. 1986;140(8):829–32.
8. Shephard R, Greenough A, Johnson K, Gerada C. Hyperphagia, weight gain and neonatal drug withdrawal. Acta Paediatr. 2002;91(9):951–3.
9. Dryden C, Young D, Campbell N, Mactier H. Postnatal weight loss in substitute methadone-exposed infants: implications for the management of breast feeding. Arch Dis Child Fetal Neonatal Ed. 2012;97(3):F214–6.
10. Vance JC, Chant DC, Tudehope DI, Gray PH, Hayes AJ. Infants born to narcotic dependent mothers: physical growth patterns in the first 12 months of life. J Paediatr Child Health. 1997;33(6):504–8.
11. Cohen RJ, Brown KH, Canahuati J, Rivera LL, Dewey KG. Effects of age of introduction of complementary foods on infant breast milk intake, total energy intake, and growth: a randomised intervention study in Honduras. Lancet. 1994;344(8918):288–93.
12. Fomon SJ, Filer LJ Jr, Thomas LN, Rogers RR, Proksch AM. Relationship between formula concentration and rate of growth of normal infants. J Nutr. 1969;98(2):241–54.
13. Paul IM, Bartok CJ, Downs DS, Stifter CA, Ventura AK, Birch LL. Opportunities for the primary prevention of obesity during infancy. Adv Pediatr Infect Dis. 2009;56:107–33.
14. Bergstralh DJKJ. Computerized matching of controls. Mayo Clinic: Rochester; 1995.
15. Koenker R. Quantile regression for longitudinal data. JMVA. 2004;91(1):74–89.
16. Koenker R, Ng PIN, Portnoy S. Quantile smoothing splines. Biometrika. 1994; 81(4):673–80.
17. Patrick SW, Schumacher RE, Benneyworth BD, Krans EE, McAllister JM, Davis MM. Neonatal abstinence syndrome and associated health care expenditures. JAMA. 2012;307(18):1934–40.
18. Rosenbaum S. Medicaid. NEJM. 2002;346(8):635–40.
19. Wright CM, Waterston A, Aynsley-Green A. Effect of deprivation on weight gain in infancy. Acta Paediatr. 1994;83(4):357–9.
20. Abdullah A. The double burden of undernutrition and overnutrition in developing countries: an update. Curr Obes Rep. 2015;4(3):337–49.
21. Tzioumis E, Adair LS. Childhood dual burden of under- and overnutrition in low- and middle-income countries: a critical review. Food Nutr Bull. 2014; 35(2):230–43.
22. Barriuso L, Miqueleiz E, Albaladejo R, Villanueva R, Santos JM, Regidor E. Socioeconomic position and childhood-adolescent weight status in rich countries: a systematic review, 1990-2013. BMC Pediatr. 2015;15:129.
23. Wang Y, Lim H. The global childhood obesity epidemic and the association between socio-economic status and childhood obesity. Int Rev Psychiatry. 2012;24(3):176–88.
24. Wu S, Ding Y, Wu F, Li R, Hu Y, Hou J, et al. Socio-economic position as an intervention against overweight and obesity in children: a systematic review and meta-analysis. Sci Rep. 2015;5:11354.
25. Davison KK, Birch LL. Childhood overweight: a contextual model and recommendations for future research. Obes Rev. 2001;2(3):159–71.
26. Savage JS, Fisher JO, Birch LL. Parental influence on eating behavior: conception to adolescence. J Law Med Ethics. 2007;35(1):22–34.
27. Savage JS, Birch LL, Marini M, Anzman-Frasca S, Paul IM. Effect of the INSIGHT responsive parenting intervention on rapid infant weight gain and overweight status at age 1 year: a randomized clinical trial. JAMA Pediatr. 2016;170(8):742–9.

19

Isolated neonatal bilateral vocal cord paralysis revealing a unilateral medullary defect

Camille Brotelande[1], Nicolas Leboucq[2], Mohamed Akkari[3], Thomas Roujeau[4], Massimo Di Maio[5], Christophe Milési[1], Michel Mondain[3], Charles Raybaud[6] and Gilles Cambonie[1*]

Abstract

Background: Congenital bilateral vocal cord paralysis is a rare occurrence. Approximately half the cases are associated with a major comorbidity, usually neurological, neuromuscular or malformative.

Case presentation: In a male newborn, respiratory distress syndrome and stridor were observed immediately following birth. The cause was bilateral vocal cord paralysis in the adducted position. Neuroradiological investigation revealed a unilateral discontinuity between the upper pons and the right medulla oblongata. Hypoplasia of the right posterior hemiarches of C1-C2 and the right exo-occipital bone was observed, as was a small clivus. MR angiography showed the absence of the distal right vertebral artery, with hypoplasia and parietal irregularities of the proximal segments. Respiratory autonomy was not obtained despite endoscopic laser cordotomy, corticosteroid therapy and nasal continuous positive airway pressure. The infant died at the age of 4 weeks after treatment was limited to comfort care.

Conclusions: A medullary lesion is an exceptional cause of congenital bilateral vocal cord paralysis. The strictly unilateral neurological and vascular defect and the absence of associated intracranial or extracranial malformation make this clinical case unique and suggest a disruptive mechanism. This case also highlights the help provided by advanced neuroimaging techniques, i.e. fibre tracking using diffusion tensor imaging, in the decision-making process.

Keywords: Bilateral vocal cord paralysis, Brainstem, Newborn

Background

Bilateral vocal cord paralysis (BVCP) is very rare in the neonate, with the incidence estimated at 0.75 cases per million births per year [1]. The series focused on congenital BVCP have highlighted two fairly well-balanced aetiological groups: one idiopathic and the other associated with major comorbidities [2–4]. The latter group includes mainly neonates with perinatal encephalopathy, neuromuscular diseases, chromosomal or genetic anomalies and major malformations [3, 5]. The malformations are generally intracranial in this context. Chiari 1 is the "classic" condition, but choroid plexus cysts, ventriculomegaly, hydrocephalus, myelomeningocele, and brainstem dysgenesis have also been described [3, 6]. We report an exceptional cause of isolated congenital BVCP, a unilateral medullary defect, and discuss its pathogenesis and the management strategy adopted in this specific case.

* Correspondence: g-cambonie@chu-montpellier.fr
[1]Department of Neonatology and Paediatric Intensive Care Unit, Arnaud de Villeneuve Hospital, Montpellier University Hospital, 371 Avenue du Doyen Gaston Giraud, 34295 Montpellier, Cedex 5, France
Full list of author information is available at the end of the article

Case presentation

This boy was born at 37^{+2} weeks of gestation from a 30-year-old mother. He was the first child of non-consanguineous and healthy Caucasian parents. The patient's mother received prenatal care during pregnancy. At 12 weeks, Doppler ultrasound (US) examination revealed increased resistance in the uterine arteries, and salicylic acid (100 mg daily) was prescribed. From the 23rd week, several Doppler US scans showed intrauterine growth retardation with persistent notching in the right uterine artery and increased resistance in the left. No scan revealed a malformation. Labour was spontaneous and the boy was born by vaginal delivery using Thierry's spatula because of abnormal foetal heart rate. Apgar scores were 4, 7 and 8 at 1, 5 and 10 min, respectively; arterial cord blood pH was 7.22 and cord lactate was 5.1 mmol/L. Birth weight was 2045 g (0.6th centile, according to customized French curves), length was 51 cm (91th centile), and head circumference was 32 cm (10th centile). The placenta was hypotrophic (280 g), with peripheral insertion of the cord and signs of maternal vascular hypoperfusion, but no lesion of decidual arteriopathy at pathological examination.

Respiratory distress, including suprasternal tugging and stridor, was observed immediately following birth. The neonate was bagged with air for a few minutes and then supported with nasal continuous positive airway pressure (CPAP). Prolonged apnoea associated with bradycardia required caffeine from the first postnatal day.

The first series of exams showed normal brain US and normal serum electrolytes with calcium. Flexible fibreoptic laryngoscopy (FFL) performed on day 2 revealed BVCP in the adducted position, causing severe airway obstruction and prompting transfer to a medical and surgical neonatal intensive care unit on day 3.

On admission, clinical examination revealed a wide anterior fontanel, enlarged coronal sutures, normal temperature, and persistent respiratory distress despite CPAP. Facial and ocular motricity were apparently normal, and the sucking reflex was present. The newborn was intubated a few hours later for worsening respiratory distress and severe apnoea. Rigid laryngotracheal endoscopy performed on day 4 under general anaesthesia showed neither malformation nor other obstruction below the glottis. Chest X-ray and abdominal and cardiac US were normal.

Neuroradiological investigations were performed between day 4 and day 15. The first brain MRI showed a deformation of the bulbo-medullary junction with an arched aspect in the anteroposterior direction slightly deflected to the left. Enlarged subarachnoid spaces and foramen magnum surrounded this junction. Cortical structures were normal, myelination was age-appropriate, and the pituitary axis and corpus callosum were normal (Fig. 1). Additional investigations were conducted, with MRI and CT focused on the cervico-occipital hinge. MRI showed a unilateral cavitated lesion, with discontinuity between the upper pons and the medulla oblongata. CT revealed vertebral anomalies, with hypoplasia of the right posterior hemiarches of C1-C2, hypoplasia of the right exo-occipital bone and a small clivus (Fig. 2). On day 15, MR angiography showed the absence of the distal right vertebral artery (Fig. 3). MRI with fibre tracking, using diffusion tensor imaging, confirmed hemisection of the right lateral and median sensorimotor fascicles (Fig. 4). Brainstem auditory evoked potentials and fundus examination were normal.

Patient management included a left unilateral endoscopic laser cordotomy on day 7 in order to proceed to extubation on day 8. The procedure was unsuccessful despite corticosteroid therapy and CPAP, and the infant was reintubated after 3 h due to the reappearance of stridor and major signs of respiratory distress. Mechanical ventilation was maintained until the end of the stay. The severity of this situation prompted a multidisciplinary ethics

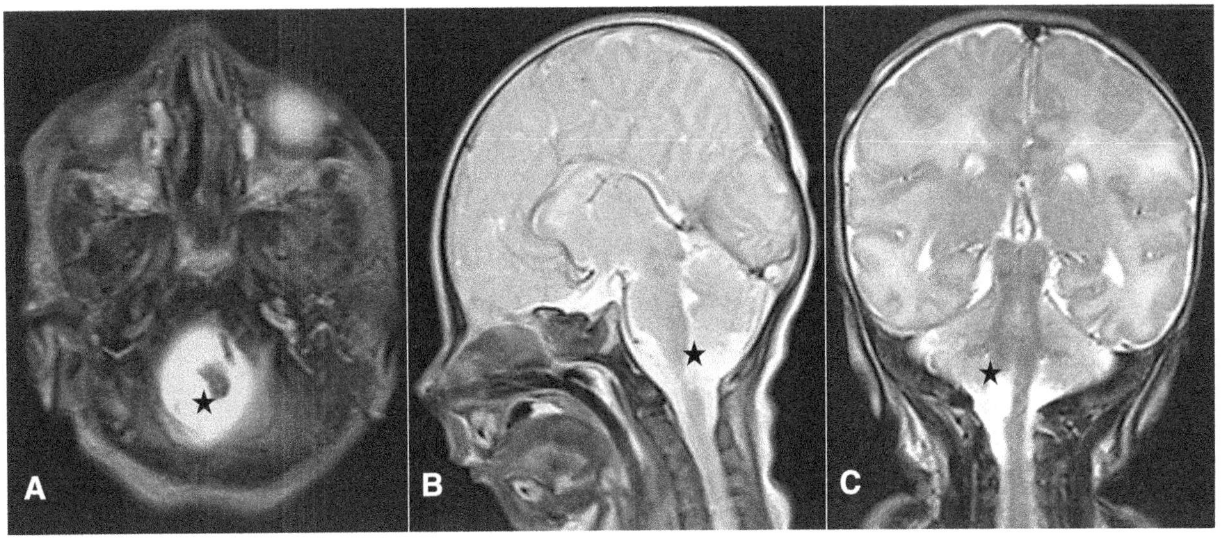

Fig. 1 Cerebral MRI. Axial (**a**), Sagittal (**b**) and Coronal (**c**) T2-weighted sequence showing deformation of the cervicomedullary junction with a focal defect within the right medulla oblongata (black stars)

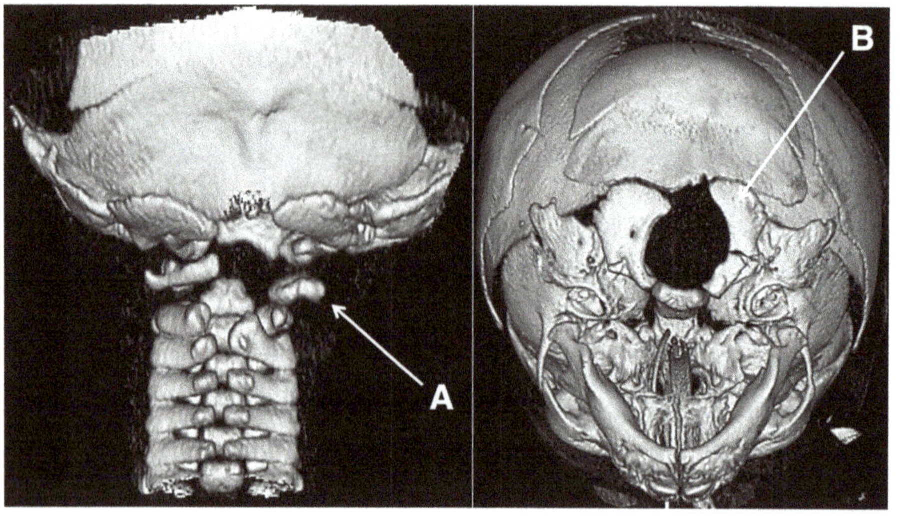

Fig. 2 3D bone CT reconstruction showing hypoplasia of the posterior hemiarches of C1-C2 (**a**) and the right exo-occipital bone (**b**) and a small clivus

consultation and the decision was made to limit care to the infant's comfort. The parents were informed and agreed with this decision, given the very poor respiratory and neurosensory prognosis. The infant died at the age of 4 weeks. An autopsy was not performed. Array comparative genomic hybridization revealed no abnormality.

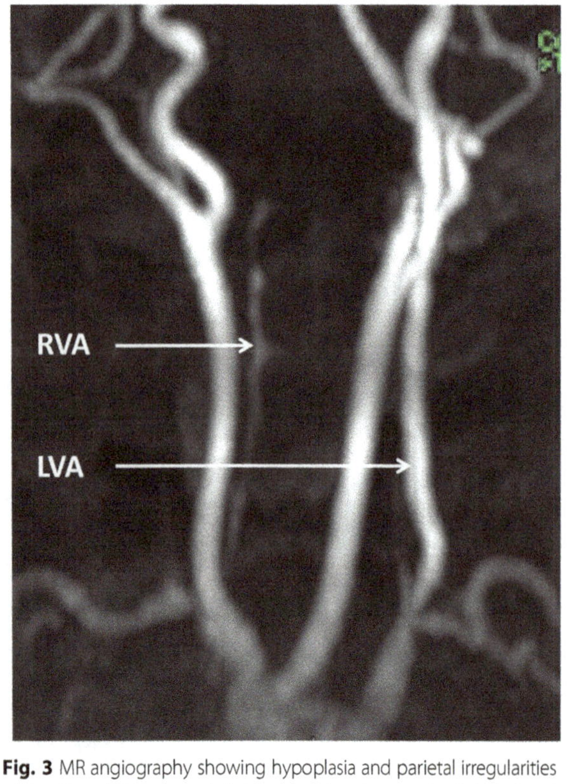

Fig. 3 MR angiography showing hypoplasia and parietal irregularities of the V1 and V2 segments (white arrow) and agenesis of the V3 and V4 segments of the right vertebral artery (RVA). LVA: left vertebral artery

Discussion

BVCP is generally diagnosed in neonates by the end of the first postnatal month [3]. Stridor is always a presenting feature, associated with respiratory difficulties of variable severity in 80–90% of the cases [7]. Direct visualization of the pharynx and larynx using FFL should be systematic to investigate stridor and enable dynamic study of vocal cord motility. This examination needs to be completed with rigid laryngotracheal endoscopy

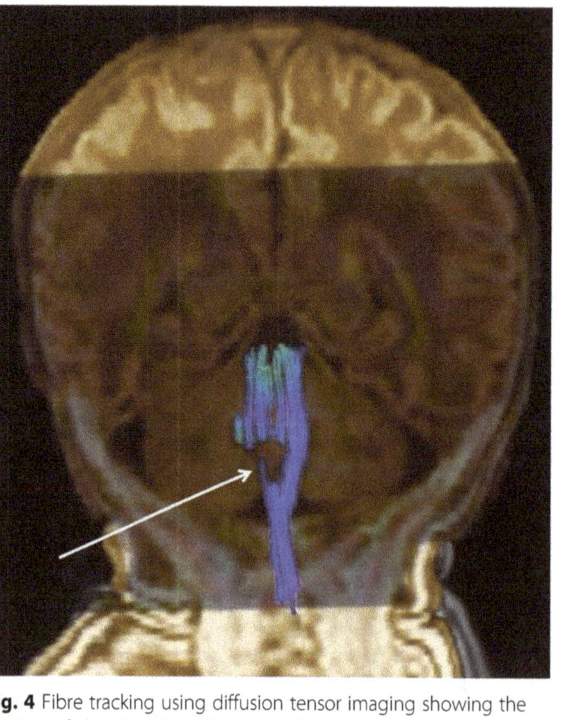

Fig. 4 Fibre tracking using diffusion tensor imaging showing the section of the right lateral and median sensorimotor fascicles (white arrow)

under general anaesthesia, for subglottic and tracheal assessment [8]. Other methods for exploring the laryngeal region have been proposed, but they are not routinely used in most centres. Laryngeal US provides dynamic morphometric parameters, and it may offer a less invasive means of evaluating vocal fold motility in critically ill neonates, which is particularly interesting for the follow-up of paralysis [9, 10]. Laryngeal electromyography can also help to better characterize laryngeal motility disorders and anticipate the prognosis of bilateral laryngeal palsies. Interpretation, however, is not fully standardized in neonates and children [11].

Unilateral or BVCP may occur in neonates following thoracic surgery, including cardiovascular surgery - mainly patent ductus arteriosus ligation [12] - and surgery for oesophageal atresia and/or tracheo-oesophageal fistula [13]. Outside of this context, additional examinations are needed to determine the underlying cause [14]. MRI of the brain, neck, mediastinum and chest provide detailed anatomical study of the brainstem, larynx, and the vagus and recurrent laryngeal nerves [15].

The central neurological disorders or anatomic abnormalities potentially associated with BVCP, including Chiari malformation alone or associated with myelomeningocele and hydrocephalus, can be detected on prenatal US examination. Williams syndrome, Moebius syndrome, congenital myasthenic syndrome, 22q deletion syndrome, and Down syndrome have occasionally been associated with BVCP in the neonatal period. Small series of familial congenital BVCP with variable inheritance patterns and chromosomal alterations have also been described [16].

In our case, MRI revealed a unilateral medullary defect, which has been referenced in the medical literature under the terms brainstem disconnection or brainstem disruption. Brainstem disconnection is a very rare congenital anomaly of the infratentorial region, defined by an absent brainstem segment. This regional discontinuity may be observed at the pontomesencephalic level but is more common at the pontomedullary level [17]. Most reports have described extensive defects, with only a thin cord of tissue between the rostral and caudal brainstem portions [18]. An asymmetrical defect or, as in our case, a unilateral defect is quite exceptional, having been reported only once within the left medulla oblongata and described by the authors as a brainstem disruption [19].

Prenatal diagnosis with foetal MRI has exceptionally been performed in cases of brainstem disconnection [20]. Polyhydramnios has been reported, probably in relation with impaired prenatal swallowing. In our patient, the sucking reflex was present, but it was difficult to determine whether deglutition was normal. In addition, the polyhydramnios may have been neutralized by the impaired uteroplacental perfusion. Cerebellar hypoplasia, sometimes detected with foetal US, has been observed in all patients with a severe defect. Other brain abnormalities have been inconsistently mentioned: absence of cerebellar peduncles, hypoplastic or absent optic nerves, absence of internal auditory canals, dilated cisterns or cerebral ventricles, periventricular nodular heterotopia, and hamartoma [20]. Extracerebral abnormalities, sometimes multiple in a single patient [21] and notably involving the axial skeleton, heart, and digestive and genitourinary tracts, have been noted in both pontomesencephalic and pontomedullary disconnections [17].

Arguments in favour of a genetic cause have mainly been raised for bilateral lesions and extensive forms associated with malformations, such as the neuronal migration disorders [22]. The absence of gliotic lesions on histological examination has also been interpreted in favour of this aetiology [23]. From this perspective, the brainstem dysgenesis results from an abnormal expression of segmentation genes or their upstream modulators at the midbrain-hindbrain boundary [17, 18]. Animal models, however, do not unequivocally reproduce segmental dysgenesis [24], and no mutation of candidate genes, such as EN2, or causative variations on whole exome sequencing have thus far been documented in humans [17, 22, 23].

Focal lesions, whether associated or not with abnormalities of the vertebrobasilar arterial system, have led to the alternative hypothesis of an acquired, i.e. disruptive, mechanism [19]. The previously described vascular abnormalities in brainstem disconnection were mainly the absence or the extreme hypoplasia of the vertebral or basilar arteries [20]. In our case, MR angiography demonstrated hypoplasia and parietal irregularities of the proximal segments and absence of the distal segments of the right vertebral artery. The unilateral, well-defined, elliptical anteroposterior lesion of the cervico-medullary junction in our patient may be consistent with intrauterine ischaemia, but the precise timing of the insult is difficult to establish. During the early embryonic period, the posterior circulation is exclusively supplied by the internal carotid arteries through a series of anastomoses that will regress with the development of the vertebrobasilar arterial system [25]. The trigeminal, otic and hypoglossal arteries intervene in the formation of the basilar artery. The cervical portion of the vertebral artery, i.e. the V1 and V2 segments, is formed by anastomoses from the first six cervical intersegmental arteries, while the proatlantal intersegmental artery contributes to the formation of the V3 and V4 segments. In our patient, the lack of visualization of the V3 and V4 segments of the right vertebral artery on MR angiography may be explained by early occlusion or agenesis of the proatlantal artery. However, the origins of these vascular abnormalities may also be dysplastic or inflammatory, in parallel with the vascular involvement observed as early as 12 weeks of gestation at the level of placenta. Moreover, the resulting ischaemia may have caused the focal defect at the medullary level, the homolateral hypoplasia of the exo-occipital bone, and the lateral mass of C1. Indeed, these last two elements probably have a common embryological origin, from the fourth occipital and the first spinal sclerotomes, and they are also perfused by the proatlantal artery [26]. The hypoplasia of the right transverse process of C2 might be related to the hypoplasia of segments V1 and V2, its blood supply being provided by the first intersegmental cervical artery [27]. Other causes of disruptions, such as alcohol or cocaine exposure during pregnancy, have also been described in brainstem disconnection [28, 29]. Nevertheless, the controversy concerning a malformative or vascular origin of this condition has not yet been resolved. The involvement of genes critical for both the formation of the brainstem and its vascularization should also not be excluded [22].

In our patient, the initial decision for endoscopic surgical treatment was taken before MRI with fibre tracking demonstrated the unilateral medullary defect. However, neither this treatment nor CPAP, which can potentiate the results of an endoscopic procedure [4], prevented rapid reintubation. Several elements were taken into account in the multidisciplinary decision to limit curative care. The prognosis of brainstem disconnection is generally very poor, with respiratory failure occurring soon after support is removed. Death generally occurs in the first 2 months following birth, but cases of prolonged survival under chronic respiratory assistance have occasionally been described [22, 30]. Indeed, functional respiratory outcome is very poor in the event of congenital BVCP associated with major underlying comorbidity, with resolution of the vocal cord immobility in only 14% of patients and decannulation after 2 to 3 years in 25% [3, 31]. More recently, survival without mechanical ventilation has also been reported; however, gastrostomy was systematically needed, as well as tracheostomy at times [17, 19]. No or minimal achievement of developmental milestones has been noted in children with large defects [17]. In our case, characterized by a rather well-circumscribed, unilateral defect, tractography was particularly useful for reconstructing the course of the fibre tracts within the brainstem [32]. This microstructural analysis highlighted a section with several bundles, including the corticospinal, spinothalamic and spinocerebellar tracts, and the medial lemniscus. In addition, the topography of the lesion suggested the involvement of parts of the spinal tract of the right trigeminal nerve, the right nucleus tractus solitarii, the right cuneiform nucleus and the medullary reticular formation. In our patient, the BVCP also expressed the involvement of the ambiguus nuclei, which intervene in the motor innervation of the laryngeal muscles and adjoin the median raphe at the lower part of the medulla. Thus, relatively small lesions of the brainstem can have dramatic consequences, as nicely expressed by Boltshauser et al.: "small lesions-big problems" [19]. These authors reported on two children, aged 19 months and 32 months, with unilateral or asymmetrical defects. The examinations confirmed the multiple and major consequences of these lesions, in particular swallowing impairment, cranial nerve deficits, hemiparesis, and motor, speech and cognitive delays [19].

Conclusion

An isolated BVCP in a neonate can be caused by a medullary defect, a very rare congenital anomaly. This case report contributes to the phenotypic description of this poorly understood entity, here characterized by a strictly unilateral neurological and vascular defect and the absence of associated malformation. It also highlights the complexity of the decision-making process and the help provided by advanced neuroimaging techniques to analyse the hindbrain region.

Abbreviations

BVCP: Bilateral vocal cord paralysis; C1: 1st cervical vertebra; C2: 2nd cervical vertebra; CPAP: Continuous positive airway pressure; CT: Computed tomography; FFL: Flexible fibreoptic laryngoscopy; MRI: Magnetic resonance imaging; US: Ultrasound

Acknowledgements

The authors thank C Stott for reviewing the manuscript and for editorial assistance.

Funding

No financial support was received.

Authors' contributions

CB reviewed the literature and prepared the manuscript; NL reviewed the literature and prepared the manuscript; MA reviewed the literature and prepared the manuscript; TR, MDM, CM and MM were involved in patient care, helped to draft the manuscript and critically read the manuscript; CR helped to draft the manuscript and critically read the manuscript; and GC reviewed the literature, prepared the manuscript and is the corresponding author. All authors read and approved the final version of the manuscript.

Competing interests

The authors declare that they have no competing interests.

Author details
[1]Department of Neonatology and Paediatric Intensive Care Unit, Arnaud de Villeneuve Hospital, Montpellier University Hospital, 371 Avenue du Doyen Gaston Giraud, 34295 Montpellier, Cedex 5, France. [2]Department of Paediatric Radiology, Arnaud de Villeneuve Hospital, Montpellier University Hospital, Montpellier, France. [3]Department of Otorhinolaryngology, Gui-de-Chauliac Hospital, Montpellier University Hospital, Montpellier, France. [4]Department of Neurosurgery, Gui-de-Chauliac Hospital, Montpellier University Hospital, Montpellier, France. [5]Neonatal Intensive Care Unit, Carémeau Hospital, Nîmes University Hospital, Nîmes, France. [6]Division of Neuroradiology, Hospital for Sick Children, University of Toronto, 555 University Avenue, Toronto, ON M5G1X8, Canada.

References

1. Murty GE, Shinkwin C, Gibbin KP. Bilateral vocal fold paralysis in infants: tracheostomy or not? J Laryngol Otol. 1994;108:329–31.
2. Miyamoto RC, Parikh SR, Gellad W, Licameli GR. Bilateral congenital vocal cord paralysis: a 16-year institutional review. Otolaryngol Head Neck Surg. 2005;133:241–5.
3. Nisa L, Holtz F, Sandu K. Paralyzed neonatal larynx in adduction. Case series, systematic review and analysis. Int J Pediatr Otorhinolaryngol. 2013;77:13–8.
4. Lesnik M, Thierry B, Blanchard M, Glynn F, Denoyelle F, Couloigner V, Garabedian N, Leboulanger N. Idiopathic bilateral vocal cord paralysis in infants: case series and literature review. Laryngoscope. 2015;125:1724–8.
5. Holinger LD, Holinger PC, Holinger PH. Etiology of bilateral abductor vocal cord paralysis: a review of 389 cases. Ann Otol Rhinol Laryngol. 1976;85: 428–36.
6. Kuo CH, Niu CK, Yu HR, Chung MY, Hwang CF, Hwang KP. Applications of flexible bronchoscopy in infants with congenital vocal cord paralysis: a 12-year experience. Pediatr Neonatol. 2008;49:183–8.
7. Jabbour J, Martin T, Beste D, Robey T. Pediatric vocal fold immobility: natural history and the need for long-term follow-up. JAMA Otolaryngol Head Neck Surg. 2014;14:428–33.
8. Daya H, Hosni A, Bejar-Solar I, Evans JN, Bailey CM. Pediatric vocal fold paralysis: a long-term retrospective study. Arch Otolaryngol Head Neck Surg. 2000;126:21–5.
9. Wang LM, Zhu Q, Ma T, Li JP, Hu R, Rong XY, Xu W, Wang ZC. Value of ultrasonography in diagnosis of pediatric vocal fold paralysis. Int J Pediatr Otorhinolaryngol. 2011;75:1186–90.
10. Ongkasuwan J, Ocampo E, Tran B. Laryngeal ultrasound and vocal fold movement in the pediatric cardiovascular intensive care unit. Laryngoscope. 2017;127:167–72.
11. AlQudehy Z, Norton J, El-Hakim H. Electromyography in children's laryngeal mobility disorders: a proposed grading system. Arch Otolaryngol Head Neck Surg. 2012;138:936–41.
12. Strychowsky JE, Rukholm G, Gupta MK, Reid D. Unilateral vocal fold paralysis after congenital cardiothoracic surgery: a meta-analysis. Pediatrics. 2014;133: e1708–23.
13. Morini F, Iacobelli BD, Crocoli A, Bottero S, Trozzi M, Conforti A, Bagolan P. Symptomatic vocal cord paresis/paralysis in infants operated on for esophageal atresia and/or tracheo-esophageal fistula. J Pediatr. 2011;158:973–6.
14. Ada M, Isildak H, Saritzali G. Congenital vocal cord paralysis. J Craniofac Surg. 2010;21:273–4.
15. Parkes WJ, Propst EJ. Advances in the diagnosis, management, and treatment of neonates with laryngeal disorders. Semin Fetal Neonatal Med. 2016;21:270–6.
16. Hsu AK, Rosow DE, Wallerstein RJ, April MM. Familial congenital bilateral vocal fold paralysis: a novel gene translocation. Int J Pediatr Otorhinolaryngol. 2015;79:323–7.
17. Poretti A, Denecke J, Miller DC, Schiffmann H, Buhk JH, Grange DK, Doherty D, Boltshauser E. Brainstem disconnection: two additional patients and expansion of the phenotype. Neuropediatrics. 2015;46:139–44.
18. Barkovich AJ, Millen KJ. Dobyns WB. A developmental and genetic classification for midbrain-hindbrain malformations. Brain. 2009;132:3199–230.
19. Boltshauser E, Bauder F, Giarrana M, Hackenberg A, Lebon S, Roulet-Perez E, Schmid R, Schmitt-Mechelke T, Poretti A. Prenatal brainstem disruptions: small lesions-big problems. Neuropediatrics. 2017;48:350–5.
20. Carr JR, Brandon J, Ross B, Bryant SO. Fetal MRI diagnosis of brainstem disconnection with novel inner ear anomalies. Prenat Diagn. 2014;34: 1018–21.
21. Duffield C, Jocson J, Wootton-Gorges SL. Brainstem disconnection. Pediatr Radiol. 2009;39:1357–60.
22. Okumura A, Lee T, Shimojima K, Hisata K, Shoji H, Takanashi J, Yamamoto T, Shimizu T, Barkovich AJ. Brainstem disconnection associated with nodular heterotopia and proatlantal arteries. Am J Med Genet A. 2009;149A:2479–83.
23. Sarnat HB, Benjamin DR, Siebert JR, Kletter GB, Cheyette SR. Agenesis of the mesencephalon and metencephalon with cerebellar hypoplasia: putative mutation in the EN2 gene--report of 2 cases in early infancy. Pediatr Dev Pathol. 2002;5:54–68.
24. Lumsden A. Segmentation and compartition in the early avian hindbrain. Mech Dev. 2004;121:1081–8.
25. Gregg L, Gailloud P. The role of the primitive lateral basilovertebral anastomosis of padget in variations of thevertebrobasilar arterial system. Anat Rec (Hoboken). 2017;300:2025–38.
26. Huang R, Zhi Q, Patel K, Wilting J, Christ B. Contribution of single somites to the skeleton and muscles of the occipital and cervical regions in avian embryos. Anat Embryol (Berl). 2000;202:375–83.
27. Padget DH. Designation of the embryonic intersegmental arteries in reference to the vertebral artery and subclavian stem. Anat Rec. 1954;119: 349–56.
28. Boix H, Ortega-Aznar A, Vazquez E, Salcedo S, Roig-Quilis M. Brainstem dysgenesis in an infant prenatally exposed to cocaine. Pediatr Neurol. 2010; 42:295–7.
29. Yigazu P, Kalra V, Altinok D. Brainstem disconnection in a late preterm neonate with classic features of fetal alcohol syndrome. Pediatr Neurol. 2014;51:745–6.
30. Jurkiewicz E, Dobrzańska A, Nowak K, Pleskaczyńska A. MRI findings in the young infant with brainstem disconnection and extracerebral features. Report of one case and review of the literature. Brain and Dev. 2010;32:495–8.
31. Funk RT, Jabbour J, Robey T. Factors associated with tracheotomy and decannulation in pediatric bilateral vocal fold immobility. Int J Pediatr Otorhinolaryngol. 2015;79:895–9.
32. Jissendi-Tchofo P, Severino M, Nguema-Edzang B, Toure C, Soto Ares G, Barkovich AJ. Update on neuroimaging phenotypes of mid-hindbrain malformations. Neuroradiology. 2015;57:113–38.

20

Newborn colonization and antibiotic susceptibility patterns of *Streptococcus agalactiae* at the University of Gondar Referral Hospital, Northwest Ethiopia

Mucheye Gizachew[1*], Moges Tiruneh[1], Feleke Moges[1], Mulat Adefris[2], Zemene Tigabu[3] and Belay Tessema[1]

Abstract

Background: Group B *Streptococcus* (GBS) that asymptomatically colonizing the recto-vaginal area of women is the most important cause of neonatal colonization. There is paucity of evidence about newborn colonization with GBS in Ethiopia. Thus, this study was aimed to determine the prevalence of newborn colonization with GBS, antibiotic susceptibility patterns of the isolates and associated risk factors at the University of Gondar Referral Hospital in Northwest Ethiopia

Methods: A prospective cross sectional study was conducted from December 2016 to November 2017. A total of 1,155 swabs from nasal, ear and umbilical areas of the newborns were collected from the 385 newborns. Identifications of the isolates and antibiotic susceptibility testing were done by using conventional methods.

Results: Sixty two (16.1%, 95% CI: 12.2% - 20%) of the newborns were colonized by GBS. Seven percent of the total specimens were positive for GBS. The antibiotics susceptibility rates of GBS (average of the three body sites tested) were 95.1%, 89.6%, 88.9%, 85.7%, 85.3%, 81.3%, 76.9%, 76.1%, 73.8%, and 34.4% to ampicillin, penicillin, ciprofloxacin, chloramphenicol, vancomycin, azitromycin, erythromycin, clindamycin, ceftriaxone, and tetracycline, respectively. A multilogistic regression analyses were shown that the newborns that were from mothers whose education status was below tertiary level, and newborns from mothers who were: being employed, being nullipara and multigravida were at risk for colonization with GBS.

Conclusion: Prevalence of neonatal colonization with GBS was higher than it was reported in three decades ago in Ethiopia. Ciprofloxacin, chloramphenicol, vancomycin and azithromycin were identified as the drug of choice next to ampicillin and penicillin.

Keywords: Antibiotic susceptibility pattern, Colonization, Group B Streptococcus, Newborns

Background

The 2016 Ethiopian Demographic and Health Survey (EDHS) indicates that the overall mortality rate of under five children is 67/1000 live births, with the infant mortality rate of 48% (29% neonatal and 19% post-neonatal) deaths/1,000 live births. The estimate of child mortality is 20 deaths/1000 children surviving to 12 months of age [1]. Women in the Amhara National Regional State have the fertility rate of 4.2, and infant and maternal mortality rates of 76/1000 live births and 676/100,000, respectively [2]. Asymptomatic *Streptococcus agalactiae* (Group B Streptococcus, GBS) recto-vaginal colonization of women is assumed to be one of the contributing factors. It is the most significant pathogen, although little is known about its epidemiology and risk in resource limited countries [3]. Since neonatal infections cause a significant proportion of deaths in the first week of life, more data are needed about the burden of neonatal colonization [4].

* Correspondence: muchegiza@gmail.com
[1]Department of Medical Microbiology, School of Biomedical and Laboratory Sciences, College of Medicine and Health Sciences, University of Gondar, P. O. Box 196, Gondar, Ethiopia
Full list of author information is available at the end of the article

Since 1960s, GBS has been identified as a major public health problem that causes perinatal morbidity and mortality. It also became the most prevalent causes of fatal infections in newborns [5–7]. The researchers estimated about 410,000 GBS cases and 147,000 stillbirths and infant deaths are estimated to occur every year. Despite containing 13% of the world's population, Africa had the highest burden with 54% cases and 65% of stillbirths and infant deaths [8]. GBS causes sepsis, pneumonia, and meningitis in neonates; bacteraemia, amnionitis, endometritis, and urinary tract infection in pregnant women [9–11]. The Global prevalence of GBS neonatal colonization rate ranged from 1.6% in Turkey [12] to 52.9% in Pakistan [13], and South Africa took the lion share among few African reports [14]. However, evidence on GBS colonization rate of newborns largely remains sparse in the African setting, particularly in Ethiopia.

Furthermore, provision of empiric treatment brings up antibiotic resistance and stewardship issues [8]. Reports from different countries revealed the reduced susceptibility to penicillin, and the increased rate of macrolide resistance GBS isolates for the last few decades [15]. A 2005-2007 Surveillance in Argentina showed the presence of GBS isolates resistance (in minimum inhibitory concentration; MIC range μg /L) to ciprofloxacin (32-64 μg/L), levofloxacin (16-32 μg/L), ofloxacin (32-64 μg/L), and norfloxacin (32-64 μg/L), and all were susceptible to penicillin (0.06 μg/L) (16). Of the 1160 GBS isolates in Australia, 6.4% demonstrated erythromycin resistance and 4.2% to clindamycin [16]. Another study in USA revealed that all the neonatal GBS were susceptible to penicillin, vancomycin, chloramphenicol, and cefotaxime. Its resistance rates to erythromycin was 20.2%, and 6.9% to clindamycin [17]. Another study in France revealed 38.2% erythromycin and 25.6% clindamycin resistance neonatal GBS [18]. However, as is the case in several other African countries, neonatal GBS colonization in Ethiopia has not been well documented. In addition, no preventive strategies for GBS infection have been yet formulated in the study area. Thus, this study was aimed to determine the prevalence of newborn colonization with GBS, its antibiotic susceptibility profile, and associated risk factors in University of Gondar referral hospital, Northwest Ethiopia.

Methods

Study area

The study was conducted at the University of Gondar Referral Hospital, Northwest Ethiopia. The University of Gondar Referral Hospital is one of the oldest hospitals located 737 km away from Addis Ababa, the Capital of Ethiopia with the Latitude of 12°31`N,and Longitude 37°25`E.. The Central Statistical Agency of Ethiopia population projection report and the Amhara National Regional State Health Bureau report showed that the Amhara region has a population of 20,018,988, of which, 49.92% were females, and 15.62% of the total population was urban inhabitants. The hospital serves about five million people. It has 450 to 600 delivery admission services a month. No GBS screening and provision of intrapartum antibiotic prophylaxis for pregnant women established yet in the hospital.

Study Design and Period

A prospective cross-sectional study design was conducted between December 2016 and November 2017.

Population

Source population

All newborns who were delivered at the University of Gondar Referral Hospital in Northwest Ethiopia were the source population.

Study population

The study populations were those newborns delivered from pregnant women whose gestational age was ≥ 35 weeks.

Inclusion and exclusion criteria

Inclusion criteria

Newborns whose mothers not on antibiotics during delivery and those newborns who have been delivered vaginally at ≥35 gestational weeks of pregnancy, and infants ≤ 30 minutes were included in the study.

Exclusion criteria

Newborns whose mothers; did use vaginal cream, lubricants or traditional sterilizer (vinegar) in the last 10 days prior to giving birth; were in emergency room, severely ill, current vaginal bleeding, use of an intra-vaginal product in the past 24hours (douche, antifungal products), mentally unstable pregnant women; those who were in multiple birth and refusal for study participation from mothers or guardians were excluded.

Sample size determination

The sample size was calculated using the single population proportion estimation formula by taking 5% as the prevalence of neonatal GBS colonization [19].

$n = \frac{z^2{}_{\alpha/2} \times p(1-P)}{d^2}$ Where; n= sample size, p = prevalence of neonatal colonization with GBS in Ethiopia (p = 5%), d= maximum allowable error (margin of error) = 0.05, Z = value of standard normal distribution (Z-statistic) at 95% confidence level (z=1.96) and it became 73 newborns; however, to increase the precision/validity of the findings, the sample size was increased to 385 by taking p = 50%.

Variables

Dependent variable

Colonization of newborns with Group B Streptococcus (GBS), Antibiotic susceptibility patterns of GBS.

Independent variables

Maternal age, residence, education, and occupation, gestational age, parity, history of still birth, history of abortion, gravidity, antenatal care (ANC) visit, contraceptive use, history of preterm delivery, length of premature rupture of membrane (ROM), human immune deficiency virus (HIV) status, sex of newborn, Appearance, Pulse, Grimace, Activity, and Respiration (APGAR) score, history of neonatal death, newborn`s weight (Kg), resuscitation required, Newborn to mother immediate close contact (baby with the mother soon following delivery or baby not in the neonatal intensive care unit), duration of labor (hours).

Data collection, sampling technique and laboratory procedures

Demographic and biological data were collected from the newborns immediately following birth pregnant women with ≥ 35 gestational weeks of pregnancy by trained midwives at the maternity ward in the hospital until the pre-determined sample size was reached.

Questionnaire

A pre-tested questionnaire (Additional file 1) 5% (20) was used to collect the data for the assessment of the study participants` (pregnant women with ≥ 35 gestational weeks) demographic situations and to investigate the associated risk factors to newborn GBS colonization. Questionnaire were prepared in English using published studies with certain change and translated into the local language (Amharic). The response of each participant re-translated into English for analysis and report.

Biological Specimen collection

Three body surface site (nasal, umbilical and ear) swabs of newborns were collected and analyzed at the University of Gondar Microbiology Laboratory by using the recommended methods [10, 20].

Swab culture

Using the Centers for Disease Control and prevention (CDC) guidelines, nasal, umbilical and ear swabs were collected from each newborn and placed in the non nutritive Amies transport medium. Within 2 to 4 hours of collection, the swabs were placed in Todd-Hewitt selective enrichment broth supplemented with colistin (10μg/ml) and naldixic acid (15μg/mL) (Cart Roth GmbH + Co. KG-Schoemperlensrr. 3-5-D-76185 Karisruhe, Germany). The inoculated selective medium was incubated at 37 °C in 5% CO_2 for 24hours. The growth (turbidity) was sub-cultured in 5% defibrinated sheep-blood agar and incubated for 24 hours at 37 °C in 5% CO_2 atmosphere. All suspected colonies (with narrow hemplysis) were sub-cultured on nutrient agar and subjected to gram stain and catalase test. All gram positive cocci and catalase negative isolates were tested for CAMP factor for presumptive identification.

CAMP (Christie–Atkins–Munch-Petersen) test

CAMP test was used to differentiate GBS (CAMP positive) from *Streptococcus pyogene* (beta-hemolytic CAMP negative) by inoculating the known *Staphylococcus aureus* onto 5% defibrinated sheep blood agar down the center of the plate with a wire loop. Group B Streptococcus (test bacterium) was then streaked in a straight line perpendicular to the *S. aureus* within 2mm far. The plate was then incubated at 35 °C for 24 hours. A positive CAMP result was indicated by an arrowhead-shaped enhanced zone of beta-hemolysis in the area between the test organism and *S. aureus* with the arrow-point towards the *S. aureus* streak. The CAMP test positive colonies were presumptively considered as GBS

Antibiotic susceptibility testing of Group B Streptococcus

Susceptibility of GBS isolates were tested against 10 antibiotics (Oxoid, Basingstoke, UK):penicillin G (P, 10 IU), ampicillin (AMP, 10μg), clindamycin (CLY, 2μg), erythromycin (E, 15μg), chloramphenicol (C,30μg), ciprofloxacin (CIP,5μg), ceftriaxone (CRO, 30μg), vancomycin (VA, 30μg), Azithromycin (AZM, 15 μg), and tetracycline (TE, 30 μg) on Mueller-Hinton agar (MHA) containing 5% sheep blood according to the Kirby-Bauer method (disk diffusion) and the CLSI criteria. An inoculum was ready by suspending 4 -5 freshly grown GBS colonies in 3-5 ml sterile physiological saline. The turbidity was adjusted to a 0.5 McFarland standard [20, 21] used as a reference to adjust the bacterial suspension for antibiotic susceptibility test. The suspension was then swabbed over the entire surface of the Muller Hinton agar containing 5% defibrinated sheep blood by using sterile cotton tip applicator. Antibiotics disks were placed in the plate and incubated in 5% CO_2 atmosphere at 37 °C for 24 hours. Zone of inhibition around antibiotic disks was measured by calibrated ruler and interpreted as sensitive, intermediate or resistant by comparing it with the standard chart [20].

Double disc diffusion

Clindamycin and erythromycin susceptibility tests and determination of different phenotypes of macrolide-lincosamide-streptogramin B (MLS_B) resistance were performed by the double-disk test on Mueller-Hinton agar (Biokar, France) containing 5% sheep blood as previously described [20, 22–24]. Erythromycin (15 μg) and clindamycin (2 μg) disks (Oxoid, UK) were placed 12mm apart edge to edge [20]. After 24 hours of incubation at 37°C, blunting of the clindamycin inhibition zone proximal to the erythromycin disk was taken as inducible clindamycin resistance. Constitutive clindamycin resistance was the resistance to both clindamycin and erythromycin without blunting of the clindamycin inhibition zone. Susceptibility to clindamycin but resistance to erythromycin without blunting of the inhibition zone around the clindamycin disk was the efflux mechanism (the M-phenotype). Eventually, resistance to clindamycin but susceptible to erythromycin was referred to as L phenotype as previously described [24, 25].

Quality control

Half day training was given to the data collectors and they were closely supervised during data collection. Pre-test was done before the actual work to check the protocol for isolation of GBS and the questionnaire for collection of demography and clinical factors of the study participants. Data cleaning were done daily. *Streptococcus agalactiae* (ATCC 12386), *Enterococcus faecalis* (ATCC 29212); *Streptococcus pyogenes* (ATCC 19615), *Staphylococcus aureus* (ATCC 29213) and *Escherichia coli* (ATCC 25922) were used as quality control throughout the study.

Data analysis and interpretation

A total of 385 newborns were enrolled in the study and the collected data were entered into excel spread sheet and exported to SPSS 20 (Chicago, IL, USA) and analyzed. Association between the outcome variable (colonization of newborns with GBS) and each independent variable (demography and clinical factors) was analyzed using bi-variable and multi-variable logistic regression model. All the variables were entered into the multivariable logistic regression using backward LR method to control the confounding effect. Explanatory variables which had significant association with the newborn GBS colonization at a p-value ≤ 0.2 in the bivariable binary logistic regression model were entered to the multivariable logistic regression model to identify the factors associated to the colonization of newborns with GBS. Association between the outcome and the independent variables was calculated by using the adjusted odds ratio at a p-value ≤ 0.05 and 95% confidence interval. Assumption of goodness of the model was checked by Hosmer-lemeshow test (p = 0.828).

Ethical considerations

The study was reviewed and approved by the Ethical Review Committees of the University of Gondar (IRB) before data collection. Permission was obtained from the Hospitals administrative bodies. The study participants were informed about the study before collecting any data or samples. Written informed consent and/or assent obtained from the study participants. Ear, nasal and umbilical swabs were collected by experienced midwives and processed in the bacteriology laboratory using conventional methods. Participants (mothers) had full right to continue or withdraw their newborns from the study. Confidentiality of all participants' information was maintained throughout the study.

Results

Demographic, obstetric characteristics and Group B Streptococcus colonization of newborns

As shown in Table 1, among the total of 385 newborns tested, 56.1% were males, 99.2% were delivered at > 37 gestational weeks of pregnancy, 89.6% newborns were weighed 2.5kg or more, and 82.1% of the newborn were delivered within 12 hours of labor. Most of the newborns` mothers (74.3%) were housewives and 35.6% of the mothers had secondary educational status followed by primary school level (34%).

A total of 1,155 swabs from three body surface sites were collected and 81 (7.0%) of the specimens were positive for GBS. Among the newborns participated in this study, 62 (16.1%; 95% CI: 12.2-20.0) newborns were colonized with GBS and 56.5% of the GBS positive newborns were males. Among the newborns positive for GBS, 77.1% were delivered from those mothers whose age was < 25 years old.

A multivariable logistic analysis indicated that the newborns who were born to mothers whose educational status was below tertiary level; none (AOR = 4.800, 95% CI: 2.752, 8.372), primary (AOR = 8.371, 95% CI: 4.701, 14.909), and secondary (AOR = 2.928, 95% CI: 1.851, 4.630); were associated with an increased risk of colonization of newborns with GBS. Some of the maternal factors such as being employed (AOR = 2.244, CI: 1.162, 4.331), being nullipara (AOR = 3.641, 95% CI: 2.320, 5.714) and being multigravida (AOR = 3.507, 95% CI: 2.296, 5.355) were also at risk for newborn colonization with GBS. Moreover, we found that two neonatal factors, for instance, newborns who were in need of resuscitation (AOR = 3.982, 95% CI: 1.113, 14.239) and those newborns who did not have immediate contact (baby not with the mother soon following delivery or baby in the neonatal intensive care unit) with their mothers (AOR = 4.219, 95% CI: 3.058, 5.823) were associated with increased risk of newborns being colonized with GBS (Table 1).

Colonization of newborns with Group B Streptococcus by the body surface sites

As noted above, 16.1% of the total newborns tested in this study were GBS colonized and of the total swabs processed, 81/1,155 (7.01%) were positive for GBS.

Table 1 Newborns GBS colonization by demographic and obstetrics characteristics including multivariable analysis, Northwest Ethiopia

Characteristics	Response	GBS+	GBS-	COR[a]; 95% CI	AOR[b], 95% CI[c]	*p-value*
Maternal age (yrs) Median = 25	<25	48	249	1	-	-
	≥25	14	74	1.019 (0.532, 1.951)	-	-
Maternal Residence	Urban	51	268	1	-	-
	Rural	11	55	0.951 (0.466, 1.942)	-	-
Maternal education	None	15	72	1.200 (0.418, 3.441)	4.800 (2.752, 8.372)	0.000004
	Primary	13	118	2.269 (0.784, 6.565)	8.371 (4.701, 14.909)	0.000004
	Secondary	28	109	0.976 (0.363, 2.609)	2.928 (1.851, 4.630)	0.000004
	Tertiary	6	24	1	1	
Maternal occupation	House wife	46	240	1	1	
	Employed	13	61	0.899 (0.457, 1.769)	2.244 (1.162, 4.331)	0.016
	Others	3	22	1.406 (0.404, 4.890)	2.102 (0.587, 7.530)	0.254
Gestational Age	<37wks	1	2	0.681 (0.061, 7.590)	NA	NA
	> /=37wks	61	321	1	NA	NA
Parity	multipara	32	164	1	1	
	nulipara	30	159	0.967 (0.561, 1.666)	3.641 (2.320, 5.714)	0.000
History of still birth	No	59	308	1	-	-
	Yes	3	15	0.958 (0.269, 3.412)	-	-
History of abortion	No	58	294	1	-	-
	Yes	4	29	1.430 (0.484, 4.223)	-	-
History of neonatal death	No	60	316	1	-	-
	Yes	2	7	0.665 (0.135, 3.277)	-	-
Gravidity	Primigravida	28	156	1	1	
	Multigravida	34	167	0.882 (0.511, 1.522)	3.507 (2.296, 5.355)	0.000
ANC visit	0 - 3	16	108	1.444 (0.782, 2.669)	-	-
	4 - 5	46	215	1	-	-
Contraceptive use	No	7	61	1	-	-
	Yes	55	262	0.547 (0.237, 1.259)	-	-
History of preterm delivery	No	60	317	1	-	-
	Yes	2	4	0.379 (0.068, 2.113)	-	-
Length of Premature ROM	≤1hr	48	223	1	-	-
	>1hr	14	100	1.537 (0.810, 2.917)	-	-
HIV status	No	59	313	1	-	-
	Yes	3	10	0.628 (0.168, 2.352)	-	-
Sex of newborn	Male	35	181	0.983 (0.568, 1.701)	-	-
	Female	27	142	1	-	-
APGAR[d] Score at 1 minute	<7	5	50	2.088 (0.797, 5.467)	-	-
	7 - 10	57	273	1	-	-
APGAR Score at 5 minutes	<7	2	28	2.847 (0.661, 12.275)	-	-
	7 - 10	60	295	1	-	-
Newborn`s weight (Kg) median =3.0	<2.5	6	34	1.098 (0.440, 2.738)	-	-
	≥2.5	56	289	1	-	-
	Yes	16	307	1	-	-
Resuscitation required	No	58	287	1	1	
	Yes	4	36	1.819 (0.623, 5.307)	3.982 (1.113, 14.239)	0.034

Table 1 Newborns GBS colonization by demographic and obstetrics characteristics including multivariable analysis, Northwest Ethiopia *(Continued)*

Characteristics	Response	GBS+	GBS-	COR[a]; 95% CI	AOR[b], 95% CI[c]	*p-value*
Newborn to mother immediate close contact	No	12	76	1.282 (0.649, 2.532)	4.219 (3.058, 5.823)	0.000
	Yes	50	247	1	1	
Duration of labor(hour)	4 - 12	54	262	1	-	-
	13 - 24	8	61	1.572 (0.711, 3.473)	-	-

[a]crude odds ratio, [b]adjusted odds ratio, [c]confidence interval, [d]Appearance, Pulse, Grimace, Activity, and Respiration

Among the three newborn body surface sites swabbed, the nasal swabs accounted for more (8.1%, 95% CI: 5.2-11.3) colonization followed by the umbilical surface swabs (7.5%, 95% CI: 5.1-10.6). Fourteen (22.6%) of the newborns colonized with GBS in this study had more than one body surface site colonization, and 8.1% had three body surface site GBS colonization (Table 2).

Antibiotic susceptibility patterns of Group B Streptococcus isolates

All the isolates were tested for 10 commonly prescribed antibiotics by using the recommended methods. Of the GBS identified from the different body surface sites of the newborns, the antibiotics susceptibility ratess (an average of the three body sites tested) were 95.1%, 89.6%, 88.9%, 85.7%, 85.3%, 81.3%, 76.9%, 76.1%, 73.8%, and 34.4% to ampicillin, penicillin, ciprofloxacin, chloramphenicol, vancomycin, azitromycin, erythromycin, clindamycin, ceftriaxone, and tetracycline respectively (Table 3). The least susceptibility rate (average of the three body surface sites) was reported in tetracycline (34.3%). Ciprofloxacin, chloramphenicol, vancomycin and azithromycin were found to be the drug of choice next to ampicillin and penicillin in our study.

Table 2 Newborns GBS* colonization by their body surface sites, Northwest Ethiopia (*n* = 62)

Newborn body site colonized	No. of GBS positive	Percentage (%)
Nasal swab[a]	31	8.1
Ear swab[a]	21	5.5
Umbilicus swab[a]	29	7.5
Total	62	16.1
Nasal swab only	19	30.6
Ear swab only	14	22.6
Umbilicus swab only	15	24.2
Nasal and ear swabs	0	0.0
Nasal and umbilicus swabs	7	11.3
Ear and umbilicus swabs	2	3.2
Nasal , ear and umbilicus	5	8.1
Total	62	100.0

*Group B Streptococcus/*Streptococcus agalactiae*, [a]*overall prevalence (62; 16.1%) without combining body sites*

Inducible and constitutive resistance Group B Streptococcus isolates to clindamycin

The phenotypic analysis of GBS isolates identified from the three body surfaces sites of the newborns was done by using erythromycin and clindamycin double disc diffusion (D-zone testing) method as per the CLSI 2017 guideline. Among the 32 GBS isolates resistant and/or intermediate resistant to erythromycin and clindmaycin, 34.4% harboured L phenotype, 31.3% had M phenotype, 21.9% had constitutive Macrolide, Lincosamide-Streptogramin (B) (cMLSB) and 12.5% contained inducible Macrolide, Lincosamide-StreptograminB (iMLSB) (Fig. 1 Legend, and Table 4). We found 12.5% inducible and 21.9% constitutive resistance GBS to clindamycin.

Discussion

Our study showed that 62 (16.1%; 95% CI: 12.2-20.0) of the newborns participated in the study were colonized with GBS, which could be the possible causes to the high morbidity and mortality of neonates in the study area. This prevalence of colonization was in agreement with different studies conducted worldwide such as: France (13.9%) [26], Turkey (17.3%) [27]), South Africa (15.8%) [14] and Gambia (12.0%) [28]. Contrary to our study, other studies showed the lower prevalence of newborn colonization with GBS and some of these were Iran (1.7% to 5.5%) [29–31], Saudi Arabia (1.0%) [32], Turkey (1.6% to 8.0%) [12, 33], Pakistan (6.0%) [13], China (4.9%) [34], India (1.3% to 3.2%) [35, 36], Korea (1.5%) [37], Bangladesh (6.3% to 7.4%; in which, the finding from umbilicus is in agreement with ours) [38, 39], Lithuania (6.4%; where 5.3% GBS were isolated from the ear swab of the newborns as it was observed in our study and 4.6% from the throat) [40], Greek (2.4%) [41], Nigeria (6.8%) [42], Tanzania (8.9%) [43] and Ethiopia (5%) [19]. The discrepancies might be associated with the Global variability of maternal colonization with GBS (differences in geography, season, IAP provision), the mode of delivery (in which newborns born by spontaneous vaginal delivery had usually more GBS colonization), and the availability of laboratory facilities and experiences of laboratories to detect GBS.

Inconsistent to our result, a lot of studies showed higher neonatal colonization with GBS, for example, studies in

Table 3 Antibiotic susceptibility patterns of GBS isolated from the newborns` body surfaces, Northwest Ethiopia

Antibiotics	Disc potency		Colonizing GBS isolates		
		Newborn`s body sites	Susceptible, n(%)	Intermediate, n(%)	Resistant, n(%)
Penicillin	10units	Nasal nare (*n*=31)	29 (93.5)	0 (0.0)	2 (6.5)
		Umbilicus (*n*=29)	26 (89.7)	0 (0.0)	3 (10.3)
		Ear (*n*=21)	18 (85.7)	0 (0.0)	3 (14.3)
Ampicillin	10µg	Nasal nare (*n*=31)	29 (93.5)	0 (0.0)	2 (6.5)
		Umbilicus (*n*=29)	28 (96.6)	0 (0.0)	1 (3.4)
		Ear (*n*=21)	20 (95.2)	0 (0.0)	1 (4.8)
Erythromycin	15µg	Nasal nare (*n*=31)	24 (77.4)	2 (6.5)	5 (16.1)
		Umbilicus (*n*=29)	21 (72.4)	1 (3.4)	7 (24.2)
		Ear (*n*=21)	17 (80.9)	0 (0.0)	4 (19.1)
Clindamycin	2µg	Nasal nare (*n*=31)	24 (77.4)	1 (3.2)	6 (19.4)[a]
		Umbilicus (*n*=29)	22 (75.9)	2 (6.9)	5 (17.2)[a]
		Ear (*n*=21)	16 (76.2)	2 (9.5)	3 (14.3)[a]
Azitromycin	15µg	Nasal nare (*n*=31)	27 (87.1)	1 (3.2)	3 (9.7)
		Umbilicus (*n*=29)	22 (75.9)	4 (13.8)	3 (10.3)
		Ear (*n*=21)	17 (80.9)	3 (14.3)	1 (4.8)
Vancomycin	30µg	Nasal nare (*n*=31)	26 (83.9)	0 (0.0)	5 (16.1)
		Umbilicus (*n*=29)	25 (86.2)	0 (0.0)	4 (13.8)
		Ear (*n*=21)	18 (85.7)	0 (0.0)	3 (14.3)
Ceftriazone	30µg	Nasal nare (*n*=31)	23 (74.2)	0 (0.0)	8 (25.8)
		Umbilicus (*n*=29)	22 (75.9)	0 (0.0)	7 (24.1)
		Ear (*n*=21)	15 (71.4)	0 (0.0)	6 (28.6)
Ciprofloxacin	5µg	Nasal nare (*n*=31)	29 (93.5)	0 (0.0)	2 (6.5)
		Umbilicus (*n*=29)	24 (82.8)	0 (0.0)	5 (17.2)
		Ear (*n*=21)	19 (90.5)	0 (0.0)	2 (9.5)
Chloramphenicol	30µg	Nasal nare (*n*=31)	26 (83.9)	3 (9.6)	2 (6.5)
		Umbilicus (*n*=29)	24 (82.8)	3 (10.3)	2 (6.9)
		Ear (*n*=21)	19 (90.4)	1 (4.8)	1 (4.8)
Tetracycline	30µg	Nasal nare (*n*=31)	8 (25.8)	3 (9.7)	20 (64.5)
		Umbilicus (*n*=29)	10 (34.5)	3 (10.3)	16 (55.2)
		Ear (*n*=21)	9 (42.9)	0 (0.0)	12 (57.1)

[a]Excluding the inducible clindamycin resistant isolates (iMLSB)

Poland (26.7% to 34.5%) [44, 45] and Bangladesh (38%) [39]. The regional differences, variability in the sample size, methods employed for GBS detection, availabilities of laboratory facilities, experiences of laboratory technologists, newborn body surface sites swabbed and time of sample collection (soon after birth or later) might be possibly explained the disparities. The differences could also be explained by the presence or absence of the IAP administration, variations of maternal colonization and density of GBS colony and mode of delivery.

In our study, the antibiotics susceptibility rates of GBS were 95.1%, 89.6%, 88.9%, 85.7%, 85.3%, 81.3%, 76.9%, 76.1%, 73.8%, and 34.4% to ampicillin, penicillin, ciprofloxacin, chloramphenicol, vancomycin, azitromycin, erythromycin, clindamycin, ceftriaxone, and tetracycline respectively. We identified that ciprofloxacin, chloramphenicol, vancomycin and azithromycin were the drug of choice next to ampicillin and penicillin. The GBS in the current study showed better sensitivity to azithromycin than erythromycin and clindamycin. Thus, given the recent interest in the azithromycin, it is wise to do more study on this drug and consider it as the alternative prophylaxis for the penicillin allergic laboring mothers to reduce the carriage of GBS in mothers and newborns and then to lower the risk of neonatal diseases beyond the trachoma control.

In agreement with our findings, a study in Egypt showed that 29.4% of the GBS isolated from the neonates were

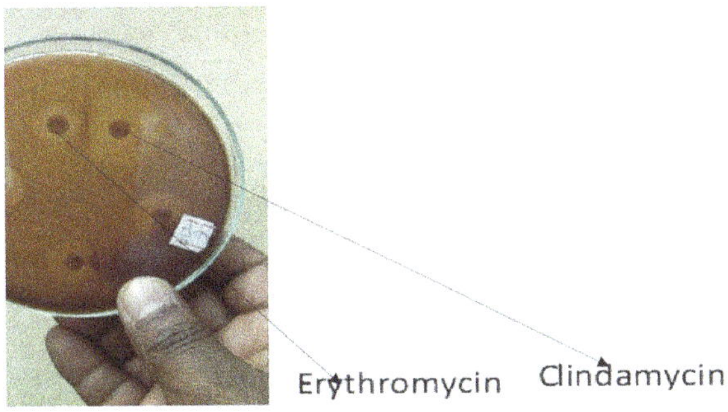

Fig. 1 Inducible Clindamycin resistance (D-zone) of GBS isolated from a newborn ear swab, Northwest Ethiopia. Legend: A *S. agalactiae* isolated from a newborn ear swab from the University of Gondar referral hospital in Northwest Ethiopia showed Inducible MLS_B phenotype (erythromycin-resistant and clindamycin sensitive) determined by means of an antibiotic disk diffusion test or D-test (the blunting of the clear circular area of no growth around the *clindamycin* disk on the side adjacent to the erythromycin disk and was designated as D-test positive)

resistance to erythromycin and 17.6% were resistance to clindamycin [46]. Another studies conducted in different parts of the world such as, in France showed that 25.6% were resistance to clindamycin and 38.2% to erythromycin [18] and 21.4% to macrolide [47], in the USA, 20.2% to 32% were resistance to erythromycin and 6.9% to 15% to clindamycin [17, 48, 49], and in Italy, 17% were resistance to erythromycin and 15.3 % to clindamycin [50]. Another report from Tanzania revealed that the neonatal GBS were 100% susceptible to penicillin, ampicillin, vancomycin and ciprofloxacin whereas susceptibility to ceftriaxone, clindamycin and erythromycin were 93.8%, 87.5% and 81.3% respectively [43]. A study in Germany also reported that all the isolates were susceptible to beta-lactams and vancomycin while 10.1% were resistance to erythromycin and 5.7% to clindamycin [51] which are lower than our reports. This variation might be explained by the fact that the laboratory facilities and health literacy of the people in our setting are different from other developed countries.

Contrasting to the results of our study, a Chinese report revealed that all the GBS isolated from the neonates were susceptible to penicillin, but the rates of resistance to clindamycin and erythromycin were 84.0% and 88.0% [52]. These discrepancies may dictate that the rates of resistance to erythromycin and clindamycin varied among geographic regions and were notably the highest in China. Additionally, a study explained that antibiotics currently prevent an estimated 29,000 cases of early onset GBS disease per year. This approach may challenge in the low-income countries where many births take place at home, and laboratory capacity for the screening of GBS is limited [8]. The provision of antibiotics to pregnant women without screening may also contribute to the emergence of antibiotic resistance. An alternative prophylaxis failure is becoming more likely to the increasing of macrolide resistance rates among the GBS isolates. Therefore, in cases when considering these antibiotics, including azithromycin as alternatives for prophylaxis and treatment for GBS, susceptibility test should be done before the prescriptions. We also reported that among the GBS tested for MLS_B by using the double disk diffusion technique, 34.4%, 31.3%, 21.9% and 12.5% isolates had L- and M- phenotypes, $cMLS_B$ and $iMLS_B$, respectively. The inducible and constitutive resistance reported in our study is lower than a study from Canada, where 40.0% of the isolates were inducible and 47.3% were constitutive resistance to clindamycin [24].

Of the possible factors associated for the colonization of the newborns that were investigated in our study, the newborns born to mothers whose education status was below tertiary level and from employed mothers had the increased risk of colonization with GBS. It could be justified by the fact that keeping personal hygiene is likely better among those people who have more education status than their counterparts. In addition, employment may increase mobility of women and expose them for different causal partnerships with different people who could be the risks for them, later becomes a source for

Table 4 Macrolide, Lincosamide-StreptograminB (MLSB) and D-shape of the GBS isolates in Northwest Ethiopia

Double disc diffusion[a]								
GBS phenotypes	Erythromycin (n)			Clindamycin (n)			Total (*n* = 32)	Percent (%)
	R, </=15mm	I, 16-20mm	S, >/=21mm	R,</ =15mm	I,16-18mm	S,>/ =19mm		
constitutive macrolide, lincosmide-streptogramin B (cMLSB)	7	0	-	6	1	-	7	21.9
inducible macrolide, lincosmide-streptogramin B (iMLSB)	4	0	-	0	0	4	4	12.5
M-phenotype	6	4	-	-	-	10	10	31.3
L-Phenotype	-	-	11	7	4	-	11	34.4
D – Shape positive	4	0	0	-	-	4	4	12.5
D – Shape negative	-	-	-	-	-	-	28	87.5

[a]CLSI (2017) disk diffusion breakpoints [57]. For erythromycin: ≥21 mm, susceptible (S); 16 to 20 mm, intermediate (I); ≤15 mm, resistant (R). For clindamycin: ≥19 mm, susceptible (S); 16 to 18 mm, intermediate (I); ≤15 mm, resistant (R)

their neonatal colonization. Being nulliparity and multigravida are among the maternal factors, and newborns who were in resuscitation and who didn`t have immediate contact with their mothers (in the neonatal intensive care unit) had also the increased risk of newborn colonization.

Congruently, different literatures presented that women with less (or no formal,/lack of) education, women of lower parity, multigravid, young maternal age (< 20 yrs), vaginal mode of delivery, intrapartum fever, prolonged premature rupture of membrane, preterm gestational age, low birth weight (< 2.5kg), and neonatal intensive care admission were associated with neonatal colonization with GBS [43, 46, 53–56]. Likewise, a study in Tanzania showed that prolonged duration of labour had the significant association with colonization of the newborns with GBS, possibly due to the extended exposure of the newborns in the birth canal [43]. This calls for the screening of pregnant women for GBS at their 35 to 37 weeks of pregnancy and provision of IAP for those women who have been positive for GBS to reduce the chances of later neonatal colonization.

We found that maternal age, obstetric history, gestational age, sex of the newborn, HIV infection, Appearance, Pulse, Grimace, Activity, and Respiration (APGAR) score, preterm delivery, number of antenatal care (ANC) visit, and duration of labour did not show a significant association with neonatal colonization. In agreement to this, Joachim and his co-workers in Tanzania [43] presented that prolonged premature rupture of membrane, intrapartum fever, mode of delivery and low birth weight did not influence neonatal colonization with GBS. Tsolia et al. [41] in their study reported that the multiparity (≥2 previous births) is associated with a low risk for maternal colonization with GBS. It might be explained by the numbers of participants in our study with these risk factors were small. It is useful to know that GBS could be transferred from pregnant women to newborns, and was evidenced by the fact that after the Caesarean section was done (before rupture of the membrane), molecular strain identification demonstrated that same GBS strain was found in mothers and their newborns [45]. So to prevent neonatal colonization with GBS and to increase newborn health conditions, prevention strategies should be developed and promoted in the study area.

Limitations

This study has main limitations in terms of small sample size, non-probability sampling method, and using only disc diffusion for antibiotic susceptibility test.

Conclusion

Prevalence of newborn colonization with GBS in this study was higher than the findings reported three Decades ago in the same area. We identified that ciprofloxacin, chloramphenicol, vancomycin and azithromycin were the drug of choice next to ampicillin and penicillin. In addition, 12.5% of the isolates in our study showed inducible clindamycin resistance. Lower education status, being employed, and being nullipara and multigrapvida were the maternal factors associated with the increased risk of newborn colonization. Resuscitation and denial of the newborn`s immediate contact with their mothers were the neonatal factors which showed the increased risk of newborn colonization. So to prevent neonatal colonization with GBS, continuous health education, screening of pregnancy for GBS at the 35 to 37 weeks of gestation and provision of IAP for those positive cases for GBS should be promoted in the study area. GBS surveillance and their antibiotic susceptibility testing should also be conducted in the country by using advanced laboratory technologies.

Abbreviations

ANC: Antenatal Care; AOR: Adjusted Odds Ratio; APGAR: Appearance, Pulse, Grimace, Activity, and Respiration; ATCC: American Type Culture Collection; CAMP: Christie–Atkins–Munch-Petersen; CI: Confidence Interval; CLSI: Clinical Laboratory Standard Institute; CO_2: Carbon dioxide; GBS: Group B Streptococcus; HIV: Human Immune deficiency Virus; IAP: Intrapartum Antibiotics Prophylaxis; MLS_B: Macrolide-Lincosamide-Streptogramin B; PROM: Premature Rupture of Membrane; *S. agalactiae*: *Streptococcus agalactiae*; *S. aureus*: *Staphylococcus aureus*; SPSS: Statistical Package for Social Sciences; μg/L: Microgram per liter

Acknowledgment

The authors would like to acknowledge the financial and material support from the College of Medicine and Health Sciences, University of Gondar, Northwest Ethiopia, the German Academic Exchange Service (DAAD), Germany, and the Institute of Virology, Leipzig University, Germany. The authors are also grateful to the study participants and data collectors.

Funding

Financial and material support were from the University of Gondar, Ethiopia, the German Academic Exchange Service (DAAD) In-Country scholarship and the Institute of Virology, Leipzig University, Germany for salary, material procurement, data collection, analysis, and interpretation and in writing the manuscript, printing and copying services.

Authors' contributions

MG participated in conception and design of the study, acquisition of data, analysis and Interpretation of findings. BT participated in conception and design of the study, and interpretation of data; he also participated in revision of the manuscript. MT participated in design of the study, acquisition and interpretation data; in revision of the manuscript. FM participated in conception of the study; and revision of the manuscript. MA participated in design of the study, and revision of the manuscript. ZT participated in interpretation of data, drafting and revision of the manuscript. All authors read and approved the final manuscript.

Ethics approval and consent to participate

It is done after we secured ethical approval from the institutional review board of the University of Gondar (R.No.O/V/P/RCS/05/478/2015 Mega project and O/V/P/RCS/05/471/2018). Permission was obtained from the University of Gondar Referral Hospitals administrative bodies. After giving a brief description about the purpose of the study, eligible mothers gave informed written consent for their participation in the questionnaire of this study and for their newborns to be a part of such a study. Confidentiality was ensured using code numbers than names and keeping the data locked

Competing interests

The authors declare that they have no competing interests

Author details

[1]Department of Medical Microbiology, School of Biomedical and Laboratory Sciences, College of Medicine and Health Sciences, University of Gondar, P. O. Box 196, Gondar, Ethiopia. [2]Department of Gynecology and Obstetrics, School of Medicine, College of Medicine and Health Sciences, University of Gondar, P. O. Box 196, Gondar, Ethiopia. [3]Department of Pediatrics, School of Medicine, College of Medicine and Health Sciences, University of Gondar, P. O. Box 196, Gondar, Ethiopia.

References

1. Central Statistical Agency (CSA) [Ethiopia], ICF. Ethiopia Demographic and Health Survey 2016: Key Indicators Report. AAddis Ababa, Ethiopia, and Rockville, Maryland: CSA and ICF; 2016. p. 21–2.
2. Amhara National Regional State Bureau of Health. Health Research Thematic Areas of Amhara Regional Health Bureau: Amhara Regional Health Bureau Health Research and Technology Transfer Core Process in collaboration with Ethiopan Network for HIV/AIDS Treatment Care and Support (ENHAT-CS) Amhara Region Program. First Edition, Bahir dar, Ethiopia. 2013:1- 41.
3. Rick AM, Aguilar A, Cortes R, Gordillo R, Melgar M, Samayoa-Reyes G, et al. Group B Streptococci Colonization in Pregnant Guatemalan Women: Prevalence, Risk Factors, and Vaginal Microbiome. Open Forum Infect Dis. 2017;4(1):ofx020.
4. Chan GJ, Lee ACC, Baqui AH, Tan J, Black RE. Prevalence of early-onset neonatal infection among newborns of mothers with bacterial infection or colonization: a systematic review and meta-analysis. BMC Infect Dis. 2015;15:118.
5. Kulkarni R, Randis TM, Antala S, Wang A, Amaral FE, Ratner AJ. β-Hemolysin/Cytolysin of Group B Streptococcus Enhances Host Inflammation but Is Dispensable for Establishment of Urinary Tract Infection. PLoS ONE. 2013;8(3):e59091.
6. Schrag SJ, Zywicki S, Farley MM, Reingold AL, Harrison LH, Lefkowitz LB, et al. Group B streptococcal disease in the era of intrapartum antibiotic prophylaxis. N Engl J Med. 2000a;342(1):15–20.
7. Valkenburg-van den Berg AW, Sprij AJ, Oostvogel PM, Mutsaers JA, Renes WB, Rosendaal FR, et al. Prevalence of colonization with group B Streptococci in pregnant women of a multi-ethnic population in The Netherlands. Eur J Obstet Gynecol Reprod Biol. 2006;124(2):178–83.
8. Seale AC, Bianchi-Jassir F, Russell NJ, Kohli-Lynch M, Tann CJ, Hall J, et al. Estimates of the Burden of Group B Streptococcal Disease Worldwide for Pregnant Women, Stillbirths, and Children. Clin Infect Dis. 2017;65(suppl_2): S200–S19.
9. Mohammed M, Asrat D, Woldeamanuel Y, Demissie A. Prevalence of group B Streptococcus colonization among pregnant women attending antenatal clinic of Hawassa Health Center, Hawassa. Ethiopia. Ethiop J Health Dev. 2012;26(1):36–42.
10. Centers for Disease Control and Prevention. Prevention of perinatal group B streptococcal disease: revised guidelines from CDC. MMWR. 2010;59(RR-10): 1–36.
11. Regan JA, Klebanoff MA, Nugent RP, Eschenbach DA, Blackwelder WC, Lou Y, et al. Colonization with group B streptococci in pregnancy and adverse outcome. VIP Study Group Am J Obstet Gynecol. 1996;174(4):1354–60.
12. Eren A, Küçükercan M, Oğuzoğlu N, Unal N, Karateke A. The carriage of group B streptococci in Turkish pregnant women and its transmission rate in newborns and serotype distribution. Turk J Pediatr. 2005;47(1):28–33.
13. Chaudhry BY, Akhtar N, Balouch AH. Vaginal carriage rate of Group B Streptococcus in pregnant women and its transmission to neonates. J Ayub Med Coll Abbottabad. 2010;22(4):167–70.
14. Madzivhandila M, Adrian PV, Cutland CL, Kuwanda L, Schrag SJ, Madhi SA. Serotype Distribution and Invasive Potential of Group B Streptococcus Isolates Causing Disease in Infants and Colonizing Maternal-Newborn Dyads. PLoS ONE. 2011;6(3):e17861.
15. Schrag SJ, Whitney CG, Schuchat A. Neonatal group B streptococcal disease: how infection control teams can contribute to prevention efforts. Infect Control Hosp Epidemiol. 2000b;21(7):473–83.
16. Garland SM, Cottrill E, Markowski L, Pearce C, Clifford V, Ndisang D, et al. Antimicrobial resistance in group B streptococcus: the Australian experience. Journal of Medical Microbiology. 2011;60(Pt 2):230–5.
17. Lin FC, Azimi PH, Weisman LE, Philips JB III, Regan J, Clark P, et al. Antibiotic Susceptibility Profiles for Group B Streptococci Isolated from Neonates, 1995–1998. Clinical Infectious Diseases. 2000;31(1):76–9.
18. Hays C, Louis M, Plainvert C, Dmytruk N, Touak G, Trieu-Cuot P, et al. Changing Epidemiology of Group B Streptococcus Susceptibility to Fluoroquinolones and Aminoglycosides in France. Antimicrob Agents Chemother. 2016;60(12):7424–30.
19. Schmidt J, Halle E, Halle H, Mohammed T, Gunther E. Colonization of pregnant women and their newborn infants with group B Streptococci in the Gondar College of Medical Sciences. Ethiop Med J. 1989;27(3):115–9.
20. Clinical Laboratory Standard Institute. Performance Standards for Antimicrobial Susceptibility Testing. 27th ed, CLSI supplement M100 Wayne, PA: Clinical and Laboratory Standards Institute;. 2017;37(1):84-87.
21. Bauer AW, Kirby WM, Sherris JC, Turck M. Antibiotic susceptibility testing by a standardized single disk method. Am J Clin Pathol. 1966;45(5):493–6.
22. Seppala H, Skurnik M, Soini H, Roberts MC, Huovinen P. A novel erythromycin resistance methylase gene (ermTR) in Streptococcus pyogenes. Antimicrob Agents Chemother. 1998;42(2):257–62.
23. Quiroga M, Pegels E, Oviedo P, Pereyra E, Vergara M. Susceptibility patterns and prevalence of GBS isolated from pregnant women in Misiones. Argentina. Braz J Microbiol. 2008;39(2):245–50.
24. Desjardins M, Delgaty KL, Ramotar K, Seetaram C, Toye B. Prevalence and mechanisms of erythromycin resistance in group A and group B streptococcus: implications for reporting susceptibility results. J Clin Microbiol. 2004;42(12):5620–3.
25. Khan AS, Walsh A, Crowleyet B. Role of efflux in macrolide resistance in β-hemolytic streptococci of groups A, B, C and G collected in an Irish teaching hospital. J Med Microbiol. 2011;60(Pt 2):262–4.
26. Jost C, Bercot B, Jacquier H, Raskine L, Barranger E, Mouchnino G, et al. Xpert GBS Assay for Rapid Detection of Group B Streptococcus in Gastric Fluid Samples from Newborns. J Clin Microbiol. 2014;52(2):657–9.
27. Kadanali A, Altoparlak U, Kadanali S. Maternal carriage and neonatal colonisation of group B streptococcus in easternTurkey: prevalence, risk factors and antimicrobial resistance. Int J Clin Pract. 2005;59(4):437–40.
28. Roca A, Bojang A, Camara B, Oluwalana C, Lette K, West P, et al. Maternal colonization with Staphylococcus aureus and Group B streptococcus is associated with colonization in newborns. Clinical Microbiology and Infection. 2017;23(12):974–9.
29. Hamedi A, Akhlaghi F, Seyedi SJ, Kharazmi A. Evaluation of group B Streptococci colonization rate in pregnant women and their newborn. Acta Med Iran. 2012;50(12):805–8.
30. Nahaei MR, Ghandchilar N, Bilan N, Ghahramani P. Maternal carriage and neonatal colonization of Streptococcus agalactiae in Tabriz. Northwest Iran. Iran J Med Sci. 2015;32(3):177–81.
31. Jahromi BN, Poorarian S, Poorbarfehee S. The prevalence and adverse effects of group B streptococcal colonization during pregnancy. Arch Iran Med. 2008;11(6):654–7.
32. Al-Sunaidi M, Al-Shahrani M, Damole IO, Bello CSS. Prevalence of Group B Streptococcus Colonization in Mothers and Babies at Abha General Hospital, Kingdom of Saudi Arabia. Med J Cairo Univ. 2011;79(2):163–5.
33. Barbaros I, Murat C, Mehmet V, Ismet TA, Can K, Sukufe D, et al. The colonization incidence of group B streptococcus in pregnant women and their newborns in Istanbul. Pediatr Int. 2005;47(1):64–6.
34. Yang J, Xu D, Yin LQ, Zhu BQ, Wang AH. Neonatal group B streptococcus infection in the Children's Hospital of Gansu Province through PCR array. Zhonghua Er Ke Zhi. 2013;51(9):688–91.

35. Kulkarni AA, Pawar SG, Dharmadhikari CA, Kulkarni RD. Colonization of pregnant women and their newborn infants with Group B Streptococci. Indain Journal Medical Microbiology. 2001;19(2):97–100.
36. Shah D, Saxena S, Randhawa VS, Nangia S. Dutta Prospective analysis of risk factors associated with group B streptococcal colonisation in neonates born at a tertiary care centre in India. Paediatr Int Child Health. 2014;34(3):184–8.
37. Uh Y, Kwon JY, Jang IH, Yoon KJ, Kim HG. Colonization rate of Group B Streptococcus in pregnant women and neonates. Korean J Clin Pathol. 1994;14(4):447–53.
38. Islam MS, Saha SK, Islam M, Modak JK, Shah R, Talukder RR, et al. Prevalence, Serotype Distribution and Mortality Risk Associated With Group B Streptococcus Colonization of Newborns in Rural Bangladesh. Pediatr Infect Dis J. 2016;35(12):1309–12.
39. Saha SK, Ahmed ZB, Modak JK, Naziat H, Saha S, Uddin MA, et al. Group B Streptococcus among Pregnant Women and Newborns in Mirzapur, Bangladesh: Colonization, Vertical Transmission, and Serotype Distribution. J Clin Microbiol. 2017;55(8):2406–12.
40. Barcaite E, Bartusevicius A, Tameliene R, Maleckiene L, Vitkauskiene A, Nadisauskiene R. Group B streptococcus and Escherichia coli colonization in pregnant women and neonates in Lithuania. Int J Gynaecol Obstet. 2012; 117(1):69–73.
41. Tsolia M, Psoma M, Gavrili S, Petrochilou V, Michalas S, Legakis N, et al. Group B streptococcus colonization of Greek pregnant women and neonates: prevalence, risk factors and serotypes. Clin Microbiol Infect. 2003;9(8):832–8.
42. Elikwu CJ, Oduyebo O, Ogunsola FT, Anorlu RI, Okoromah CN, König B. High group B streptococcus carriage rates in pregnant women in a tertiary institution in Nigeria. Pan Afr Med J. 2016;25:249.
43. Joachim A, Matee MI, Massawe FA, Lyamuya EF. Maternal and neonatal colonisation of group B streptococcus at Muhimbili National Hospital in Dar es Salaam, Tanzania: prevalence, risk factors and antimicrobial resistance. BMC Public Health. 2009;9:437.
44. Kowalska B, Niemiec KT, Drejewicz H, Polak K, Kubik P, Elmidaoui A, et al. Prevalence of group B streptococcal colonization in pregnant women and their newborns based on the results of examination of patients in the Obstetric and Gynecology Department of the National Research Institute of Mother and Child--a pilot study. Ginekol Pol. 2003;74(10):1223–7.
45. Strus M, Pawlik D, Brzychczy-Włoch M, Gosiewski T, Rytlewski K, Lauterbach R, et al. Group B streptococcus colonization of pregnant women and their children observed on obstetric and neonatal wards of the University Hospital in Krakow, Poland. J Med Microbiol. 2009;58(Pt 2):228–33.
46. Sultan AM, Mahfouz RA, Ali MM, Taher S. Virulence Factors of Streptococcus agalactiae in Neonatal Sepsis. Egyptian Journal of Medical Microbiology. 2012;21(2):1–10.
47. Mouy DD, Cavallo J, Leclercq R, Fabre R. The Aforcopi-Bio Network. Antibiotic Susceptibility and Mechanisms of Erythromycin Resistance in Clinical Isolates of Streptococcus agalactiae: French Multicenter Study. Antimicrob Agents Chemother. 2001;45(8):2400–2.
48. Phares CR, Lynfield R, Farley MM, Mohle-Boetani J, Harrison LH, Petit S, et al. Epidemiology of invasive group B streptococcal disease in the United States, 1999-2005. JAMA. 2008;299(17):2056–65.
49. Castor ML, Whitney CG, Como-Sabetti K, Facklam RR, Ferrieri P, Bartkus JM, et al. Antibiotic resistance patterns in invasive group B streptococcal isolates. Infect Dis Obstet Gynecol. 2008;2008:727505.
50. Creti R, Imperi M, Berardi A, Pataracchia M, Recchia S, Alfarone G, et al. Neonatal Group B Streptococcus Infections: Prevention Strategies, Clinical and Microbiologic Characteristics in 7 Years of Surveillance. Pediatr Infect Dis J. 2017;36(3):256–62.
51. Fluegge K, Supper S, Siedler A, Berner R. Antibiotic Susceptibility in Neonatal Invasive Isolates of Streptococcus agalactiae in a 2-Year Nationwide Surveillance Study in Germany. Antimicrob Agents Chemother. 2004;48(11):4444–6.
52. Dong Y, Jiang S, Zhou Q, Cao Y. Group B Streptococcus causes severe sepsis in term neonates: 8 years experience of a major Chinese neonatal unit. World Journal of Pediatrics. 2017;13(4):314–20.
53. Schuchat A, Zywicki SS, Dinsmoor MJ, Mercer B, Romaguera J, O'Sullivan MJ, et al. Risk factors and opportunities for prevention of early-onset neonatal sepsis: a multicenter case-control study. Pediatrics. 2000;105(1 Pt 1):21–6.
54. Patil KP, Singla SS, Nagmoti MB, Swamy MK. Group B Streptococci Colonization in Pregnant women: is Screening a Necessary? J South Asian Feder Obst Gynae. 2013;5(2):64–7.
55. Regan JA, Klebanoff MA, Nugent RP. The epidemiology of group B streptococcal colonization in pregnancy. Vaginal Infections and Prematurity Study Group. Obstet Gynecol. 1991;77(4):604–10.
56. Orrett FA. Colonization with Group B streptococci in pregnancy and outcome of infected neonates in Trinidad. Pediatr Int. 2003;45(3):319–23.
57. Clinical and Laboratory Standards Institute. Performance Standards for Antimicrobial Susceptibility Testing. 27th ed. CLSI supplement M100. Way n e, PA: Clinical and Laboratory Standards Institute. 2017;37(1):84-7.

21

Relationship between asymptomatic rotavirus infection and jaundice in neonates

Nu Ri Hwang[1] and Jin Kyu Kim[1,2*]

Abstract

Background: Rotavirus (RV) infection in neonates can be mild or even asymptomatic. In RV infection, jaundice is often reported, but the relationship between jaundice and RV infection has not been studied. This study aimed to determine the importance of asymptomatic RV screening in neonates with jaundice.

Methods: Neonates from the neonatal intensive care unit (NICU) of Chonbuk National University Hospital, those transferred from local obstetrics and gynecology hospitals and outpatient clinics were selected from 2014 to 2017. The study included only infants aged between 3 and 28 days. Jaundice was defined according to gestational age and birth age, in accordance with the American Academy of Pediatrics guidelines criteria. RV infection was confirmed by a stool test, and RV screening and laboratory tests were performed at admission.

Results: Among 596 patients, 166 patients had jaundice. RV infection was observed in 70 (42%) jaundice patients. There were 36 (22%) jaundice patients with asymptomatic RV infection. Patients with onset of jaundice 3–7 days after birth had a high incidence of RV infection. When the RV test was positive, the risk of jaundice was significantly high [odds ratio (OR) 1.89; 95% confidence interval (CI), 1.20–2.98; $p = 0.006$].

Conclusions: Infants with the onset of jaundice > 3 days after birth were likely to have RV infection. Therefore, we suggest that screening tests for RV infection be included as part of the evaluation of jaundiced infants presenting to NICU.

Keywords: Jaundice, Neonatal intensive care unit, Rotavirus infection

Background

Rotavirus (RV) is the most common cause of viral gastroenteritis in children, and 43–78% of asymptomatic neonatal infections have been described [1]. Despite being predominantly asymptomatic, neonatal RV infection has received considerable attention, because some studies have reported that natural infection in the neonatal period has been shown to confer protection against subsequent severe diseases [2]. Although it is known that jaundice occurs in premature infants due to RV infection, studies on whether RV infection causes jaundice in neonates are lacking [3, 4].

Jaundice itself is not a disease but rather a symptom or sign of a disease [5]. Many conditions may clinically present as prolonged neonatal jaundice, including neonatal hepatitis and extrahepatic biliary atresia. These conditions have numerous infectious, metabolic, and genetic causes [6]. Multiple studies have described patients with proven bacterial infections who developed jaundice during the course of their illness [7, 8]. In previous studies, urinary tract infection was observed in 12.5% of asymptomatic jaundiced neonates, with the onset of unconjugated hyperbilirubinemia in the first week of life [9]. Although studies on jaundice due to bacterial infections have progressed, there are limited studies on jaundice caused by viral infections. Therefore, we investigated the relationship between asymptomatic RV infection and jaundice in neonates.

* Correspondence: kyunim99@gmail.com
[1]Department of Pediatrics, Chonbuk National University Medical School, 20, Geonjiro Deokjin-gu, Jeonju-si, Jeollabuk-do 54907, South Korea
[2]Research Institute of Clinical Medicine of Chonbuk National University–Biomedical Research Institute of Chonbuk National University Hospital, Jeonju, Korea

Methods

Study participants

A retrospective study of 1755 patients admitted to the neonatal intensive care unit (NICU) of Chonbuk National University Hospital through local obstetrics and gynecology hospitals and outpatient clinics was conducted from June 2014 to June 2017. Only patients aged 3–28 days at the time of admission were included in the study, to exclude patients within the incubation period of rotavirus and early jaundice due to blood type incompatibility. Patients were excluded from the study if they died within 3 days of admission or if there were no test results or records after admission. Finally, 596 patients were included in the analysis. During the study period, all admitted patients underwent RV screening tests and were screened daily for gastrointestinal symptoms. The demographic features that were evaluated included gestational age (GA), birth weight, small for gestational age, sex, age at admission, hospital day, mode of delivery, Apgar score (1 min/5 min), perinatal problems, and breastfeeding. Jaundice was diagnosed according to total bilirubin level and GA, in accordance with the American Academy of Pediatrics criteria [10]. Diarrhea was defined as the passage of unusually loose or watery stools, at least three times in a 24-h period (≥3 times/day or ≥ 2-fold increase in the number of stools per 8 h) [11]. Diarrhea was ascertained by the nurse at the time of admission, and by the nurse and doctor if the symptoms occurred after admission. Frequent passing of formed stools was not considered diarrhea. Babies fed only breast milk often pass loose, "pasty" stools; this was also not considered diarrhea. Vomiting was defined as the forceful expulsion of gastric contents occurring at least once in a 24-h period and without a respiratory or structural gastrointestinal tract cause [12]. Fever was defined as an axillary temperature of ≥38 °C. Perinatal problems included premature rupture of membranes, maternal diabetes mellitus, maternal thyroid disease, and maternal infection. Antibiotics were used during the period of hospitalization. Late-onset sepsis was considered when infection was detected in blood and cerebrospinal fluid cultures 7 days after delivery, caused by postnatal acquisition (with nosocomial or community sources) of the pathogen. In addition, respiratory viral polymerase chain reaction (PCR) was screened at the time of admission. Patients who tested positive for rotavirus were maintained on conservative therapy, such as fluid therapy and phototherapy until the stool test yielded negative findings in the isolation room.

Clinical procedures

All patients underwent stool examination, respiratory viral PCR, and blood tests on admission. The stool test was performed within 24 h of admission. The RIDASCREEN® (R-Biopharm AG, An der Neuen Bergstraße 17, Germany) RV test is an enzyme immunoassay for the qualitative determination of RV in stool samples. The stool test was performed using enzyme-linked immunosorbent assay (ELISA), and the clinical records were retrospectively analyzed. The RIDASCREEN® Rotavirus was validated by comparison with three commercial rotavirus ELISAs. The sensitivity was 82.1% and specificity was 100% [13]. Blood tests included reticulocyte count, total bilirubin, direct bilirubin, hemoglobin (Hb) level, Coombs test, ABO incompatibility, C-reactive protein (CRP), and blood culture. The cut off value of total bilirubin was 15 mg/dL and that of CRP was 5 mg/L in this study [14, 15]. The respiratory viral PCR panel consists of multiple tests for respiratory virus influenza A/B, respiratory syncytial virus A/B, parainfluenza virus 1/2/3, coronavirus 229E/OC43/HKU1, rhinovirus A/B, adenovirus, human metapneumovirus, parainfluenza virus 4, bocavirus 1/2/3/4, enterovirus, coronavirus NL63, and Flu A-H1/H3/H1N1.

Statistical analysis

Continuous variables are expressed as mean ± standard deviation, while categorical variables are expressed as number and percentage. Comparisons between continuous variables were performed using the Mann–Whitney *U* test or Student's *t*-test, while comparisons between categorical variables were performed using the chi-squared test or Fisher's exact test. Logistic regression analysis was performed to control for all variables and to determine the significant independent factors associated with jaundice. Adjusted odds ratios (ORs) and 95% confidence intervals (CIs) were calculated for each possible associated factor. Nominal values, such as sex, mode of delivery, presence or absence of RV infection, ABO incompatibility, blood culture, perinatal problems, and breastfeeding pattern, were compared using the χ^2 test. Continuous variable parameters, such as GA, birth weight, age on admission, levels of serum total bilirubin, Hb level, reticulocyte count, Apgar score, CRP, and antibiotic use days were compared using an independent sample *t*-test. Statistical analyses were performed using SPSS version 18.0 (SPSS Inc., Chicago, IL, USA) and statistical significance was set at a p value of < 0.05.

Results

A total of 596 patients were included in the study. Among these, 90% of infants were born at term (37–42 weeks of gestation) and 357 (60%) were born via vaginal delivery. The mean age of the study population was 11.4 ± 0.3 days. The mean birth weight was 3230.6 ± 508.3 g, and 338 (56%) infants were male and 258 (44%) were female. Among all patients, 166 (27.9%) were diagnosed with jaundice. The number of patients diagnosed with RV infection was 177 (29.7%). There was no significant seasonal variation in this study period.

Table 1 presents the demographic characteristics of patients with and without jaundice. There was no significant difference between the two groups for GA, birth weight, small for gestational age (SGA), sex, Apgar score, and perinatal problems. Perinatal problems included two cases of maternal diabetes mellitus, two cases of maternal thyroid disease, and 32 cases of premature rupture of membranes (PROM). At the time of admission, the mean ages of the jaundice and non-jaundice groups were 8.3 ± 0.4 days and 12.6 ± 0.4 days, respectively ($p = 0.001$). Hospital stay was shorter in the jaundice group than in the non-jaundice group (5.1 ± 0.6 days vs. 7.1 ± 0.4 days, respectively, $p = 0.007$. The rate of vaginal delivery in the jaundice group was significantly higher than that in the non-jaundice group [117 (70.5%) vs. 240 (55.8%), respectively, $p = 0.001$]. The rate of exclusive breastfeeding was significantly higher in the jaundice group than in the non-jaundice group [29.5% (49/166) vs. 16.5% (71/430), respectively, $p = 0.001$].

Table 2 presents a comparison of the factors that may affect jaundice. Reticulocyte counts demonstrated a significant difference of 2.3% ± 0.2% in the jaundice group and 1.9% ± 0.1% in the non-jaundice group ($p = 0.029$). Total bilirubin, direct bilirubin, and Hb levels were significantly higher in the jaundice group than in the non-jaundice group ($p = 0.001$). CRP level was significantly different in the jaundice group at 2.1 ± 0.4 mg/L and non-jaundice group at 7.2 ± 0.9 mg/L ($p = 0.001$). In the jaundice group, the RV infection rate was 70 (42%) and that of asymptomatic RV infection was 36 (21%), which was significantly different from the non-jaundice group ($p = 0.001$). There was no statistically significant difference in late-onset sepsis between the two groups. Respiratory PCR demonstrated a significant difference of 6 (3.6%) in the jaundice group and 61 (14.2%) in the non-jaundice group ($p = 0.001$). Among the 166 patients with jaundice, 63 (37.9%) used antibiotics.

Table 3 present the jaundice and bilirubin levels in neonates with positive and negative RV infection. There was no difference in direct bilirubinemia with the presence of RV infection in the jaundice group. The total bilirubin level at ≤15 mg/dL was higher in the rotavirus positive group than in the rotavirus negative group (27.1% vs. 13.5%, respectively; $p = 0.028$).

Table 4 presents the results of the logistic regression analysis performed with all factors, seven of which demonstrated statistically significant differences. The risk of jaundice increased when the patient was older than 37 weeks, when the mode of delivery was vaginal, when the newborn was exclusively breastfed, when the Hb level was ≥15 mg/dL, and when tests for RV infection were positive (all $p < 0.05$). The risk of jaundice decreased when the age at admission was ≥7 days compared to that when age at admission was < 7 days [OR = 0.29; 95% CI, 0.16–0.51; $p = 0.001$]. The risk of jaundice decreased

Table 1 Demographic characteristics of patients with and without jaundice

Characteristics	Jaundice (+) (*n* = 166)	Jaundice (−) (*n* = 430)	*p* value
Gestational age (weeks)	38.5 ± 0.1	39.0 ± 0.1	0.140
< 37 weeks (%)	8 (4.8)	53 (12.3)	
Birth weight (g)	3287.4 ± 38.4	3208.7 ± 24.7	0.090
Small for gestational age, n (%)	2 (1.2)	9 (2.1)	0.473
Male (%)	73 (44.0)	184 (42.8)	0.817
Age at admission (days)	8.3 ± 0.4	12.6 ± 0.4	0.001
Hospital days (days)	5.1 ± 0.6	7.1 ± 0.4	0.007
Vaginal delivery, n (%)	117 (70.5)	240 (55.8)	0.001
Apgar score (1 min)	8.8 ± 0.1	8.8 ± 0.1	0.741
Apgar score (5 min)	9.6 ± 0.2	9.8 ± 0.1	0.417
Perinatal problem, n (%)	14 (8.4)	22 (5.1)	0.131
Exclusive breastfeeding, n (%)	49 (29.5)	71 (16.5)	0.001

Table 2 Associated factors of patients with and without jaundice

Characteristics	Jaundice (+) (*n* = 166)	Jaundice (−) (*n* = 430)	*p* value
Reticulocyte count (%)	2.3 ± 0.2	1.9 ± 0.1	0.029
Total bilirubin level (mg/dL)	18.7 ± 0.4	7.0 ± 0.2	0.001
Direct bilirubin level (mg/dL)	1.3 ± 0.1	0.8 ± 0.01	0.001
Hemoglobin level (mg/dL)	16.3 ± 0.2	14.6 ± 0.1	0.001
Coombs test positive, n (%)	5 (3.0)	1 (0.2)	0.560
ABO incompatibility, n (%)	2 (1.2)	1 (0.2)	0.133
C-reactive protein (mg/L)	2.1 ± 0.4	7.2 ± 0.9	0.001
Rotavirus positive, n (%)	70 (42.2)	107 (24.9)	0.001
Asymptomatic rotavirus positive, n (%)	36 (21.7)	31 (7.2)	0.032
Antibiotic use (days)	2.1 ± 3.5	3.0 ± 4.3	0.015
Late-onset sepsis, n (%)	1 (0.6)	4 (0.9)	0.695
Respiratory viral PCR, n (%)	6 (3.6)	61 (14.2)	0.001

PCR polymerase chain reaction

Table 3 Jaundice and bilirubin levels in neonates with positive and negative RV infection

Characteristics	Rotavirus (+) (*n* = 70)	Rotavirus (−) (*n* = 96)	*p* value
Direct bilirubinemia (≥2 mg/dL)	3 (4.3)	9 (9.4)	0.211
Jaundice diagnosed			0.001
3–6 days old, n (%)	51 (72.9)	39 (40.6)	
≥7 days old, n (%)	19 (27.1)	57 (59.4)	
Total bilirubin level			0.028
≤15 mg/dL, n (%)	19 (27.1)	13 (13.5)	
> 15 mg/dL, n (%)	51 (72.9)	83 (86.5)	
C-reactive protein (mg/L)	1.9 ± 0.4	2.2 ± 0.5	0.604

Table 4 Multivariate analysis of the risk factors for jaundice

Association factors		Univariate analysis		Multivariate analysis	
		Odds ratio	*P* value	Odds ratio	*P* value
Gestational age	≥37 weeks	2.78 (1.29–5.97)	0.009	2.82 (1.23–6.49)	0.015
	< 37 weeks	1.00 (reference)		1.00 (reference)	
Birth weight	≥3.2 kg	1.06 (0.74–1.52)	0.746		
	< 3.2 kg	1.00 (reference)			
Sex	Male	0.96 (0.67–1.38)	0.833		
	Female	1.00 (reference)			
Age at admission	≥7 days	0.35 (0.24–0.51)	0.001	0.29 (0.16–0.51)	0.001
	< 7 days	1.00 (reference)		1.00 (reference)	
Vaginal delivery	Yes	1.89 (1.29–2.78)	0.001	1.83 (1.20–2.8)	0.005
	No	1.00 (reference)		1.00 (reference)	
Perinatal problem	Yes	1.37 (0.77–2.46)	0.288		
	No	1.00 (reference)			
Exclusive breastfeeding	Yes	2.12 (1.39–3.22)	0.001	3.91 (2.36–6.49)	0.001
	No	1.00 (reference)		1.00 (reference)	
Reticulocyte count	≥2%	1.51 (1.04–2.19)	0.029		
	< 2%	1.00 (reference)			
Hemoglobin level	≥15 mg/dL	3.56 (2.39–5.30)	0.001	3.05 (1.96–4.74)	0.001
	< 15 mg/dL	1.00 (reference)		1.00 (reference)	
C-reactive protein	≥5 mg/L	0.39 (0.23–0.65)	0.001	0.34 (0.20–0.61)	0.001
	< 5 mg/L	1.00 (reference)		1.00 (reference)	
Rotavirus test	Positive	2.20 (1.51–3.21)	0.001	1.89 (1.20–2.98)	0.006
	Negative	1.00 (reference)		1.00 (reference)	
Late-onset sepsis	Yes	0.65 (0.07–5.82)	0.645		
	No	1.00 (reference)			

when the CRP level was ≥5 mg/dL compared to that when the CRP level was < 5 mg/dL [OR = 0.34; 95% CI, 0.20–0.61; $p = 0.001$].

Discussion

An important finding of our study is that RV infection was associated with neonatal jaundice. The prevalence of jaundice was 27.8% among all patients admitted to NICU, and among jaundiced patients, 42.2% had positive tests for RV infection. In addition, 22% of jaundiced patients demonstrated asymptomatic RV infection. The incidence of jaundice was higher in the RV-positive group.

RV is now known to be an important causative agent of hospital infections. An electrophoretic analysis revealed that 41% of RV infections occur during winter and 30% of asymptomatic infections occur in other seasons [16]. In addition, other reports on RV infection in neonates suggested a high infection rate with few signs or symptoms [17]. Only 14 (23%) infants infected with RV experienced fever, vomiting, and diarrhea [12]. Several factors have been proposed to be responsible for asymptomatic RV infection observed in neonates, including host features such as physiological immaturity of the neonatal gut, the role of maternal antibodies, and virulence characteristics of the unique neonatal strains. It is known that asymptomatic infants usually develop asymptomatic infections due to the newborn strain, which is completely different from the RV strain found in pediatric patients, but it is known to cause diarrhea, dehydration, jaundice, metabolic acidosis, necrotizing enteritis, and even death [18]. Identifying neonates who are infected with RV is important for infection control in the NICU. The prevalence of RV in hospitals is high, but once mass incidence occurs, it is difficult to block transmission, despite proper patient isolation [19]. Moreover, most infected neonates have no specific enteritis symptoms and go through an incubation period. Therefore, infants with asymptomatic jaundice caused by RV infection should be screened for rapid isolation.

Jaundice is common and is associated with a variety of physiological and pathological conditions. It is the main reason for hospital readmission during the neonatal period and has long been recognized as a clinical manifestation of infection in the neonate and early infancy [7]. It is known that various infections such as neonatal sepsis, congenital infection, and hepatitis are risk factors for neonatal jaundice. Previous studies have demonstrated that urinary tract infections were associated with jaundice, but there is no such study on RV [8, 9, 20, 21]. In our study of the jaundice group, total bilirubin levels were less than 15 mg/dL in the rotavirus infection group. Rotavirus-induced jaundice did not increase the total bilirubin level more than in other causes. In addition, rotavirus infection is diagnosed early in the disease because it can be screened before other causes.

Besides RV infection, neonates born at term, born via vaginal delivery, those who are exclusively breastfed, and who have high Hb were at high risk in this study. Breastfeeding was associated with neonatal jaundice that lasted longer and reached higher peak levels than milk feeding [21]. Jaundice in breastfed babies usually appears between 24 and 72 h after birth, peaks by 5–15 days of life, and disappears by the third week of life; high bilirubin levels have been reported in such infants [22]. While exclusive breastfeeding has historically been an important predictor for jaundice, the mechanism underlying the association is not well understood. Our results demonstrate that vaginal delivery was associated with jaundice. The present findings indicate that naturally delivered neonates were more likely to have jaundice than those born via cesarean section. Previous studies have shown that the risk of jaundice increases in children delivered via cesarean section [5]. Similar to our study, Bulbul et al. [23] reported a statistically significant correlation between the severity of jaundice and mode of delivery. However, other studies have yielded controversial results regarding the relationship between labor and jaundice. Some studies demonstrated a lack of significant relationship between mode of delivery and jaundice [24].

Our study has several limitations owing to its retrospective nature. It did not include healthy infants and was targeted toward infants admitted to the NICU. Although the RIDASCREEN® RV test has high sensitivity to RV infection, there is a possibility of false positives in the RV test results. Therefore, asymptomatic RV-positive patients can have false-positive results. In addition to the exclusion of 1159 (66%) patients, we excluded patients in the incubation period of rotavirus; this difference may lead to selection bias of the included patients or incorrect risk estimates. However, our study was also meaningful in that all patients admitted to the NICU were screened for RV infection.

Conclusions

RV infection can occur in asymptomatic neonates presenting with jaundice. Jaundice may be the first sign of RV infection before other signs become evident. Thus, we suggest that RV screening tests be considered as a part of the diagnostic evaluation of neonates older than 3 days presenting with hyperbilirubinemia.

Abbreviations

CRP: C-reactive protein; GA: Gestational age; Hb: Hemoglobin; NICU: Neonatal intensive care unit; PCR: Polymerase chain reaction; PROM: Premature rupture of membrane; RV: Rotavirus; SGA: Small for gestational age

Acknowledgments

The authors thank the nurses and doctors of the neonatal intensive care unit.

Funding

Not applicable.

Authors' contributions

Study conception and design: JKK. Acquisition of data: NRH. Analysis and interpretation of data: NRH, JKK. Preparation, critical revision and final approval of the manuscript: both authors.

Competing interests

The authors declare that they have no competing interests.

References

1. Cicirello HG, Das BK, Gupta A, Bhan MK, Gentsch JR, Kumar R, et al. High prevalence of rotavirus infection among neonates born at hospitals in Delhi, India: predisposition of newborns for infection with unusual rotavirus. Pediatr Infect Dis J. 1994;13:720–4.
2. Ramani S, Sowmyanarayanan TV, Gladstone BP, Bhowmick K, Asirvatham JR, Jana AK, et al. Rotavirus infection in the neonatal nurseries of a tertiary care hospital in India. Pediatr Infect Dis J. 2008;27:719–23.
3. Chung KO, Lee DS, Kim DK, Choi SM, Kim WT, Yu SH. Study of nosocomial infection of rotavirus in preterm and full-term neonates. Korean J Pediatr. 1999;42:332–8.
4. Baek JM, Kim HY, Lee JH, Choi BM, Lee J, Lee KC, et al. Incidence and clinical manifestations of rotaviral infections in a neonatal intensive care unit. J Korean Soc Neonatol. 2009;16:55–63.
5. Brits H, Adendorff J, Huisamen D, Beukes D, Botha K, Herbst H, et al. The prevalence of neonatal jaundice and risk factors in healthy term neonates at National District Hospital in Bloemfontein. Afr J Prim Health Care Fam Med. 2018;10:e1–6.
6. Goedhals D, Kriel J, Hertzog ML, Janse van Rensburg MN. Human cytomegalovirus infection in infants with prolonged neonatal jaundice. J Clin Virol. 2008;43:216–8.
7. Bernstein J, Brown AK. Sepsis and jaundice in early infancy. Pediatrics. 1962;29:873–82.
8. Ng SH, Rawstron JR. Urinary tract infections presenting with jaundice. Arch Dis Child. 1971;46:173–6.
9. Shahian M, Rashtian P, Kalani M. Unexplained neonatal jaundice as an early diagnostic sign of urinary tract infection. Int J Infect Dis. 2012;16:e487–90.
10. Subcommittee on Hyperbilirubinemia. Management of hyperbilirubinemia in the newborn infant 35 or more weeks of gestation. Pediatrics. 2004;114:297–316.
11. Sharma R, Hudak ML, Premachandra BR, Stevens G, Monteiro CB, Bradshaw JA, et al. Clinical manifestations of rotavirus infection in the neonatal intensive care unit. Pediatr Infect Dis J. 2002;21:1099–105.

12. Staat MA, Azimi PH, Berke T, Roberts N, Bernstein DI, Ward RL, et al. Clinical presentations of rotavirus infection among hospitalized children. Pediatr Infect Dis J. 2002;21:221–7.
13. Gautam R, Lyde F, Esona MD, Quaye O, Bowen MD. Comparison of premier™ Rotaclone®, ProSpecT™, and RIDASCREEN® rotavirus enzyme immunoassay kits for detection of rotavirus antigen in stool specimens. J Clin Virol. 2013;58:292–4.
14. Kovacs A, Chan L, Hotrakitya C, Overturf G, Portnoy B. Rotavirus gastroenteritis: clinical and laboratory features and use of the Rotazyme test. Am J Dis Child. 1987;141:161–6.
15. Hisamuddin E, Hisam A, Wahid S, Raza G. Validity of C-reactive protein (CRP) for diagnosis of neonatal sepsis. Pak J Med Sci. 2015;31:527–31.
16. Sukumaran M, Gowda K, Maiya PP, Srinivas TP, Kumar MS, Aijaz S, et al. Exclusive asymptomatic neonatal infections by human rotavirus strains having subgroup I specificity and "long" RNA electropherotype. Arch Virol. 1992;126:239–51.
17. Rodriguez WJ, Kim HW, Arrobio JO, Brandt CD, Chanock RM, Kapikian AZ, et al. Clinical features of acute gastroenteritis associated with human reovirus-like agent in infants and young children. J Pediatr. 1977;91:188–93.
18. de Villiers FP, Driessen M. Clinical neonatal rotavirus infection: association with necrotising enterocolitis. S Afr Med J. 2012;102:620–4.
19. Santos N, Riepenhoff-Talty M, Clark HF, Offit P, Gouvea V. VP4 genotyping of human rotavirus in the United States. J Clin Microbiol. 1994;32:205–8.
20. Garcia FJ, Nager AL. Jaundice as an early diagnostic sign of urinary tract infection in infancy. Pediatrics. 2002;109:846–51.
21. Omar C, Hamza S, Bassem AM, Mariam R. Urinary tract infection and indirect hyperbilirubinemia in newborns. N Am J Med Sci. 2011;3:544–7.
22. Alcock GS, Liley H. Immunoglobulin infusion for isoimmune haemolytic jaundice in neonates. Cochrane Database Syst Rev 2002. https://doi.org/10.1002/14651858.CD003313.
23. Bulbul A, Cayonu N, Sanli ME, Uslu S. Evaluation of risk factors for development of severe hyperbilirubinemia in term and near term infants in Turkey. Pak J Med Sci. 2014;30:1113–8.
24. Garosi E, Mohammadi F, Ranjkesh F. The relationship between neonatal jaundice and maternal and neonatal factors. Iran J Neonatol. 2016;7:37–40.

22

C-Reactive Protein (CRP) levels in neonatal meningitis in England: an analysis of national variations in CRP cut-offs for lumbar puncture

Jonathan P. Sturgeon*, Beatrice Zanetti and Dwight Lindo

Abstract

Background: Recent National Institute for Health and Care Excellence (NICE) CG149 guidelines suggest considering performing a lumbar puncture (LP) to investigate for meningitis in early-onset sepsis in a neonate when a C-reactive protein (CRP) level >10mg/L, but the evidence for this recommendation is poorly defined.

Methods: Data on trust-wide LP protocols, neonatal meningitis incidence, lumbar punctures, and CRP levels seen in cases of neonatal meningitis were asked of all 137 trusts in England that recorded a birth in 2017. Our local Kingston Hospital data on every LP performed was obtained to estimate the specificity of CRP rises.

Results: 73/123 (59.3%) of trusts follow the NICE CG149 recommendation of considering an LP if the CRP >10mg/L. The national incidence of neonatal meningitis was 0.467/1,000 births, and an LP was performed in 1.37% of all babies, which was significantly higher in trusts considering the CRP > 10mg/L cut-off. A CRP > 10mg/L cut-off sensitivity was 88.9% based on the highest CRP level 4 days around the LP from national data of 199 cases; specificity was 78.8% based on our single-unit analysis.

Conclusions: Proposing a universal CRP > 10mg/L cut-off for a lumbar puncture has been counter-productive in England. Following it generates significantly more LPs, to the point that 40.7% of trusts have chosen not to follow it. It also has poor sensitivity missing over 11% of meningitis. We therefore do not recommend a universal cut-off, rather considering the whole clinical picture (including prematurity) when considering whether to do an LP.

Keywords: meningitis, neonatal, CG149, C-reactive protein, CRP, cut-off, neonatal meningitis, lumbar puncture, cerebrospinal fluid

Background

Neonatal meningitis is a potentially serious infection which occurs in around 0.25 – 1.0 per 1000 live births [1, 2]. Although the case-fatality rate of neonatal meningitis has fallen to around 6.6% for all-cause meningitis [1] or 12.4% for GBS meningitis [3], the morbidity associated with the disease remains unchanged over the last 30 years [2, 4].

A lumbar puncture (LP) is required to investigate for meningitis by sampling cerebrospinal fluid (CSF) for microscopy, bacterial culture, and protein and glucose levels. The decision of when to perform an LP in a neonate can be a difficult one. For those with early onset sepsis (usually <72h old), the American Academy of Pediatrics (AAP) recommend performing an LP if the blood culture is positive, the 'clinical course or laboratory data strongly suspect bacterial sepsis,' or if the infant does not respond to antimicrobial therapy [5]. In England and Wales, the National Institute for Health and Care Excellence (NICE) have published CG149 guidance suggesting an LP be 'considered' if the blood culture is positive, the baby does not respond to antimicrobial therapy, or if the baby has a 'C-reactive protein concentration of 10 mg/litre or greater' [6]. This decision to name a specific cut-off CRP of 10mg/L has been criticised by some, with a previous study carried out in 2014 finding that when only the 59 regional referral neonatal units were examined just 14% (10/56) of them followed this CRP guidance [7].

* Correspondence: jonathan.sturgeon@nhs.net
Department of Paediatrics, Kingston Hospital, Kingston, London KT2 7QB, UK

This study therefore aimed to determine the compliance of all neonatal units in England with this NICE CG149 guidance, the number of LPs performed and the number of neonatal meningitis cases seen, as well as the CRP levels seen in these cases in order to estimate a sensitivity for a CRP cut-off of 10mg/L in neonatal meningitis. A recent evaluation of all the lumbar punctures performed at our local unit (Kingston Hospital, London) is also included.

Methods

Assessment of national picture of neonatal meningitis for all NHS trusts across England

A list of all 137 NHS trusts at which a birth had taken place in England in the most recent maternity report was obtained from NHS Digital [8]. Requests were made under the Freedom of Information Act (2000).

CRP Level for lumbar puncture

Each trust was asked for their neonatal sepsis and lumbar puncture protocol as of 13/2/2018, and whether there was a specific CRP which would warrant a lumbar puncture. Responses were assessed as to whether any 'consideration' was given to a lumbar puncture because the CRP was >10mg/L, and whether there were any additional levels stated at which a lumbar puncture should be done. If different numbers for different hospitals in the same trust were given, the highest number was captured.

Lumbar puncture and meningitis incidence

For the period between 01/10/2015 (when some ICD10 codes were changed) and 31/3/2018 each trust was asked for the number of episodes with Z38.*, representing any live birth by any mode of delivery, the number of these which also had a lumbar puncture procedure code A55.9, and finally which of these received a G00.*, G01.*, G02.*, or G03.* code for meningitis.

Maximal CRP in meningitis

Each trust that had >5 episodes of neonatal meningitis was asked to provide the highest CRP level seen in the 4 days before or 4 days after the positive lumbar puncture for each patient (defined as culture positive, WCC > 20/mm^3, or PCR positive) – only providing a result if there were a positive CSF.

Assessment of local lumbar puncture results at Kingston Hospital

Every CSF sample received from the neonatal or post-natal wards at Kingston Hospital by the laboratory between 15/12/2014 – 31/1/2018 was included. Kingston rigidly interpreted the NICE CG149 guidelines, with the trust's guidelines introduced in June 2013, aiming to perform an LP on every neonate with a CRP > 10mg/L, as well as if any positive culture or clinical concern.

The CSF protein, glucose, cell count, and CSF culture result were noted, as well as the maximal blood CRP in the first three days after starting antibiotics, and blood culture result. The baby's age and gestation were also noted. A lumbar puncture was considered culture positive if the CSF grew an organism, and 'cell count' positive if there were more than 20 WCC/mL in the CSF sample.

Data analysis

Data were analysed using SPSS (v24, IBM Corp); graphs were prepared using Graphpad Prism (v7.0c, Graphpad software); trusts were mapped using Tableau Desktop (v10.5, Tableau Software). Groups were compared using Mann-Whitney U test with significance being considered at $p<0.05$, having confirmed the data was not normally distributed.

Results

National data

Out of the 137 trusts listed in England that recorded a birth in 2016-7, because of three mergers and two trusts only providing community care with no inpatient facilities, at the time of the requests there were 132 trusts that could provide treatment to a potentially sick neonate. All were successfully contacted to request the desired information.

CRP level for lumbar puncture

A total of 123/132 (93.2%) of trusts responded. 73/123 (59.3%) of trusts gave some degree of consideration to a lumbar puncture when the CRP was over 10mg/L, therefore directly following the NICE CG149 guidelines. The remainder either did not give any CRP value – leaving the decision for a lumbar puncture up to treating clinician (20/123, 16.3%), or gave a higher CRP level at which lumbar punctures would be considered (30/123, 24.4%, range 20 – 50 mg/L, median 20mg/L). Data shown on the map in Fig. 1.

Of the 73 trusts that did give some form of consideration to an LP with a CRP of >10mg/L, 32 gave a further de facto higher level for babies who were asymptomatic, usually on the postnatal ward (range 20 – 60 mg/L, median 20mg/L).

Lumbar puncture and meningitis rates

101/132 trusts (76.5%) provided full data on lumbar punctures and meningitis rates. On top of this, eight trusts provided their number of cases of meningitis in the period as 'under five' over concerns over identification of patients, and three trusts inadvertently provided the diagnosis code of A55.9, rather than the procedure code, and did not respond to requests to correct it. These data were excluded from analysis. There were

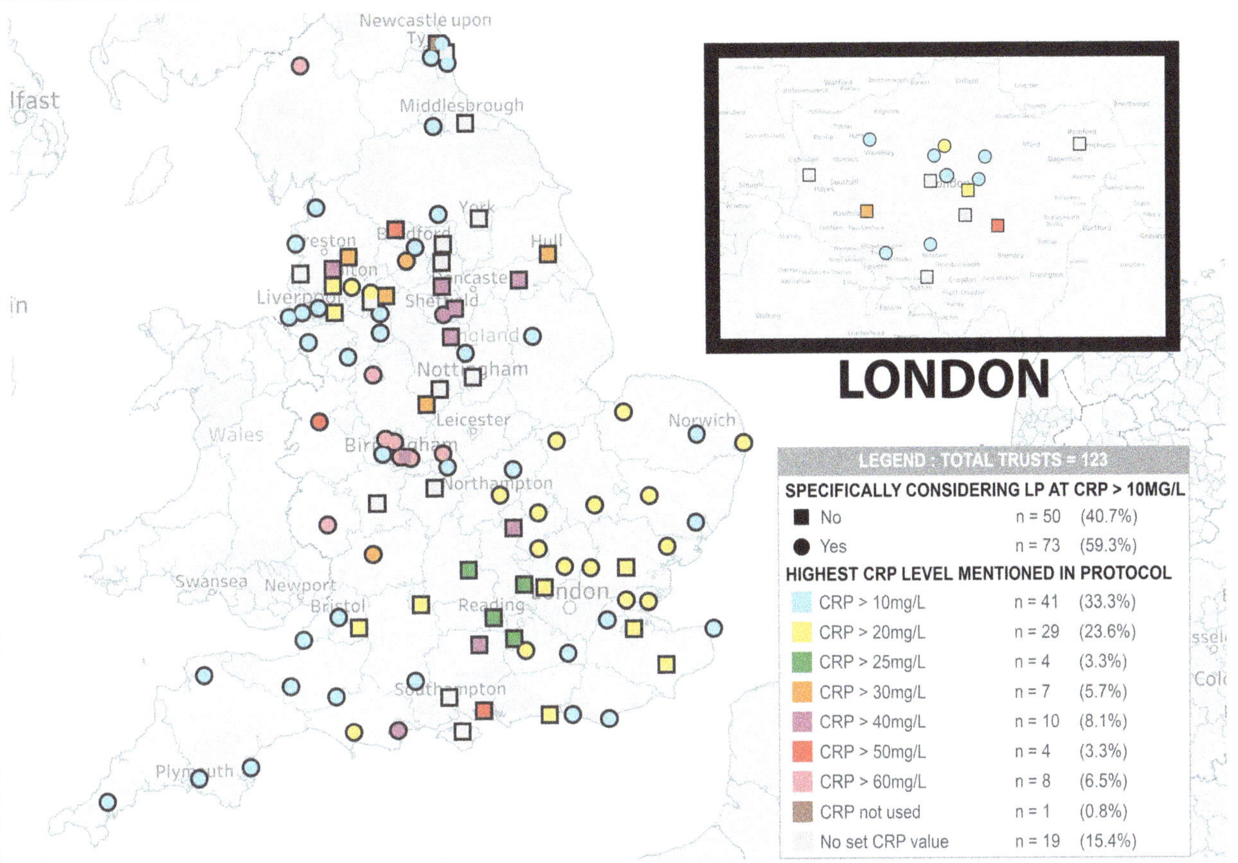

Fig. 1 Map of England showing the trusts which consider a neonatal LP at CRP > 10mg/L, as well as the maximum CRP cut-off for an LP mentioned in their protocol. Map background © OpenStreetMap contributors, and is reproduced under the Open Database Licence; information is available from openstreetmap.org

1,233,485 live births between 1/10/15 and 31/3/18. Of these 16,963 (1.37%) also received a lumbar puncture coding, and 576 also received a meningitis diagnosis in the same episode, representing a nationwide incidence of 0.467/1000 live births. Trusts considering an LP at CRP > 10mg/L carry out a significantly higher number of LPs compared with trusts that do not specifically mention this cut-off (median 1.07%, IQR 0.65 – 2.3%, of live births v 0.85%, IQR 0.34 – 1.31%, p=0.042), without a corresponding significant increase in meningitis cases (0.27/1,000 live births, IQR 0.00 – 0.87, v 0.20/1,000, IQR 0.04 – 0.64, p=0.54), as shown in Fig. 2.

CRP rises in neonates with meningitis

CRP levels were provided for 199 cases of neonatal meningitis out of a possible 393 cases, representing a response rate of 50.6% of cases from trusts with over 5 cases. The mean maximum CRP was 56.7mg/L, with 22 cases (11.1%) having a maximum CRP level of <10mg/L in their meningitis infection; this represents a sensitivity of 88.9% for that cut-off in all neonatal meningitis. The breakdown of the maximum CRPs seen is shown in Fig. 3.

Local (Kingston Hospital) lumbar puncture data

511 CSF samples were sent from the neonatal unit or postnatal ward at Kingston Hospital between 15/12/2014 – 31/01/2018. There was an LP frequency of 2.76% of live births. The mean maximal CRP seen in the babies was 36.9mg/L. The breakdown of all LPs by neonatal maximal CRP are shown in Fig. 4.

There were 12 CSF samples that were positive on bacterial culture, 11 of these were commensal organisms and on consideration of the whole clinical picture of the baby the attending physician considered them contaminants. The culture-positive CSF sample was *Enterobacteriaceae* growth in a premature baby who had a maximum CRP of < 10 mg/L, with the LP done because they also grew the same organism in their blood culture. A total of 224 samples were also tested for virology, and 1 was positive with an enterovirus with a maximal CRP of between 20 - 29.9 mg/L.

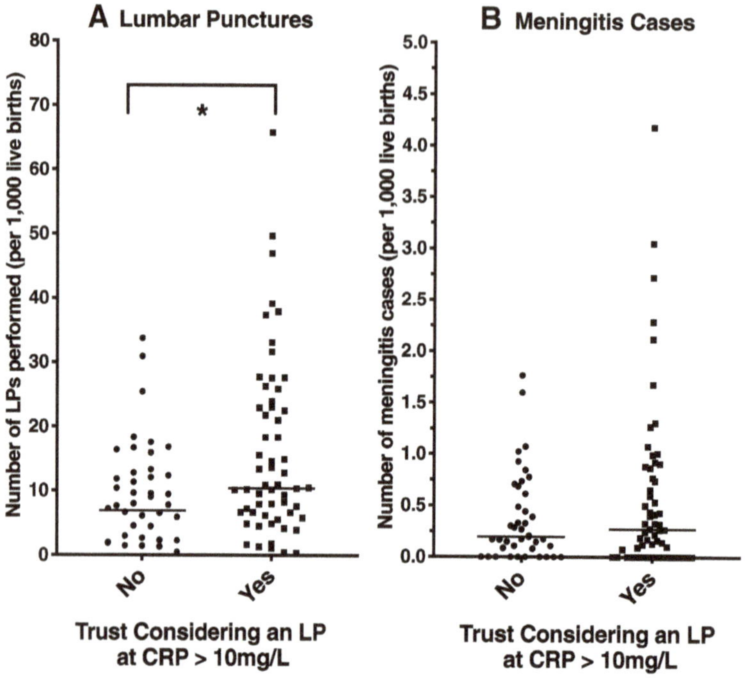

Fig. 2 Graphs showing **a** the number of LPs done per 1000 live births by trust and **b** the number of meningitis cases diagnosed per 1000 live births. Each dot represents an individual trust, separated in to trusts which consider a lumbar puncture (LP) at CRP >10mg/L or not. The bars represent the median values. * = $p<0.05$

Four further babies were treated as meningitis because of a significant pleocytosis, with a white cell rise to >20/mm^3 in the CSF. Two additional cases of mild pleocytosis (20-35/mm^3) were considered by the attending physician to be because of a traumatic tap, and were not treated as meningitis.

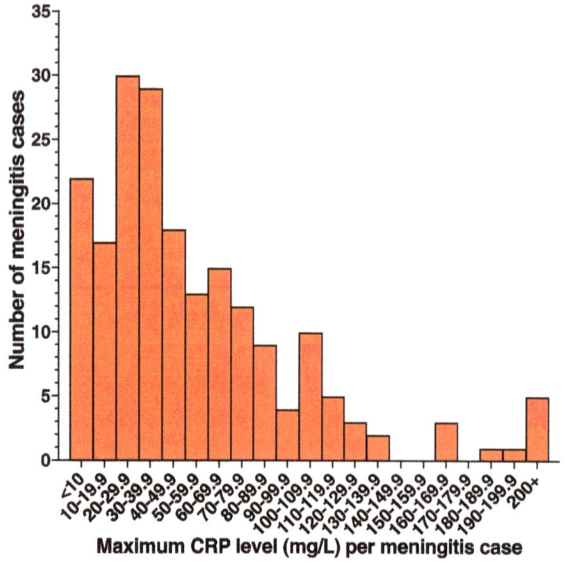

Fig. 3 The maximal CRP levels seen in cases of neonatal meningitis, using the national data

There were 2273 incidences of babies being screened and treated for sepsis, making them potentially eligible for an LP. As no baby with CRP <10mg/L was subsequently re-admitted with a positive CSF, it is reasonable to assume they are likely not to have had meningitis. With this assumption, this represents a local specificity for the CRP >10mg/L cut-off of 78.8%. The local positive predictive value (PPV) of CRP > 10mg/L cut-off was 1.0% overall, but broken down was 0.4% for babies over 37 weeks' gestation, and 5.6% for pre-term babies.

Discussion

This study looked at the adoption of the NICE CG149 CRP >10mg/L cut-off for considering an LP in neonatal units in England, the number of LPs and cases of neonatal meningitis diagnosed, the CRP rises seen in these cases, as well as the breakdown of all neonatal LPs performed at our local unit.

The observed neonatal meningitis incidence rate of 0.467/1,000 live births fits well with the 0.25 – 1.0/1,000 values already reported in the literature [2]. The national neonatal LP rate of 1.37% is slightly lower than the 1.7% previously quoted from a single-centred study from 1995, [9] which was before the introduction of the 2012 CG149 guideline, and lower than the Kingston LP incidence of 2.76% which rigidly used a CRP >10mg/L cut-off. This suggests following the release of the CG149

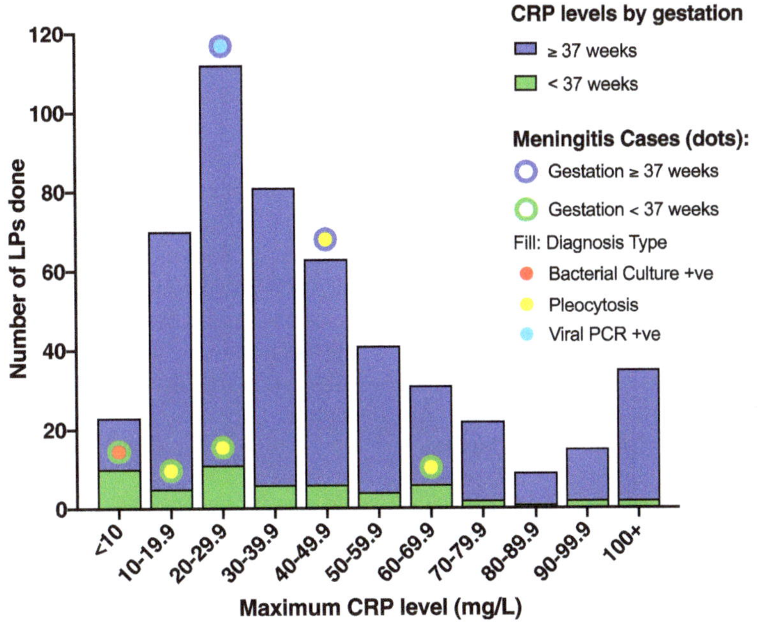

Fig. 4 Graph showing the maximal CRP levels seen in those babies who had a lumbar puncture (LP) at Kingston Hospital, along with the cases that had meningitis

guideline, the number of LPs had not increased, perhaps reflecting the level of its adoption.

Only 59.3% of the 123 local trusts who responded have guidelines that specifically follow the NICE CG149 CRP >10mg/L cut-off for 'considering' an LP in a neonate, with the remainder either not having a level, or having a higher cut-off. The CRP level is just one of the three NICE CG149 criteria for consideration of an LP, but because of the low incidence of either positive blood cultures [10] or poor response to antibiotics, it is the criteria that most considerations for an LP would fall under. Several trusts expand in their protocol why their CRP cut-off does not follow the national guidance, with one trust simply putting 'it has been admitted this number is not evidence based', another saying it was 'too low', and there has been concerns that adopting the CRP cut-off increases the number of LPs done [11]. This is seen in this study in the significantly higher rate of LPs done in trusts who have adopted the CG149 CRP criteria in their protocols.

When looking at their explanation for why they chose a CRP < 10mg/L cut-off for an LP, the NICE guideline development group (GDG) based their CRP > 10mg/L recommendation looking at evidence of CRP rises seen in neonatal sepsis. For a sepsis diagnosis their evidence looked at different CRP cut-offs from 2.5mg/L [12] to 10mg/L [13] for diagnosis of sepsis in babies aged under 12 hours [12] to up to 10 days old [14], therefore making their final recommendation based on the increased likelihood of sepsis rather than specifically meningitis. The GDG were no doubt considering that in bacteraemic infants, the meningitis incidence can be as high as 23% [15, 16].

However, CRP rises do not necessarily mean bacteraemia, and vice-versa. CRP responses in neonatal infection are heterogenous: CRP synthesis is delayed during the early inflammatory response therefore CRP has low sensitivity during early phases of the disease, necessitating repeat measurements [17]. Severity of illness, hypoxia, prematurity, and co-morbidities can all blunt a CRP response [18]. In addition, the CRP can also rise secondary to non-infective conditions including respiratory distress syndrome, meconium aspiration syndrome, stressful delivery, perinatal asphyxia or intraventricular haemorrhage [19] meaning it is poorly specific. Although CRP cannot cross the placenta, maternal pro-inflammatory cytokines such as IL-6 can cross the placenta, potentially inducing CRP production in the neonate [20]. Consequently, studies have shown that maternal fever and prolonged labour can increase CRP in uninfected neonates [21]. These non-infectious rises can be significant – one study of 859 well neonates showed a mean CRP rise to 4.1mg/L by 48 hours, with the 95% centile of the results rising to 13.3mg/L [22].

Because of the low incidence of neonatal meningitis, few studies have been done on the CRP rises in neonatal meningitis, and those done have small numbers: the sensitivity of a CRP > 10mg/L cut-off has been suggested to be 76.3% in one study, [23] and a CRP > 40mg/L to be 72.7% at 24h [24]. This study is therefore able to add a significant body of data representing the CRP rises in neonatal meningitis with a positive CSF (either culture positive, WCC > 20/mm3, or PCR positive), with poor sensitivity and specificity for a CRP > 10mg/L cut-off. Being the highest recorded CRP value 4 days around the positive LP, the timings of the CRPs in this study do not match the initial and 18-24h timings of the NICE CG149 guideline. This wider timeframe was chosen to ensure the highest CRP rise was captured when an LP could have been done at any time during the course of the illness. If the CRP rise could have been restricted to the CG149 initial and 18-24h repeat values of the septic episode, the sensitivity is likely to have been even lower.

Limitations of this study are related to how the data was obtained, through Freedom of Information Act (2000) requests. As well as the administrative burden it places on trusts, no personally identifiable information could be obtained, so information such as the neonate's gestation could not be requested. Gestation is significant with neonatal sepsis: premature babies below 33 weeks' gestation, and low-weight infants are more likely to get infections, [1] and their CRP rises are likely to be less. Reflecting the likely different response to meningitis in term babies, several one-centre reports [25–27] as well as one review question, [28] suggest no asymptomatic term baby had meningitis regardless of CRP level. This is reflected in our local results with the CRP > 10mg/L cut-off demonstrating a significantly lower PPV at 0.4% for term babies, but 5.6% for pre-term babies. Finally, because Hospital Episode Statistics were used to identify cases of neonatal meningitis, and each case required a Z38.* birth code given once only, any neonate who had meningitis after discharge or transfer would not be included.

Finally, because there is no coding differentiation between early- and late-onset sepsis meningitis, both are included in this study. Although the organisms causing late-onset sepsis may be different, CRP responses in early- and late- onset sepsis are similar with potentially more sensitivity for sepsis in late-onset sepsis [29].

Conclusions

With the dissimilar causes and responses of CRP rises in different-gestation neonates, and the lack of evidence of CRP changes in neonatal meningitis, it is easy to see why the AAP did not recommend a laboratory-marker cut-off for doing an LP [5]. The NICE GDG may well have been attempting to ensure all neonates with meningitis were included by selecting a specific CRP for their LP criteria. Recognising these criteria were poorly specific they included the instruction to only 'consider' an LP if CRP > 10mg/L or one of the other criteria were filled – allowing for physician discretion to reduce unnecessary LPs. This approach has practically been counter-productive when considering its adoption, on both sensitivity and specificity grounds. Because physician discretion is not conducive to black-and-white instructions on local protocols, 40.7% trusts have not adopted it presumably due to the number of LPs it would require given the test's low specificity on the background of low-incidence disease. It also fails to include 11.1% of neonatal meningitis cases. Because of both of these failures, it does not seem prudent to assign a universal CRP cut-off for consideration of an LP, rather the decision should be multi-faceted taking in to account the gestation, clinical assessment, microbiology results, strength of concern, as well as any blood results such as CRP.

Abbreviations

AAP: American Academy of Pediatrics; CRP: C-reactive protein; CSF: cerebrospinal fluid; GDG: guideline development group; LP: lumbar puncture; NICE: National Institute for Health and Care Excellence; PPV: positive predictive value

Acknowledgements

Many thanks to Sarah Furrows who helped to collect the local data on cerebrospinal fluid samples. We would like to acknowledge and thank all the trusts responding to the requests for data. Additional thanks to Jenny Crooks in the trust Research and Development office for helping to confirm ethical and regulatory requirements for this project.

Funding

Nil.

Authors' contributions

Project idea by DL and JS; Data collection by JS and BZ; JS, BZ, and DL helped to write and review the manuscript, which was approved by all authors.

Ethics approval and consent to participate

As the national data involved is anonymised publicly-available data, no ethical opinion from an ethics committee was sought, which is in line with current views on ethical requirements of freedom of information act data[30]. The local Kingston data was collected by the clinical care team and then anonymised for the purposes of this project. The local Research & Development office has confirmed that no ethical approval or consent was required for this project; the local data released has been approved by the trust's Caldecott guardian.

Competing interests

JS is an Academic Clinical Fellow in paediatrics, which is funded by the NIHR.

References

1. Holt D, Halket S, de Louvois J, Harvey D. Neonatal meningitis in England and Wales: 10 years on. Archives of disease in childhood Fetal and neonatal edition. 2001;84(2):F85–9.
2. Heath PT, Okike IO, Oeser C. Neonatal Meningitis: Can We Do Better? In: Curtis N, Finn A, Pollard AJ, editors. Hot Topics in Infection and Immunity in Children VIII. New York: Springer New York; 2011. p. 11–24.

3. Heath PT, Balfour G, Weisner AM, Efstratiou A, Lamagni TL, Tighe H, O'Connell LA, Cafferkey M, Verlander NQ, Nicoll A, et al. Group B streptococcal disease in UK and Irish infants younger than 90 days. Lancet. 2004;363(9405):292–4.
4. Polin RA, Harris MC. Neonatal bacterial meningitis. Seminars in neonatology : SN. 2001;6(2):157–72.
5. Polin RA. Management of Neonates With Suspected or Proven Early-Onset Bacterial Sepsis: Pediatrics; 2012.
6. Neonatal infection (early onset): antibiotics for prevention and treatment. Clinical guideline [CG149] [https://www.nice.org.uk/guidance/cg149/]
7. Mukherjee A, Ramalingaiah B, Kennea N, Duffy DA. Management of neonatal early onset sepsis (CG149): compliance of neonatal units in the UK with NICE recommendations. Archives of disease in childhood Fetal and neonatal edition. 2015;100(2):F185.
8. NHS Maternity Statistics, England 2016-17 [https://digital.nhs.uk/data-and-information/publications/statistical/nhs-maternity-statistics/2016-17]
9. Wiswell TE, Baumgart S, Gannon CM, Spitzer AR. No lumbar puncture in the evaluation for early neonatal sepsis: will meningitis be missed? Pediatrics. 1995;95(6):803–6.
10. Cailes B, Kortsalioudaki C, Buttery J, Pattnayak S, Greenough A, Matthes J, Bedford Russell A, Kennea N, Heath PT. Epidemiology of UK neonatal infections: the neonIN infection surveillance network. Archives of Disease in Childhood - Fetal and Neonatal Edition. 2017;103(6):F547–53.
11. Mukherjee A, Davidson L, Anguvaa L, Duffy DA, Kennea N. NICE neonatal early onset sepsis guidance: greater consistency, but more investigations, and greater length of stay. Archives of Disease in Childhood - Fetal and Neonatal Edition. 2015;100(3):F248–9.
12. Resch B, Gusenleitner W, Muller WD. Procalcitonin and interleukin-6 in the diagnosis of early-onset sepsis of the neonate. Acta paediatrica. 2003;92(2):243–5.
13. Benitz WE, Han MY, Madan A, Ramachandra P. Serial serum C-reactive protein levels in the diagnosis of neonatal infection. Pediatrics. 1998; 102(4):E41.
14. Franz AR, Kron M, Pohlandt F, Steinbach G. Comparison of procalcitonin with interleukin 8, C-reactive protein and differential white blood cell count for the early diagnosis of bacterial infections in newborn infants. The Pediatric infectious disease journal. 1999;18(8):666–71.
15. Isaacs D, Barfield CP, Grimwood K, McPhee AJ, Minutillo C, Tudehope DI. Systemic bacterial and fungal infections in infants in Australian neonatal units. Australian Study Group for Neonatal Infections. The Medical journal of Australia. 1995;162(4):198–201.
16. May M, Daley AJ, Donath S, Isaacs D. Early onset neonatal meningitis in Australia and New Zealand, 1992-2002. Archives of disease in childhood Fetal and neonatal edition. 2005;90(4):F324–7.
17. Hengst JM. The role of C-reactive protein in the evaluation and management of infants with suspected sepsis. Advances in neonatal care : official journal of the National Association of Neonatal Nurses. 2003;3(1):3–13.
18. Chiesa C, Natale F, Pascone R, Osborn JF, Pacifico L, Bonci E, De Curtis M. C reactive protein and procalcitonin: reference intervals for preterm and term newborns during the early neonatal period. Clinica chimica acta; international journal of clinical chemistry. 2011;412(11-12):1053–9.
19. Mathai E, Christopher U, Mathai M, Jana AK, Rose D, Bergstrom S. Is C-reactive protein level useful in differentiating infected from uninfected neonates among those at risk of infection? Indian pediatrics. 2004;41(9):895–900.
20. Chan GJ, Lee AC, Baqui AH, Tan J, Black RE. Risk of early-onset neonatal infection with maternal infection or colonization: a global systematic review and meta-analysis. PLoS medicine. 2013;10(8):e1001502.
21. Chiesa C, Signore F, Assumma M, Buffone E, Tramontozzi P, Osborn JF, Pacifico L. Serial measurements of C-reactive protein and interleukin-6 in the immediate postnatal period: reference intervals and analysis of maternal and perinatal confounders. Clinical chemistry. 2001;47(6):1016–22.
22. Perrone S, Lotti F, Longini M, Rossetti A, Bindi I, Bazzini F, Belvisi E, Sarnacchiaro P, Scapellato C, Buonocore G. C reactive protein in healthy term newborns during the first 48 hours of life. Archives of Disease in Childhood - Fetal and Neonatal Edition. 2018;103(2):F163–6.
23. GC D, Tony K, Despina K, BD P, Kenneth T. C-reactive protein and immature-to-total neutrophil ratio have no utility in guiding lumbar puncture in suspected neonatal sepsis. Journal of paediatrics and child health. 0(0):848–54.
24. Dapaah-Siakwan F, Mehra S, Lodhi S, Mikhno A, Cameron G. White Cell Indices and CRP: Predictors of Meningitis in Neonatal Sepsis? International Journal of Pediatrics. 2016;4(2):1355–64.
25. Abdelrhim H, Heaton P. G410(P) Is what we do rationale? Is lumbar puncture indicated in well looking term newborns < 72 hours age with high CRP values? Archives of Disease in Childhood. 2014;99(Suppl 1):A172.
26. Johnson CE, Whitwell JK, Pethe K, Saxena K, Super DM. Term newborns who are at risk for sepsis: are lumbar punctures necessary? Pediatrics. 1997;99(4):E10.
27. Kumar P, Sarkar S, Narang A. Role of routine lumbar puncture in neonatal sepsis. Journal of paediatrics and child health. 1995;31(1):8–10.
28. Ray B, Mangalore J, Harikumar C, Tuladhar A. Is lumbar puncture necessary for evaluation of early neonatal sepsis? Archives of Disease in Childhood. 2006;91(12):1033–5.
29. Loni R, Sengupta A, Jaganathan G, Singh PK. The evaluation of C-reactive protein as a screening tool for neonatal sepsis. International Journal of Contemporary Pediatrics. 2016;3(4):1329–33.
30. Savage A, Hyde R. Using freedom of information requests to facilitate research. International Journal of Social Research Methodology. 2014;17(3): 303–17.

Hospitalisation after birth of infants: cross sectional analysis of potentially avoidable admissions across England using hospital episode statistics

Eleanor Jones[1*], Beck Taylor[1], Gavin Rudge[1], Christine MacArthur[1], Deepthi Jyothish[2], Doug Simkiss[3] and Carole Cummins[1]

Abstract

Background: Admissions of infants in England have increased substantially but there is little evidence whether this is across the first year or predominately in neonates; and for all or for specific causes. We aimed to characterise this increase, especially those admissions that may be avoidable in the context of postnatal care provision.

Methods: A cross sectional analysis of 1,387,677 infants up to age one admitted to English hospitals between April 2008 and April 2014 using Hospital Episode Statistics and live birth denominators for England from Office for National Statistics. Potentially avoidable conditions were defined through a staged process with a panel.

Results: The rate of hospital admission in the first year of life for physiological jaundice, feeding difficulties and gastroenteritis, the three conditions identified as potentially preventable in the context of postnatal care provision, increased by 39% (39.55 to 55.33 per 1000 live births) relative to an overall increase of 6% (334.97 to 354.55 per 1000 live births). Over the first year the biggest increase in admissions occurred in the first 0–6 days (RR 1.26, 95% CI 1.24 to 1.29) and 85% of the increase (12.36 to 18.23 per 1000 live births) in this period was for the three potentially preventable conditions.

Conclusions: Most of the increase in infant hospital admissions was in the early neonatal period, the great majority being accounted for by three potentially avoidable conditions especially jaundice and feeding difficulties. This may indicate missed opportunities within the postnatal care pathway and given the enormous NHS cost and parental distress from hospital admission of infants, requires urgent attention.

Keywords: Infant admission, Avoidable readmission, Postnatal care

Background

Hospital admissions, especially emergency ones place a huge cost on health services [1, 2] and there is evidence from studies using Hospital Episode Statistics (HES) data for England that emergency admissions of children have increased substantially. In children under 15 between 1999 and 2010 in England all emergency admissions increased with the greatest increase in infants: in 2010 over a third of infants had an admission some time in their first year [3].

* Correspondence: exj480@student.bham.ac.uk
[1]Institute of Applied Health Research, University of Birmingham, Edgbaston, Birmingham B15 2TH, England
Full list of author information is available at the end of the article

While emergency admissions between 2006 and 2016 increased in all age categories 0–24, this was greatest in those under one [4]. Short-stay (< 2 days) unplanned admissions among children up to age 10 increased between 1996 to 2006, again with the greatest increase in children less than one [4]. A study of infant admission in England using HES data showed that between 2005 and 2014, 5.2% of infants were readmitted unexpectedly within 30 days of postnatal discharge and that the risk of readmission increased by 4.4% annually from 4.4% in 2005 to 6.3% in 2014 [5]. Whilst similar trends have been observed in Scotland [6] in the United States and Canada the proportion of hospital stays for children has decreased or remained relatively unchanged over the period 2000–2012 [5, 7].

Over the last 30 years, the postnatal length of stay in hospital in the UK has reduced considerably: in 1989–90, only 44% women were discharged within two days of giving birth compared to 81% women in 2016–17 [8]. Over the last decade, the number of women going home on the same calendar day that they gave birth has increased considerably from (16.5% in 2005/06 to 19.8% in 2016/17 [8]. Following discharge from hospital, women and babies also have fewer visits from community midwifery services before being discharged to the care of the community health visitor and GP [9, 10].

We wanted to know whether the changes to postnatal care provision coincided with the increase in infant admissions which in some cases may have been potentially avoided. We sought to investigate whether the increase in infant admissions was predominantly in the early neonatal period and whether it was confined to a sub-group of conditions more sensitive to the quantity and quality of postnatal care, and therefore amenable to intervention earlier in the care pathway. If findings showed this to be the case, the current five year national maternity review programme in England [11] would provide an opportunity to consider the potential for intervention.

Methods

Data on all admissions to hospital in the first year of life across England from 1st April 2008 to 31st March 2014 from Hospital Episode Statistics (HES) were included. We developed clinical definitions of potentially avoidable conditions. Admission rates were calculated with denominator data on all live births from Office for National Statistics (ONS). Main outcomes were admissions to hospitals for potentially preventable conditions across different ages within the first year and overall admissions.

An anonymised extract of inpatient data from Hospital Episode Statistics (HES) for all NHS hospitals in England from 1st April 2008 to 31st March 2014 was obtained. HES collects routine demographic data, administrative information and clinical information based on World Health Organisation (WHO) ICD 10 (2008, 2010 and 2014 versions) and OPCS4 and is suitable for research purposes [12]. All admissions (planned and unplanned) of infants less than one year old at the start of their admission episode were extracted. Since the vast majority of infant admissions are unplanned, that is, emergencies, it was decided to include all admissions in these analyses. An inpatient admission was defined as a 'continuous inpatient spell' which is the continuous time spent in hospital from admission to discharge regardless of any within-hospital transfers [12]. This may have included several 'episodes of care' under different medical teams at various NHS care providers. Clinical diagnosis data were obtained from the final discharge episode of the spell. This method was chosen because using the diagnosis from the admission episode might underestimate the case-mix severity in multi-episode spells. The majority of inpatient spells only have one episode which is both the admission and discharge episode. Duplicate cases and cases with an implausible admission/discharge date were removed and readmissions were explored using the HES identification variable.

To avoid capturing routine admissions to the postnatal ward which frequently occur with a hospital birth, based on the HES data dictionary [12] cases with method of admission codes of '31 (admitted antenatally)', '32 (admitted postnatally)', i.e. immediately following delivery, '82 (the birth of a baby in this healthcare provider)'; or '83 (baby born outside the healthcare provider except when born at home as intended)' were excluded. Also excluded were cases with episode type given as 'Birth episode'; diagnosis ICD10 coded as 'Z37-Z38' (Singleton, born in Hospital) or admission source coded as '79' (Babies born in or on the way to hospital) (Additional file 1).

The data recorded in HES for each admission included a code for infant age category on admission. Codes for gender, region of admission and ethnicity were also included and a score for social deprivation was assigned, allowing exploration of rate variations by these characteristics. Ethnicity within HES is self-reported and the 16 Census ethnic groups [13] were merged into 5 groups to avoid risk of de-anonymisation for any very small groups when merged with the ONS data: White (British, Irish, Any other white background), Asian (Indian, Pakistani, Bangladeshi, Any other Asian Background), Black (Caribbean, African, Any other black background), Other (White and Black Caribbean, White and Black African, White and Asian, Any other mixed Background, Chinese, Any other ethnic group), Not stated (not stated, missing/null).

Each infant admitted was assigned a Local Authority District and Government Office Region (GOR) of residence based on their lower super output area (LSOA) of residence. A LSOA is a small unit of United Kingdom census geography [14] and contains a mean resident population of approximately 1600 individuals [14]. An index of multiple deprivation 2010 score was assigned to each individual based on the LSOA [15]. The index of multiple deprivation (IMD) is an area based score that combines housing, social and economic indicators to indicate the level of deprivation in each area. The income domain score is the one that most accurately reflects material deprivation as it is based on the Government definition of poverty. These were converted into quintiles by subdividing the ranks of the 32,480 areas in England, quintile 1 being most deprived and quintile 5 least deprived.

Denominator data on all live births across England was provided by Office for National Statistics (ONS), providing frequencies of live births by financial year of birth, Region (mothers' area of usual residence), gender, ethnicity (White, Black, Asian, Other, Not stated) and IMD quintile.

Pre-specified definitions of ICD-10 codes of potentially avoidable admissions were produced before analysis of admission rates. The definition of potentially avoidable in this context was a condition or illness which could have been identified before postnatal discharge from hospital or in the community and adequately treated during birth hospitalisation or through community care services. The process for identifying conditions/illness that could be considered potentially avoidable within the HES dataset was undertaken with an advisory panel comprising a consultant general paediatrician, a consultant community paediatrician/professor of child health and a clinical coding manager at a specialist children's hospital. The selection of conditions/illnesses and corresponding coding framework was developed in a four stage approach (Fig. 1). Firstly, frequencies of common illnesses/conditions with the relevant ICD-10 codes by age on admission were produced from the dataset and the paediatricians considered the clinical care pathways, in addition to the physiological and aetiological factors associated with the conditions. Secondly, the list of potentially avoidable conditions and corresponding coding framework was refined. Thirdly, discussion with an expert clinical paediatric coder identified specific HES diagnosis coding rules and standards relevant to the dataset. Finally, a formal list of conditions and corresponding ICD-10 codes was agreed (Additional file 2). Conditions identified as potentially avoidable were physiological jaundice, feeding difficulties and gastroenteritis and these were pre-specified as the main outcomes prior to data analysis. Potentially avoidable implies that although the infant may require admission to hospital at the point of contact with secondary care services, the risk of developing the illness or the severity of the illness may have been reduced had the problem been identified and an intervention taken place earlier.

Patient involvement was via the National Institute for Health Research Collaboration for Leadership in Applied Health Research and Care West Midlands Patient and Public Involvement Supervisory Committee.

Analyses

SPSS (V.22) was used to analyse all infant admissions. Summary statistics were used to describe the proportion of avoidable infant admissions in 0–6 days and 7–28 days, 1 to under 3 months, 3 to under 6 months, 6 to under 9 months and 9 to 12 months after birth by condition/illness, ethnicity, deprivation indices, region in England and year of admission. Frequency of admissions by hospital trust was also explored in addition to exploring readmission rates. Unadjusted annual infant admission rates and annual rates for specific conditions and 95% confidence intervals were calculated by (N admissions for each year/N live births 2008–09) × 100. Change in admission rates were

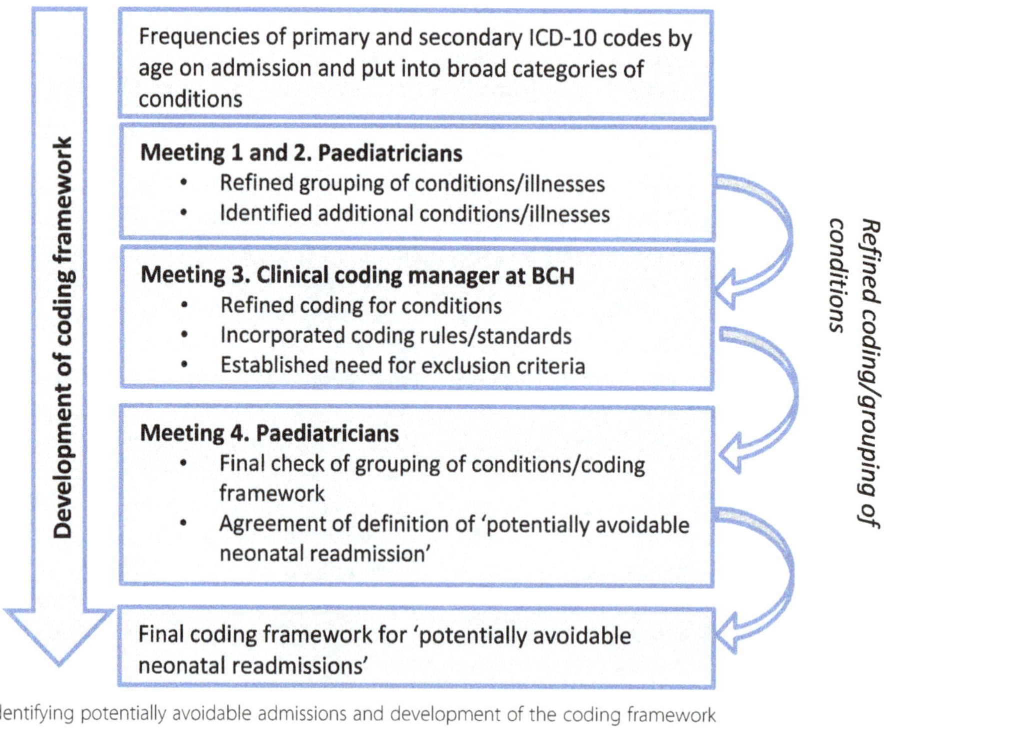

Fig. 1 Process for identifying potentially avoidable admissions and development of the coding framework

calculated as follows: (rate in 2013–14/rate in 2008–09) × 100. Where appropriate, Cochrane Armitage tests for trend were conducted to assess significance of the year on year trend over the 6 year period. A sample size calculation was not necessary due to the exploratory and descriptive nature of the study. The following sensitivity analyses were conducted: comparison of the rates of admissions by episodes of care versus spells of care and selecting the primary diagnosis code versus all diagnostic codes.

Results

There were 1,387,677 admissions in the first year of life and 4,063,050 live births from 1st April 2008 to 31st March 2014. The overall rate of admission increased significantly over the period from 335·0 (95% CI 333·8–336·1) to 354·6 (95% CI 353·6–355·9) per 1000 live births (Table 1). Infants born in 2013/14 had 1·06 times the risk of being admitted to hospital within the first year of life compared to infants born in 2008/09 (Relative risk 1·06, 95% CI 1·05–1·06). Infants who had one admission were 47% more likely to be readmitted at least once more within the first year of life. The increase in admissions was most marked for the 0–6 day age category where admission rate increased from 26·39 per 1000 live births (95% CI 26·01–26·78) in 2008/09 to 33·31 per 1000 live births in 2013/14 (95% CI 32·88–33·74) ($P < 0.0001$). Infants born in 2013/14 had 1·26 times the risk of being admitted within the first 6 days of life compared with infants born in 2008/09 (Relative risk 1·26, 95% CI 1·24–1·29) (Fig. 2).

Admission rates also varied considerably by ethnicity where the highest rate of admission was in the 'not stated' ethnicity category (528·22 per 1000 live births (95% CI 525·93–530·52) compared to 216·85 per 1000 live births (95% CI 215·11–218·60) in the Black ethnicity category.

The rate of admission for the *potentially avoidable conditions* increased by 39% from 39·79 to 55·33 per 1000 live births (Table 2). In the 0–6 day age category the increase in admissions to hospital for these three conditions from 12·36 to 18·23 per 1000 live births contributed 85% of the increase in admission rate. The rate of admission for infants under 7 days increased by 6·92 per 1000 live births (RR 1·26, 95% CI 1·24–1·29) however, once the potentially avoidable admissions were removed the rate only increased by 1·05 per 1000 live births (RR 1·07 95% CI 1·04–1·10) (Table 2).

For *physiological jaundice* there were a total of 73,403 admissions over the study period, the rate of admission increasing from 16·30 (95% CI 16·00–16·61) to 22·35 (95% CI 21·99–22·70) admissions per 1000 live births ($P < 0.0001$) (Table 3). The admission rate in 2013/14 was 1·37 times the risk of being admitted in 2008/09 (RR 1·37 95% CI 1·34–1·.40), an absolute risk increase of 6 per 1000 live births. The increase was concentrated in the 0–6 day category where the admission rate rose from 8.40 to 12·45 per 1000 with statistically significant increases confined to the first 28 days. (Table 3) The duration of hospital admission for physiological jaundice was short with a median length of stay of 1·6 days. The vast majority of infants (94%) admitted for physiological jaundice had a hospital duration of ≤3 days.

The admission rate for physiological jaundice differed significantly by gender: 44,153 male infants (21·20 per 1000 live births (95% CI 21·03–21·37) were admitted over the period compared to 29,251 female infants (14·77 per 1000 live births (95% CI 14·63–14·92). The infant admission rate for physiological jaundice varied by IMD quintile (Table 4), the lowest in the most deprived quintile (16·97 per 1000 live births, 95% CI 16·73–17·21)). The rate of admission for physiological jaundice differed by ethnicity (Table 4). The lowest rate was for black infants where the rate was 6·97 per 1000 live births (95% CI 6·62–7·33) and the rate of admission was four times higher for infants with an ethnicity code 'not stated' (26·14 per 1000 live births, 95% CI 25·41–26·87).

The admission rate for *feeding difficulties* rose from 11·35 (95% CI 11·10–11·60) per 1000 live births in 2008/09 to 13·12 (12·85–13·40) in 2013/14 ($P < 0.0001$). The age specific admission rate for feeding difficulties varied considerably over the period. The largest increase in risk of admission over the period was in the 0–6 day age category where there was a 46% increase in 2013/14 compared with 2008/09 (RR 1·46, 95% CI 1·39–1·54) ($P < 0.0001$). Admissions to hospital for feeding difficulties after one month of age were much less common and the rate consistently decreased with age up to one year (Table 3). The median length of admission for feeding difficulties was 1 day and the majority of infants (91·7%) had an admission of 3 days or under.

There was no significant difference in the rate of admission by gender: the rate for male infants was 12·57 per 1000 live births (95% CI 12·42–12·72) compared to 12·37 per 1000 live births (95% CI 12·22–12·53) for females. There was a small but significant difference in the admission rate for feeding difficulties by IMD quintile with the lowest rate in the most deprived quintile 11·31 per 1000 live births, (95% CI 11·11–11·50). The lowest rate of admission was observed for black infants (6·59 per 1000 live births, 95% CI 6·26–6·94) compared to 16·69 in the 'not stated' ethnicity category (95% CI 16·10–17·28).

For *gastroenteritis* the rate of infant admission per 1000 live births rose from 12·14 in 2008/09 (95% CI 11·88–12·40) to 19.86 (95% CI 19·52–20·19) ($P < 0.0001$). The rate of admission for gastroenteritis significantly increased across all age categories but admission was least frequent in infants in the first 28 days. It was greatest in the 9–12 month age category, although infants aged 1–3 months had the largest relative increase in risk of admission (RR 2·04, 95% CI 1·90–2·19) from 2008/09–2013/14

Table 1 Number and incidence (per 1000 live births) of infants admitted by year of birth and age group in England 2008/09–2013/14

YEAR	Total No. admissions	No. Live births	Rate* (95% CI)	Age specific rates of admissions per 1000 population (95% CI)					
				0–6 days	7–28 days	1–3 months	3–6 months	6–9 months	9–12 months
2008/09	223,735	667,932	334·97 (333·83–336·10)	26·39 (26·01–26·78)	47·96 (47·44–48·47)	77·38 (76·74–78·02)	65·56 (64·97–66·15)	58·43 (57·86–58·99)	59·25 (58·69–59·82)
2009/10	225,130	674,949	333·55 (332·43–334·68)	27·96 (27·56–28·35)	46·81 (46·30–47·31)	77·11 (76·47–77·74)	65·04 (64·45–65·63)	58·20 (57·65–58·76)	58·44 (57·88–59·00)
2010/11	235,288	682,892	344·55 (343·42–345·67)	30·07 (29·66–30·47)	48·82 (48·31–49·33)	80·69 (80·05–81·34)	67·49 (66·89–68·08)	58·27 (57·72–58·83)	59·20 (58·64–59·76)
2011/12	228,534	689,582	331·41 (330·30–332·52)	28·95 (28·55–29·34)	48·03 (47·52–48·53)	78·20 (77·56–78·83)	63·81 (63·24–64·39)	55·78 (55·24–56·32)	56·64 (56·09–57·18)
2012/13	240,090	685,174	350·41 (349·28–351·54)	31·14 (30·73–31·55)	50·66 (50·14–51·18)	82·94 (82·29–83·59)	67·46 (66·86–68·05)	57·91 (57·36–58·47)	60·59 (60·03–61·16)
2013/14	234,900	662,521	354·55 (353·59–355·89)	33·31 (32·88–33·74)	51·49 (50·96–52·02)	84·40 (83·73–85·07)	68·77 (68·16–69·38)	58·19 (57·63–58·76)	58·39 (57·82–58·93)
Cochran Armitage test for trend			775·7362 ($P < 0·0001$)	611·4452 ($P < 0·0001$)	166·0960 ($P < 0·0001$)	959·3922 ($P < 0·0001$)	58·8150 ($P < 0·0001$)	3·7260 ($P = 0·0536$)	0·0190 ($P = 0·8904$)

***per 1000 live births**

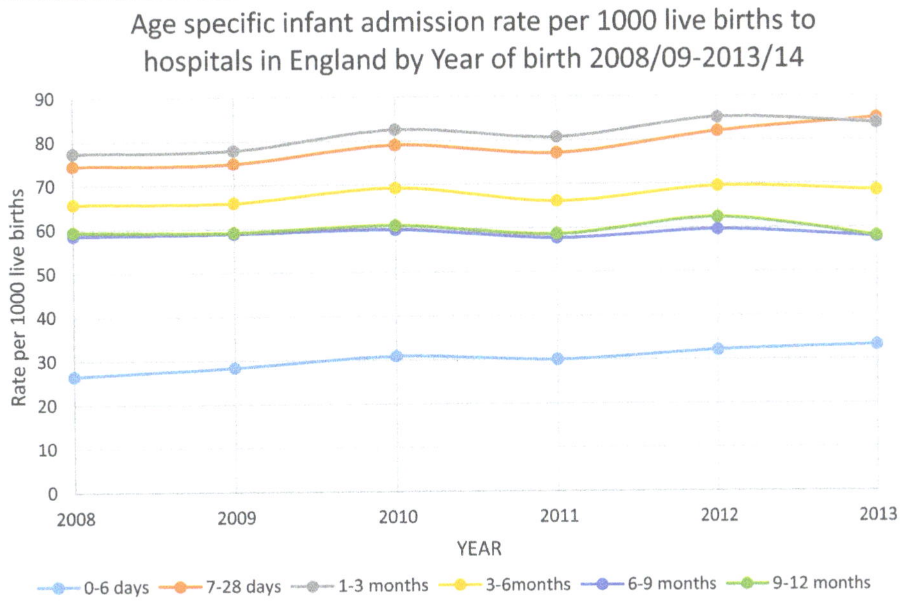

Fig. 2 Age specific infant hospital admission rates in England per 1000 live births by year of birth 2008/09 to 2013/14

(Table 3). The median length of stay was less than one day and 96.8% infants were discharged within 3 days.

There was a small but significant difference in rate of admission for gastroenteritis by gender; the rate for male infants was 15·73 per 1000 live births (95% CI 15·56–15·90) and 14.07 (95% CI 13·90–14·23) for female infants. The highest rate was noted in the most deprived IMD quintile (17·01 per 1000 live births, 95% CI 16·77–17·25) (Table 4). There was also considerable variation by ethnicity, where the rate of admission per 1000 live births was more than double for infants with 'not stated' ethnicity, 18·04 per 1000 live births, (95% CI 17·43–18·65) compared to 8·31 per 1000 live births (95% CI 7·92–8·69).

The number of admissions for the conditions identified as potentially avoidable varied considerably with high numbers of admissions to bigger paediatric hospitals.

Discussion

The rate of hospital admission in the first year of life for the three conditions identified as potentially preventable increased by 39% relative to an overall increase of 6%. Over the first year the biggest increase in admissions occurred in the first 0–6 days and 85% of the increase in this period was for the identified potentially preventable conditions of jaundice, feeding difficulties and gastroenteritis for which admissions rose from 12·36 to 18·23 per 1000 live births.

This study used a large routinely collected national dataset and a robust method to develop a working definition of 'potentially avoidable' infant admissions in the context of postnatal care provision, drawing on the expertise of paediatricians, research data analysts and clinical coders. The potentially avoidable conditions were pre-specified prior to calculation of admission rates. The

Table 2 Frequency and rate (per 1000 live births) of admission for infants aged 0–6 days (overall and potentially preventable conditions (physiological jaundice, feeding difficulties and gastroenteritis))

YEAR	overall No. admissions	No. avoidable conditions	No. live births	rate[a] overall admission	admission rate[a] for potentially avoidable conditions
2008/09	17,629	8257	667,932	26·39	12·36
2009/10	18,869	8798	674,949	27·96	13·04
2010/11	20,534	9932	682,892	30·07	14·54
2011/12	19,962	10,313	689,582	28·95	14·96
2012/13	21,334	11,373	685,174	31·14	16·60
2013/14	22,067	12,079	662,521	33·31	18·23

[a]per 1000 live births

Table 3 Number and incidence (per 1000 live births) of infant admissions for potentially preventable conditions for infants by Year and Age group on admission 2008/09–2013/14

YEAR	No. admissions	Rate [a] (95% CI)	Age specific rates of admissions per 1000 live births (95% CI)					
			0–6 days	7–28 days	1–3 months	3–6 months	6–9 months	9–12 months
Gastroenteritis								
2008/09	8108	12·14 (11·88–12·40)	0·02 (0·01–0·03)	0·38 (0·33–0·43)	1·77 (1·67–1·87)	2·48 (2·36–2·60)	3·37 (3·23–3·51)	4·11 (3·96–4·26)
2009/10	8257	12·23 (11·97–12·50)	0·01 (0·00–0·02)	0·35 (0·31–0·40)	1·80 (1·70–1·90)	2·43 (2·31–2·54)	3·53 (3·39–3·68)	4·11 (3·95–4·26)
2010/11	7785	11·40 (11·15–11·65)	0·01 (00·00–0·010	0·28 (0·24–0·32)	1·56 (1·46–1·65)	2·46 (2·34–2·58)	3·20 (3·07–3·34)	3·89 (3·75–4·04)
2011/12	7859	11·40 (11·15–11·65)	0·01 (0·00–0·01)	0·26 (0·22–0·30)	1·55 (1·46–1·64)	2·34 (2·23–2·45)	3·27 (3·14–3·41)	3·96 (3·81–4·11)
2012/13	15,451	22·55 (22·20–22·90)	0·04 (0·03–0·06)	0·58 (0·53–0·64)	3·61 (3·47–3·76)	4·58 (4·42–4·74)	6·24 (6·06–6·43)	7·49 (7·29–7·69)
2013/14	13,155	19·86 (19·52–20·19)	0·03 (0·02–0·05)	0·56 (0·50–0·61)	3·61 (3·47–3·75)	4·32 (4·16–4·47)	5·30 (5·12–5·47)	6·04 (5·86–6·23)
Cochran Armitage test for trend:		3170·9178 ($P < 0·0001$)	10·2750 ($P = 0·013$)	57·4530 ($P < 0·0001$)	805·7172 ($p < 0·0001$)	748·2772 ($P < 0·0001$)	742·1982 ($P < 0·0001$)	779·7762 ($P < 0·0001$)
Physiological jaundice								
2008/09	10,890	16·30 (16·00–16·61)	8·40 (8·18–8·62)	6·14 (5·95–6·32)	1·66 (1·56–1·76)	0·02 (0·01–0·04)	0·05 (0·03–0·07)	0·03 (0·02–0·05)
2009/10	10,637	15·76 (15·46–16·06)	8·22 (8·01–8·44)	5·93 (5·74–6·11)	1·54 (1·45–1·64)	0·02 (0·01–0·03)	0·03 (0·02–0·02)	0·01 (0·01–0·02)
2010/11	11,305	16·56 (16·25–16·86)	8·96 (8·73–9·18)	6·16 (5·98–6·35)	1·37 (1·28–1·46)	0·02 (0·01–0·03	0·02 (0·01–0·04)	0·01 (0·02–0·02)
2011/12	11,947	17·33 (17·02–17·63)	9·35 (9·12–9·58)	6·76 (6·57–6·95)	1·42 (1·36–1·51)	0·02 (0·01–0·04)	0·04 (0·02–0·05)	0·02 (0·01–0·04)
2012/13	13,823	20·17 (19·84–20·51)	10·80 (10·59–11·05)	7·65 (7·44–7·85)	1·63 (1·53–1·72)	0·04 (0·03–0·05)	0·04 (0·03–0·06)	0·02 (0·01–0·03)
2013/14	14,806	22·35 (21·99–22·70)	12·45 (12·19–12·27)	8·22 (8·00–8·36)	1·61 (1·51–1·71)	0·02 (0·01–0·03)	0·03 (0·02–0·04)	0·02 (0·01–0·03)
Cochran Armitage test for trend:		1053·1403 ($P < 0·0001$)	800·999 ($P < 0·0001$)	430·788 ($P < 0·0001$)	0·0260 ($P = 0·8719$)	0·4890 ($P = 0·4844$)	1·4770 ($P = 0·2242$)	1·3500 ($P = 0·2453$)
Feeding difficulties								
2008/09	7581	11·35 (11·10–11·60)	3·94 (3·79–4·09)	4·14 (3·99–4·29)	2·06 (1·95–2·16)	0·77 (0·70–0·83)	0·28 (0·24–0·33)	0·16 (0·13–0·19)
2009/10	8046	11·92 (11·66–12·18)	4·80 (4·63–4·96)	4·12 (3·96–4·27)	1·93 (1·82–2·03	0·68 (0·62–0·74)	0·24 (0·21–0·28)	0·15 (0·12–0·18)
2010/11	8784	12·86 (12·60–13·13)	5·58 (5·40–5·75)	4·27 (4·15–4·43)	1·97 (1·87–2·08)	0·70 (0·64–0·77)	0·22 (0·18–0·25)	0·12 (0·10–0·15)
2011/12	8879	12·88 (12·61–13·14)	5·60 (5·43–5·78)	4·23 (4·08–4·39)	1·95 (1·8–2·05)	0·74 (0·68–0·81)	0·23 (0·19–0·26)	0·13 (0·10–0·15)
2012/13	8706	12·71 (12·44–12·97)	5·75 (5·74–5·93)	4·10 (3·95–4·25)	1·80 (1·70–1·90)	0·70 (0·64–0·77)	0·21 (0·18–0·24)	0·14 (0·11–0·17)
2013/14	8694	13·12 (12·85–13·40)	5·75 (5·56–5·93)	4·29 (4·14–4·45)	1·91 (0·81–2·02)	0·79 (0·73–0·86)	0·25 (0·21–0·29)	0·12 (0·10–0·15)
Cochran Armitage test for trend:		97·70 ($P < 0·0001$)	260·5501 ($P < 0·0001$)	54·0300 ($P < 0·0001$)	6·1920 ($P = 0·0128$)	0·6870 ($P = 0·4072$)	2·7600 ($P = 0·0966$)	3·3200 ($P = 0·0684$)

[a]per 1000 live births

Table 4 Number and incidence (per 1000 live births) of infant admissions for potentially preventable conditions by Ethnicity, Gender, and IMD quintile 2008/09–2013/14

	Feeding difficulties		Gastroenteritis		Physiological Jaundice	
	No admissions	Rate (95% CI)	No admissions	Rate (95% CI)	No admissions	Rate (95% CI)
Ethnicity[a]						
White	37,746	12·81 (12·68–12·94)	47,616	16·16 (16·01–16·30)	51,082	17·34 (17·19–17·48)
Asian	5102	12·19 (11·86–12·52)	4570	10·92 (10·60–11·23)	9517	22·74 (22·28–23·19)
Black	1415	6·59 (6·25–6·94)	1783	8·31 (7·92–8·69)	1497	6·97 (6·62–7·33)
Other	3391	11·26 (10·89–11·64)	3365	11·18 (10·80–11·55)	6556	21·78 (21·26–22·30)
Not stated	3036	16·69 (16·10–17·28)	3282	18·04 (17·43–18·65)	4756	26·14 (25·41–26·87)
Gender						
Male	26,183	12·57 (12·42–12·72)	32,761	15·73 (15·56–15·90)	44,153	21·20 (21·03–21·37)
Female	24,502	12·37 (12·22–12·53)	27,854	14·07 (13·90–14·23)	29,251	14·77 (14·63–14·92)
IMD Index[a]						
1	12,708	11·31 (11·11–11·50)	19,122	17·01 (16·77–17·25)	19,077	16·97 (16·73–17·21)
2	10,860	11·89 (11·67–12·11)	13,967	15·29 (15·04–15·55)	16,111	17·64 (17·37–17·91)
3	9899	13·14 (12·82–13·40)	10,903	14·47 (14·20–14·74)	14,084	18·69 (18·39–19·00)
4	8952	13·63 (13·35–13·91)	8953	13·63 (13·35–13·91)	12,367	18·83 (18·50–19·16)
5	7995	12·99 (12·71–13·27)	7254	11·78 (11·51–12·05)	11,245	18·27 (17·93–18·60)

[a]Missing data:
Gastroenteritis: 0.7% IMD index, 0.6% Ethnicity
Physiological Jaundice: 0.9% IMD index, 0.6% Ethnicity
Feeding difficulties: 0.8% IMD index, 0.4% ethnicity

coding framework used to identify such admissions incorporated inclusion and exclusion criteria to ensure that infants with underlying conditions were excluded from the sample population (for example, infants born with cleft lip and palate, and subsequent feeding difficulties). It is reassuring that the incidence of admissions for physiological jaundice and feeding difficulties over the age of 3 months was very small, suggesting that the selection of codes for these conditions was accurate. Although a systematic review of coding accuracy studies suggested that HES data has improved significantly over time [16], it is unlikely that this would have affected our study findings because the NHS Payment by Results system, a key driver for improving HES data accuracy, had been fully implemented by 2007 [17, 18].

HES is widely accepted as a database for health research and suitable for studies identifying trends in healthcare [19], although there are a number of limitations. The ethnicity variable was not as complete as other data fields with 7% of infant admissions having a 'missing' or 'not known' code. Previous research has indicated that missing ethnicity data may not be random and instead relates to service pressures, a lack of opportunity for health professionals enquiry or the circumstances of hospital admission [20, 21]. Additionally, the broad denominator ethnicity categories necessary to maintain confidentiality prohibited a thorough assessment of admission rates by ethnicity. It was not possible to explore hospital level admission rates because denominator data were not available at hospital level but we anticipate that variation would be affected by patient and hospital level factors. Finally, we did not have data on smoking status and breastfeeding status.

Use of age specific admission rates for infants under one year showed that the increase in admission over the period 2008 to 2014 only existed within the first 6 months of life, and had increased most in the 0–6 day category. The admission rate for infants from 6 to 12 months remained stable over the period. Our findings are consistent with those of other studies that explore unplanned infant admissions to hospital [6]. It is also consistent with the literature in the finding that the rate of admissions varied by IMD [22]. The overall admission rate to hospital by IMD quintiles supports existing evidence that admission rates are strongly correlated with measures of social deprivation [22]. For admission rates for jaundice and feeding difficulties however the admission rate was highest in the least deprived quintiles and may reflect variation in infant feeding practices with women in the least deprived quintiles more likely to breastfeed. Inability to initiate and establish breastfeeding resulting in an insufficient milk supply is a known risk factor for physiological jaundice [23]. Exclusive initial breastfeeding initially rose from 65% in 2005 to 69% in 2010 when 46% of babies were still exclusively breastfed at one week [24]. While breastfeeding may be a factor influencing the trends seen, it does not provide a sufficient explanation of them. Increases in admission rates for gastroenteritis showed a different pattern from jaundice and feeding difficulties as the increase for this was greatest in infants after the first month and may possibly be related to feeding practices and insufficient support for infant feeding.

The change in infant admission rates we observed over the period was concentrated in those under 7 days of age and for the potentially avoidable conditions, particularly jaundice and feeding difficulties. In England over a similar period of time women and infants have had less routine contact with health professionals as the length of stay in hospital after birth and the median community visits following discharge from birth has reduced [9, 10]. Over the period of this study, the average postnatal length of stay hospital reduced slightly from 1.7 days in 2008/09 to 1.5 days in 2013/14 [25]). Several large surveys of women's experiences of postnatal care have shown that a large proportion felt that they needed more support, particularly establishing breastfeeding [11, 26–29]. Although temporal association does not prove causation, the increase in admissions may in part prove to be attributed to changes in the postnatal care provision and management of neonates in the community. Other possible causes to the increase observed in this study include an increase in parents being advised by NHS 111 system to take their child straight to hospital, and a decrease in training and experience for doctors to triage neonates in primary care [3]. If the reduction in postnatal care provision does have a part to play in the increase in infant admission rate, the current National Maternity Review in England [11] aimed at transforming maternity services has the opportunity to ensure that women's needs are being met prior to discharge from hospital. It could also ensure that women are able to have more effective community provision including more frequent home visits where needed and easy access to midwifery advice in order to identify potential infant health problems to improve this situation.

Conclusion

Our findings show that most of the increase in the rate of admission to hospital for infants up to age one over the period 2008–2014 was in the early neonatal period; and the great majority of this increase is explained by the three conditions, physiological jaundice, feeding difficulties and gastroenteritis, predominantly the former two. Potential missed opportunities within the postnatal care pathway require urgent modification given current NHS capacity and resource issues.

Abbreviations

GOR: Local Authority District and Government Office Region; HES: Hospital Episode Statistics; IMD: Index of multiple deprivation; LSOA: Lower super output area; ONS: Office for National Statistics; WHO: World Health Organisation

Acknowledgements

With thanks to Paul Allen at Birmingham Children's Hospital NHS Trust for his contribution to the design of the coding framework for potentially avoidable conditions.

Funding

This paper presents independent research funded by the National Institute for Health Research (NIHR) Collaboration for Leadership in Applied Health Research and Care West Midlands. The views expressed are those of the author(s) and not necessarily those of the NHS, the NIHR or the Department of Health. Carole Cummins, Christine Macarthur and Beck Taylor report funding and Eleanor Jones a stipend from NIHR CLARHC West Midlands, during the conduct of the study.

Authors' contributions

EJ, CC, CM and BT conceived the study. GR extracted the data. EJ, CC, CM, BT, DS and DJ developed the definition of potentially avoidable infant admission and ICD 10 and OPCS 4 coding framework. EJ, CC, CM and BT were responsible for statistical analysis and interpretation. All authors contributed to the manuscript draft and critical revision of the manuscript for intellectual content. All authors read and approved the final manuscript.

Competing interests

The authors declare that they have no competing interests.

Author details

[1]Institute of Applied Health Research, University of Birmingham, Edgbaston, Birmingham B15 2TH, England. [2]Birmingham Women's and Children's NHS Foundation Trust, Steelhouse Lane, Birmingham B4 6NH, England. [3]Division of Mental Health and Wellbeing, Warwick Medical School, University of Warwick, Coventry, UK.

References

1. Blunt I. Focus on preventable admissions. Trends in emergency admission for ambulatory care sensitive conditions 2001-2013. http://www.qualitywatch.org.uk/sites/files/qualitywatch/field/field_document/131010_QualityWatch_Focus_Preventable_Admissions.pdf. Accessed 8 June 2017.
2. Purdy S. Avoiding hospital admission. What does the research say? The King's Fund. 2010. http://www.kingsfund.org.uk/sites/files/kf/Avoiding-Hospital-Admissions-Sarah-Purdy-December2010.pdf. Accessed 8 June 2017.
3. Gill P, Goldacre M, Mant D. Increase in emergency admissions to hospital for children aged under 15 in England, 1999-2010: national database analysis. Arch Dis Child. 2013;98:328–34.
4. Saxena S, Bottle A, Gilbert R, Sharland M. Increasing short-stay unplanned hospital admissions among children in England; time trends analysis '97–'06. PLoS One. 2009;4:10.

5. Harron K, Gilbert R, Cromwell D, Oddie S, Meulen J. Newborn length of stay and risk of readmission. Paediatr Perinat Epidemiol. 2017;31:221–32.
6. Al-Mahtot M, Barwise-Munro R, Wilson P, Turner S. Changing characteristics of hospital admissions but not the children admitted—a whole population study between 2000 and 2013. Eur J Pediatr. 2018;177:381–8.
7. Witt W, Weiss A, Elixhauser A. Overview of Hospital Stays for Children in the United States, 2012. HCUP statistical brief #187. Rockville, MD: Agency for Healthcare Research and Quality; 2014. https://www.hcup-us.ahrq.gov/.
8. NHS Digital. NHS maternity statistics 2016–17. 2017 https://digital.nhs.uk/data-and-information/publications/statistical/nhs-maternity-statistics. Accessed 10 Oct 2018.
9. Byrom S, Edwards G, Bick D. Essential midwifery practice. Postnatal care. 2009. [electronic resource], Chichester Ames, Iowa: Wiley-Blackwell.
10. Care Quality Commission. Maternity Survey: Quality and Methodology Report. 2017:2017 https://www.cqc.org.uk/publications/surveys/maternity-services-survey-2017. Accessed 10 June 2018.
11. NHS England. National Maternity Review: better births – improving outcomes of maternity services in England – a five year forward view for maternity care. 2016. https://www.england.nhs.uk/wp-content/uploads/2016/02/national-maternity-review-report.pdf. Accessed 8 June 2017.
12. NHS Digital. HES Data Dictionary: Admitted patient Care (APC) Hospital Episode Statistics. 2017. NHS digital. Leeds; http://content.digital.nhs.uk/media/23711/Admitted-Patient-Care/pdf/Admitted_Patient_Care_.pdf. Accessed 8 June 2017.
13. Office for National Statistics. Population estimates by Ethnic Group: methodology Paper: London: 2011. https://www.ons.gov.uk/peoplepopulationandcommunity/populationandmigration/populationestimates/methodologies/populationestimatesbyethnicgroup. Accessed 8 June 2017).
14. Office for National Statistics. Census geography. https://www.ons.gov.uk/methodology/geography/ukgeographies/censusgeography. Accessed 8 June 2017).
15. Department for communities and Local Government. The English Indices of deprivation 2010. London; 2011. https://www.gov.uk/government/uploads/system/uploads/attachment_data/file/6871/1871208.pdf. Accessed 8 June 2017.
16. Burns EM, Rigby E, Mamidanna R, Bottle A, Aylin P, Ziprin P, Faiz OD. Systematic review of discharge coding accuracy. J Public Health. 2012;34:138–48.
17. Department of Health. Reforming NHS financial flows – Introducing Payment by Results. 2002, Department of Health, London. http://webarchive.nationalarchives.gov.uk/20130107105354/http://www.dh.gov.uk/prod_consum_dh/groups/dh_digitalassets/@dh/@en/documents/digitalasset/dh_4018704.pdf. Accessed 8 June 2017.
18. Confirmation of PbR arrangements for 2007/08, Gateway reference 7539, 2006, Department of Health https://webarchive.nationalarchives.gov.uk/+/http://www.dh.gov.uk/en/Publicationsandstatistics/Publications/PublicationsPolicyAndGuidance/DH_062914. Accessed 8 June 2017.
19. Garrett E, Barnes H, Dibbin C. Health Administrative Data: exploring potential for academic research. St Andrews: Administrative Data Liaison Service. http://www.academia.edu/10325382/Health_administrative_data_Exploring_the_potential_for_academic_research. Accessed 8 June 2017.
20. Fraser LK, McKinney PA, Parslow RC, Miller M, Aldridge J, Hain R, et al. Rising national prevalence of life-limiting conditions in children in England. Pediatrics. 2012;129:923–e9.
21. Mathur R, Bhaskaran K, Chaturvedi N, Leon DA, vanStaa T, Grundy E, et al. Completeness and usability of ethnicity data in UK-based primary care and hospital databases. J Public Health. 2014;36:684–92.
22. Majeed A, Bardsley M, Morgan D, O'Sullivan C, Bindman AB. Cross sectional study of primary care groups in London: association of measures of socioeconomic and health status with hospital admission rates. BMJ. 2000;321:1057–60.
23. Lain S, Roberts C, Bowen J, Nassar N. Early discharge of infants and risk of readmission for jaundice. Pediatrics. 135:314–21.
24. McAndrew F, Thompson J, Fellow L. Large A. Infant Feeding Survey: Speed M and Renfrew M; 2010. http://content.digital.nhs.uk/catalogue/PUB08694/Infant-Feeding-Survey-2010-Consolidated-Report.pdf . Accessed 8 June 2017
25. NHS digital. NHS Maternity Statistics in England 2013-2014 [Online]. NHS digital. http://www.hscic.gov.uk/catalogue/PUB16725. Accessed 8 June 2017.
26. Redshaw M, Rowe R, Hockley C, Brocklehurst P. Recorded delivery: a national survey of women's experience of maternity care 2006. Oxford: The National Perinatal Epidemiology Unit; 2007.
27. Redshaw M, Henderson J. Safely delivered: a national survey of women's experience of maternity care 2014. Oxford: The National Perinatal Epidemiology Unit; 2015.
28. Bhavnani V, Newburn M. Left to your own devices: the postnatal care experiences of 1260 first time mothers. London: National Childbirth Trust; 2010.
29. Care Quality Commission. National findings from the. Survey of women's experiences of maternity care. London: Care Quality Commission; 2013. p. 2013.

Prevention of neonatal late-onset sepsis

Gary Alcock[1,3], Helen G. Liley[1,2], Lucy Cooke[1] and Peter H. Gray[1,2*]

Abstract

Background: Late-onset sepsis (LOS), defined as sepsis occurring after 48 h of age causes substantial mortality and morbidity in very low birth weight infants. Risk factors for LOS include immaturity, intravascular catheters, mechanical ventilation, and prolonged parenteral nutrition (PN). Little attention has been paid to studying the effects of PN administration methods. The aim of the study was to compare a bundle of measures for PN line management incorporating a strict aseptic technique with standard line management on LOS in very low birth weight infants.

Methods: Infants <1500 g birth weight who required PN were randomised to either a bundle of a strict aseptic technique for line management together with single use intravascular catheter for PN or a standard technique. The primary outcome was the incidence of LOS in the first 28 days of life. Secondary outcomes were mortality, neonatal morbidities and developmental outcome at 12 months of age.

Results: There were 126 infants in the aseptic technique group and 123 in the standard technique group. Forty (31.8%) infants in the aseptic technique group and 36 (29.3%) in the standard technique group had an episode of sepsis ($p = 0.77$). This corresponds to incidences of 15.8 and 14.2 episodes of sepsis per 1000 patient days respectively. Subgroup analyses for infants <1000 g also revealed no difference in the rate of sepsis between the intervention and control groups. ($p = 0.43$). There were no significant differences in secondary outcomes and development between the groups.

Conclusion: A bundle of measures including strict aseptic technique for parenteral nutrition line management did not result in a reduction in LOS when compared to a standard technique. There is no evidence to recommend this as routine practice.

Keywords: Preterm, Parenteral nutrition, Late-onset sepsis, Catheter associated infections

Background

Late-onset sepsis (LOS) defined as sepsis occurring after 48 h of age causes substantial mortality and morbidity in very low birth weight infants [1, 2]. The incidence of LOS varies amongst neonatal units from 11% to 27% for infants of very low birth weight (VLBW) [2, 3]. The morbidity and mortality of episodes of hospital-acquired sepsis are high [4], with morbidities including longer duration of mechanical ventilation and hospital stay, and delays in establishing feeding. Studies also implicate neonatal infections as one of the risk factors for adverse neurological outcomes [5].

Risk factors for LOS include immaturity, intravascular catheters, mechanical ventilation, and prolonged parenteral nutrition (PN) [6]. Importantly, some studies have suggested that PN is one of the most significant sepsis risk factors in VLBW infants [7–9], although the evidence is virtually all retrospective and has not been able to account for immaturity in the analyses. Furthermore,

* Correspondence: Peter.Gray@mater.org.au
[1]Newborn Services, Mater Mothers' Hospital, Raymond Tce, South Brisbane, QLD 4101, Australia
[2]Mater Research Institute-The University of Queensland, South Brisbane, QLD, Australia
Full list of author information is available at the end of the article

it remains uncertain whether PN is causal in sepsis or merely associated with the presence of a venous catheter in situ.

Strategies reported to have the most significant impact in reducing the incidence of LOS have involved bundles focussing on various combinations of hand washing, infection control practices and intravenous central line management [10–12]. Few single interventions have been reported to significantly influence LOS. Aly et al. [13] however found a reduction in LOS after the introduction of a closed medication system in comparison to a historical control group.

Little attention has been paid to studying the effects of PN administration methods. In a historical cohort study, Maas et al. [14] demonstrated a significant reduction in the incidence of catheter-related bacteraemia in neonates following the introduction of a new catheter care protocol. The protocol maximised aseptic precautions and was supported by a continuing education program. There have been randomised controlled trials investigating the use of prophylactic antibiotics to reduce the risks of PN associated sepsis [15], but we could find no randomised controlled trials investigating different methods of PN line management.

Our usual practice has been to administer PN through multiuse intravascular lines with the PN bags, syringes and tubing being changed by one nurse using a clean, no touch technique. A retrospective case-control audit in our NICU indicated that the majority of episodes of LOS in VLBW infants occurred in the first 28 days of life and after adjustment for birth weight, receiving PN was the factor associated with the greatest risk [8].

The study aimed to evaluate whether a bundle of line management measures focused on reducing the risk of contamination of PN lines would reduce the incidence of LOS in VLBW babies. The hypothesis was that the study intervention; comprised of a strict sterile technique for line changes and minimising the administration of other medications or fluids through PN lines would reduce catheter contamination and by minimising breaches would reduce the incidence of LOS when compared to the standard technique routinely used in the Neonatal Intensive Care Unit (NICU). The secondary hypothesis was that the intervention would result in an improvement in developmental outcome.

Methods

This prospective randomised controlled trial enrolled infants managed in the NICU at the Mater Mothers' Hospital (MMH), Brisbane. Ethics approval was obtained from the MMH Research Ethics Committee and the University of Newcastle Human Research Ethics Committee. The trial was registered with the Interdisciplinary Maternal Perinatal Australasian Collaborative Trials (IMPACT) Network (Trial registration number: PT0363) and with the Australian New Zealand Clinical Trials Registry (ANZCTR) (Trial registration number: ACTRN12617000455369 [retrospective registration]). Informed written consent was obtained from a parent prior to study enrolment.

Two techniques of PN line management were employed, designated - standard and study intervention techniques. Eligible babies were randomly allocated to each technique, using a web based randomisation program (Randomization.com: http://www.randomization.com). Randomisation sequence and block size were masked in blocks of 10 stratified by birth weight (500-999 g and 1000-1499 g). Allocation was sealed in sequentially numbered opaque envelopes prepared by an administrative staff member not involved in the study.

VLBW infants with a birth weight < 1500 g were eligible if they survived at least 48 h, and were considered by the clinical team to require PN. Infants were excluded if they were not expected to survive to randomisation, had major congenital anomalies (including any infant expected to need neonatal surgery in the first 28 days) or had early onset sepsis (positive blood or CSF culture at <48 h of life). Once the decision had been made to commence PN on eligible infants and after parental consent had been obtained, babies were randomized to one of the two methods of PN line management used in the study. These are described in Table 1 and in more detail in the Additional file 1. All other care was according to NICU routines or at the discretion of the medical staff.

Primary outcome

The primary outcome was the occurrence of LOS in the first 28 days of life.

Definite sepsis was pre-defined for the purposes of the study as the presence of a culture of blood or cerebrospinal fluid positive for a pathogenic bacterium or

Table 1 Methods of parenteral nutrition (PN) line management employed in the study

Standard technique	Study Intervention bundle
Parenteral nutrition (PN) line changes were performed by one nurse using a no touch sterile technique but without mask, surgical scrub, or gown and gloves	Parenteral nutrition (PN) line changes by two nurses, one performing a surgical scrub and wearing a mask, gown and gloves to prevent breach of sterility.
PN lines were used as needed for other compatible infusions such as sedatives	PN lines were not used for other infusions, unless the infusion fluids were prepared and changed using the study intervention techniques
PN lines were used for boluses of medications including antibiotics	PN lines were only used for other medications in an emergency or if no other route could reasonably be used

yeast together with two of the following: physical signs of infection (any of blood pressure instability, lethargy, temperature instability, pallor, increasing apnoea and glucose intolerance); a raised haematologic sepsis score [16] (≥ 4) from the full blood count; a C reactive protein (CRP) >10 mg/L (laboratory normal value ≤10 mg/L) or new onset thrombocytopaenia. Probable sepsis was defined as a positive blood culture plus only one of: a raised hematologic sepsis score in the absence of physical signs, new onset thrombocytopaenia or a raised CRP measurement, or physical signs of sepsis and normal laboratory investigations. For the purpose of analysis, episodes of probable sepsis and definite sepsis were combined. Blood cultures were collected by venepuncture and were not obtained from intravascular catheters already in situ.

Secondary outcomes

Mortality, chronic lung disease (oxygen requirement >36 weeks gestation), retinopathy of prematurity, duration of parenteral nutrition, duration of mechanical ventilation and respiratory support, administration of postnatal corticosteroids, duration of hospitalisation and neurodevelopmental outcome at 12 months of age.

Data other than those required for sepsis classification were collected prospectively. These included demographic data together with items needed to score the Clinical Risk Index for Babies (CRIB) [17] and Score of Neonatal Acute Physiology (SNAP) [18]. Neonatal variables collected included duration of PN, data to verify episodes of sepsis as well as mortality and late neonatal morbidities.

Following hospital discharge, the surviving infants were assessed at the Growth and Development Unit, MMH at 12 months corrected for prematurity. A psychologist who was unaware of the infant's study group allocation and sepsis history performed the Griffiths Mental Development Scales (General Quotient [GQ], Mean 100; Standard Deviation 12) [19]. For those infants who had a GQ <50, a score of 50 was arbitrarily assigned.

Sample size estimation

At the MMH between 1998 and 1999 the incidence of LOS was 30% [8]. A tertiary neonatal unit employing a PN management strategy similar to the study technique between 1990 and 2002 reported the incidence of LOS to range between 3.1% and 13.2% for infants <1500 g [20]. Based on an incidence of LOS of 30%, a sample size of 250 (125 per group) was calculated to demonstrate a clinically significant reduction in the incidence of LOS from 30% to 15% with Type I and II errors set at 5% and 20% respectively.

Statistical analyses

Demographic data were compared with categorical data being analyzed using χ^2 analyses or Fisher's exact tests. Continuous data were analysed using Student's t test if normally distributed and the Mann Whitney U test for non-parametrically distributed data. Subgroup analyses were performed for episodes of LOS in infants <1000 g birth weight and for episodes of LOS that commenced whilst receiving PN. Statistical calculations were performed using Stata version 8.0.

Results

Between May 2001 and July 2003, 444 infants of birth weight 500-1499 g were assessed for eligibility (Fig. 1). Of the 332 considered eligible, 252 infants were enrolled in the study. Of these, it was subsequently determined that three did not fulfil eligibility criteria and they were excluded post-hoc. Overall 249 randomised infants were analysed; 126 infants in the study intervention group and 123 in the standard technique group (Fig. 1). The groups were similar with respect to birth weight and gestation and other demographic characteristics (Table 2).

Four infants in the study intervention arm were withdrawn from study treatment because the protocol-driven procedures to maintain separate intravenous access for

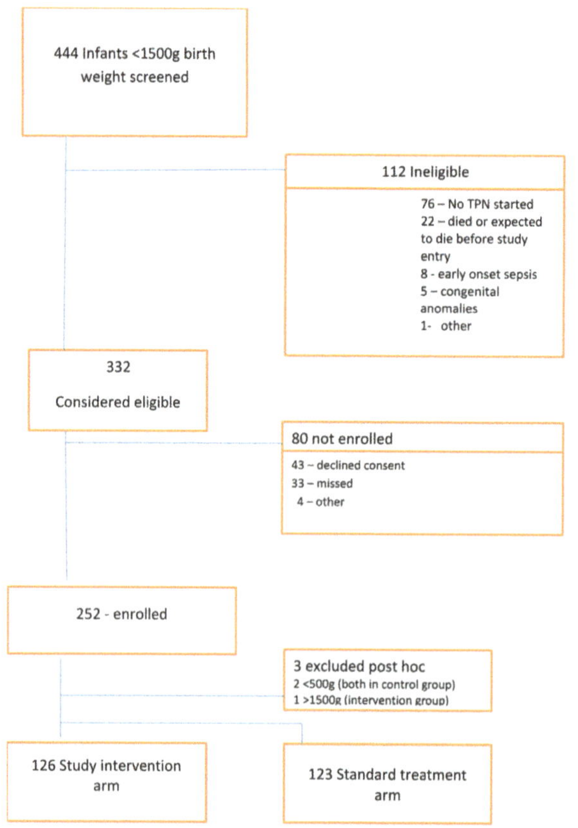

Fig. 1 Participant flow diagram

Table 2 Demographic characteristics of the study intervention bundle and standard care cohorts

	Study intervention	Standard technique
	n = 126	*n* = 123
Birth weight (g) – median [IQ range]	1024 [805, 1224]	1020 [795, 1210]
Infants <1000 g	61	60
Gestation (weeks) – mean (SD)	27.7 (2.4)	28.0 (2.2)
PROM	28 (22.2)	19 (15.5)
Antenatal steroids	114 (90.4)	114 (92.7)
Preterm labour	61 (48.4)	52 (42.3)
Vaginal delivery	27 (21.4)	20 (16.3)
Outborn	9 (7.1)	5 (4.1)
Surfactant	88 (69.8)	72 (58.5)
SNAP - median [IQ range]	15 [0, 32]	14 [0, 30]
CRIB score – median [IQ range]	2 [1, 6]	2 [1, 5]
Male gender	67 (53.6)	65 (53.3)
Apgar score at 5 min – median [IQ range]	8 [8,9]	8 [8,9]

Data presented as number n (%), median [interquartile range] or mean (standard deviation)
PROM prolonged rupture of membranes, *SNAP* Score of Neonatal Acute Physiology, *CRIB* Clinical Risk index for Babies

medications was considered too burdensome, but they were included in analyses on an intention to treat basis.

Seventy two infants had a positive blood culture with definite LOS, while three had probable sepsis. One infant with Serratia marcescens meningitis had a negative blood culture. Hence for analysis, 76 infants (31%) had LOS with sepsis in the first 28 days. Coagulase negative Staphylococci caused 69% of episodes of LOS during the study period, while 17% were due to gram negative bacilli. There was no difference in the distribution of organisms between the study intervention and standard care arms in the study (p = 0.83).

Primary outcome

Forty infants (31.8%) in the study intervention group and 36 (29.3%) in the standard group had at least one episode of LOS in the first 28 days (Table 3). This corresponds to incidences of 15.8 and 14.2 episodes of sepsis per 1000 patient days respectively.

In subgroup analyses for infants of birth weight < 1000 g, 45.9% randomised to the study intervention bundle and 38.3% receiving the standard technique had an episode of LOS. (Table 3) The incidence rates were 23.6 per 1000 patient days and 18.9 per 1000 patient days respectively. The majority of episodes of LOS (80%) occurred whilst infants were receiving PN and corresponded to rates in the study intervention and standard technique groups of 23.1 and 23.4 per 1000 patient days respectively.

Secondary outcomes are reported in Table 4, with no statistical differences between the groups. On follow-up at 12 months corrected for prematurity, 95 (82%) of the 116 survivors in the study intervention group attended together with 95 (83%) of the 115 in the standard technique group. The mean GQ in the study intervention group was 94.8 (SD, 13.2) compared to 94.4 (SD, 15.3) in the standard technique group (p = 0.85).

Table 3 Sepsis outcomes in study intervention bundle and standard technique groups

	Study intervention bundle	Standard technique	*P* value
	n = 126	*n* = 123	
Sepsis in 1st 28 days	40 (31.8)	36 (29.3)	0.77
Sepsis in 1st 28 days if birth weight < 1000 g	28 (45.9)	23 (38.3)	0.43
Sepsis in 1st 28 days whilst on parenteral nutrition	33 (26.2)	31 (25.2)	0.97

Data presented as number n (%)

Discussion

The bundle of PN line management strategies used in the current study incorporating measures that involved a strict aseptic technique to avoid contamination during line changes together with reductions in line breaches was not associated with a reduction in the incidence of LOS when compared to standard PN line management. The prespecified subgroup analyses, while having some limitations with regard to reduced statistical power showed no benefit for the study intervention while the infants were receiving PN or for those of birth weight < 1000 g. Furthermore, there was no benefit in terms of improved developmental outcome at 12 months of age. However, with the proviso that four infants had the study intervention ceased because it was construed by clinicians as too burdensome

Table 4 Secondary Outcomes for the study intervention bundle and standard care cohorts

	Study intervention bundle	Standard technique	*p*
	n = 126	*n* = 123	
Died	10 (7.9)	8 (6.5)	0.81
Chronic lung disease	40 (31.8)	31 (25.4)	0.27
Postnatal corticosteroids	6 (4.8)	3 (2.4)	0.50
ROP > stage 2	13 (10.3)	5 (4.1)	0.085
Laser treatment for ROP	7 (5.6)	6 (4.9)	1.0
Duration of PN (days)	9.9 [5.7, 16.6]	9.0 [5.8, 14.3]	0.38
Duration of ventilation (days)	3 [0, 8.6]	2.0 [0, 7.2]	0.15
Duration of respiratory support (days)	12.9 [3.0, 39.8]	9.6 [4.0, 35.7]	0.47
Length of hospital stay (days)	73.5 [55, 92]	69 [51, 85]	0.15

Data presented as number n (%), median [interquartile range]
ROP retinopathy of prematurity, *PN* parenteral nutrition

for these patients, there were no adverse effects attributed to the intervention technique.

The results of our study were unexpected and the reasons for the lack of effectiveness of the study intervention remain unclear. It is possible that awareness among staff in the NICU that management of PN lines may affect risk for LOS might have improved diligence with respect to management of all PN lines, affecting LOS incidence in the control group.

Several studies have implicated PN as an important risk factor for LOS [7–9, 21]. The present study confirmed that most episodes of LOS in premature neonates requiring PN coincide temporally while the babies are receiving PN. It is possible that the association of PN with LOS is not causative and that the need for PN is a marker of the vulnerability for these fragile infants. This may be because infants receiving PN tend to have more invasive procedures such as placement of intravascular catheters and blood sampling.

There is strong evidence that contamination of the catheter hub is an important mechanism for entry of pathogenic bacteria into the blood stream [22], which may occur during PN line changes or during injections of medication. Thus the technique used to disinfect the catheter hub may be more important than infection control measures such as sterile gowns and gloves in preventing hub contamination. In our study, in both the study intervention and standard technique groups the catheter hub was disinfected with a 70% isopropyl alcohol swab.

It has been shown that intravenous lipid emulsions, which form an essential part of PN, affect immune function [23]. Thus PN could exert an additional risk for LOS in premature neonates through its effects on the already immature immune system of the premature infant. Hence the effect of a change in line management technique might be limited. Limitation of the use of PN and the duration of its use could be more important [24] and indeed it has been suggested that PN should be ceased and long lines removed when 120 ml/kg/day of enteral nutrition is attained [25].

Recently, it has been shown that the use of bundles of measures focussed on multiple aspects of hand hygiene, infection control measures and intravascular central line management have resulted in a reduction in the incidence of LOS in neonates [11, 12, 26]. A recent multicentred study has also shown that with a bundle of quality improvement measures there was a greater than 50% reduction in infection rates in neonatal intensive care units [25]. Unfortunately, comparisons with the current study are not possible as Bowen et al. [25] reported infection rates for their total population, whereas our infection rates relate only to infants in the study who were receiving PN. The evidence from previous studies is limited in that infection rates are compared with a historical cohort, but the results are consistent and have led to recommendations for the prevention of infection in the NICU [27]. There are likely to be many sources of infection in preterm infants. Any beneficial effects of one intervention may be obscured by the other reservoirs of infection. Our bundle of measures was designed to reduce the contamination of PN line catheter hubs during line changes. However, despite best efforts, lines could become contaminated via the skin breach or by haematogenous seeding.

There was little evidence that the study intervention was harmful although the study intervention technique was abandoned in four infants (3.2%) because of difficulty in inserting peripheral intravenous lines (PIVs) for intravenous medication or infusions. The use of a PIV for medication injections in addition to the intravenous line for PN infusion however was successfully accomplished in the majority of babies.

It has been shown that preterm infants with infection during the neonatal period are more likely to have neurodevelopmental impairment including cognitive development than for uninfected infants [28, 29]. In the present study, given that there was no difference in LOS between the study arms, it was not surprising that there was no difference in developmental outcomes between the two groups of infants. The developmental assessment however occurred at 1 year of age with no opportunity for assessment at an older age. If later developmental assessments had been performed, it is possible that differences in cognitive development may have become evident.

Limitations to the study include the fact that the study was undertaken more than a decade ago during which time there have been a number of changes in practices in many neonatal units that may reduce the rate of LOS. These include the use of probiotics and the more rapid rate of enteral feed increases resulting in shorter periods of PN. Nevertheless, given that the intervention arm focussed on PN line changes, it is felt that the study provides important information relevant to current management. A difficultly in the diagnosis of neonatal infection is that it is usual practice to withdraw blood from a peripheral vein for culture and not from central catheters. Thus it is possible that rates of sepsis could be underestimated or indeed overestimated as contamination with skin organisms especially coagulase negative staphylococci is a possibility. The diagnosis of infection in our study was rigorous and required additional evidence of sepsis including physical signs and abnormal laboratory results. Thus it is considered that the rate of infection documented in the present study is likely to be accurate.

The study, however had many strengths including blinding of outcome assessment, intention to treat analysis, relatively large sample size, and the low rate of attrition. Criteria for the primary outcome measure (LOS episodes) and other outcomes were predefined. Although the study was randomised, there were some minor weaknesses. Three infants were withdrawn from the study after randomisation. This was due to mistaken recruitment of two infants <500 g birth weight and one >1500 g, who were not eligible for inclusion. The inadvertent inclusion of these three infants was not a systematic error and post randomisation exclusion was considered appropriate.

Conclusion

The bundle of PN line management employing a two-nurse sterile technique and measures to reduce breaches of lines used to infuse the PN did not reduce the incidence of LOS in infants of <1500 g birth weight. There was no evidence from this study to recommend this as a routine practice. Further research is required to assess measures that are potentially effective to reduce what is considered to be a preventable complication of prematurity.

Abbreviations

CRIB: Clinical Risk Index for Babies; CRP: C-reactive protein; GQ: General Quotient; LOS: Late-onset sepsis; MMH: Mater Mothers' Hospital; NICU: Neonatal Intensive Care Unit; PIV: Peripheral intravenous line; PN: Parenteral nutrition; ROP: Retinopathy of prematurity; SNAP: Score of Neonatal Acute Physiology; VLBW: Very low birth weight

Acknowledgements

We acknowledge the contribution of Sharyn Morris and Sue Jenkins-Manning, Clinical Nurse Research Assistants and David Sibbritt, Senior Lecturer in Biostatistics, The University of Newcastle together with the nursing and medical staff at the Department of Neonatology and the Growth and Development Unit, Mater Mothers' Hospital, Brisbane.

Funding

The study was supported by the John P Kelly Mater Research Foundation.

Authors' contributions

GA, HL, LC and PHG made substantial contributions to the design of the study. GA, HL and PHG made substantial contributions for the analysis and interpretation of the data. GA, HL and PHG were involved in the drafting of the manuscript. All authors gave final approval for the version to be published and agreed to be accountable for all aspects of the work.

Competing interests

The authors declare that they have no competing interests.

Author details

[1]Newborn Services, Mater Mothers' Hospital, Raymond Tce, South Brisbane, QLD 4101, Australia. [2]Mater Research Institute-The University of Queensland, South Brisbane, QLD, Australia. [3]Present address: The Townsville Hospital, 100 Angus Smith Drive, Douglas 4814, Australia.

References

1. Fanaroff A, Korones S, Wright L, Verter J, Poland RL, Bauer CR, et al. Incidence, presenting features, risk factors and significance of late onset septicaemia in very low birth weight infants. Pediatr Infect Dis J. 1998;17: 593–8.
2. Lean WL, Kamlin CO, Garland SM, Jacobs SE. Stable rates of neonatal sepsis in a tertiary neonatal unit. J Paediatr Child Health. 2015;51:294–9.
3. Isaacs D, Barfield C, Clothier T, et al. Late-onset infections of infants in neonatal units. J Paediatr Child Health. 1996;32:158–61.
4. Tsai MH, Hsu JF, Chu SM, Lien R, Huang HR, Chiang MC, et al. Incidence, clinical characteristics and risk factors for adverse outcome in neonates with late-onset sepsis. Pediatr Infect Dis J. 2014;33:e7–10.
5. Mitha A, Foix-L'Hélias L, Arnaud C, EPIPAGE Study Group. Neonatal infection and 5-year neurodevelopmental outcome in very preterm infants. Pediatrics. 2013;132:e372–80.
6. Dong Y, Speer CP. Late-onset neonatal sepsis; recent developments. Arch Dis Child Fetal Neonatal Ed. 2015;100:F257–63.
7. Avila-Figueroa C, Goldmann DA, Richardson DK, Gray JE, Ferrari A, Freeman J. Intravenous lipid emulsions are the major determinant of coagulase-negative staphylococcal bacteremia in very low birth weight newborns. Pediatr Infect Dis J 1998;17:10–17.
8. Alcock G, Liley H, Wodgate P, Tudehope D, Coory, M. First episodes of late onset sepsis in very low birth weight infants. A case controlled study Pediatr Res 2002;51:305A.
9. Shah J, Jeffries AL, Yoon EW, Lee SK. Shah PS. Canadian Neonatal Network Am J Perinatol. 2015;32:675–82.
10. Ng PC, Wong HL, Lyon DJ, So KW, Liu F, Lam RK, et al. Combined use of alcohol hand rub and gloves reduces the incidence of late onset infection in very low birthweight infants. Arch Dis Child Fetal Neonatal Ed. 2004;89: 336–40.
11. Schulman J, Stricof R, Stevens TP, Horgan M, Gase K, Holzman IR, et al. Statewide NICU central-line-associated blood stream infection rates decline after bundles and checklists. Pediatrics. 2011;127:436–44.
12. Butler-O'Hara MB, D'Angio CT, Hoey H, Stevens TP. An evidence-based catheter bundle alters central venous catheter strategy in newborn infants. J Pediatr. 2012;160:972–7.
13. Aly H, Herson V, Duncan A, Herr J, Bender J, Patel K, et al. Is bloodstream infection preventable among premature infants? A tale of two cities. Pediatrics. 2005;115:1513–8.
14. Maas A, Flament P, Pardou A, Deplano A, Dramaix M, Struelens M. Central venous catheter-related bacteraemia in critically ill neonates: risk factors and impact of a prevention programme. J Hosp Infect. 1998;40:211–4.
15. Lodha A, Furlan AD, Whyte H, Moore AM. Prophylactic antibiotics in the prevention of catheter-associated bloodstream bacterial infection in preterm neonates: a systematic review. J Perinatol. 2008;28:526–33.
16. Rodwell RL, Leslie AL, Tudehope DI. Early diagnosis of neonatal sepsis using a haematologic scoring system. J Pediatr. 1988;112:761–7.
17. International Neonatal Network. The CRIB (clinical risk index for babies) score: a tool for assessing initial neonatal risk and comparing performance of neonatal intensive care units. Lancet. 1993;342:193–8.
18. Richardson D, Gray J, McCormick M, Workman K, Goldmann D. Score for neonatal acute physiology. A physiologic severity index for neonatal intensive care. Pediatrics. 1993;91:617–23.
19. Griffiths R. The Griffiths Mental Development Scales. Henley on Thames: Association for Research in Infant and Child Development 1996.
20. Cartwright D. The Grantly Stable Neonatal Unit Annual Clinical Report. Brisbane: The Royal Women's hospital;2002.
21. Kawagoe JY, Segre CA, Pereira CR, Cardosa MF, Silva CV, Fukishima JT. Risk factors for nosocomial infections in critically ill newborns: a 5-year prospective cohort study. Am J Infect Control. 2001;29:109–14.
22. Garland JS, Aklex CP, Sevallius JM, Murphy DM, Good MJ, Volberding AM, et al. Cohort study of the pathogenesis and molecular epidemiology of

catheter-related bloodstream infection in neonates with peripherally inserted venous catheters. Infect Control Hosp Epidemiol. 2008;29:243–9.
23. Waitzberg DL, Lotierzo PH, Logullo AF, Torrinhas RS, Pereira CC, Meier R. Parenteral lipid emulsions and phagocytic systems. Br J Nutr. 2002; 87(Suppl1):S49–57.
24. Milstone AM, Reich NG, Advani S, et al. Catheter dwell time and CLABSIs in neonates with PICCs: a multicentre cohort study. Pediatrics. 2013;132:e1609.
25. Bowen JR, Callander I, Richards R, Lindrea KB, For the sepsis prevention in NICUs group. Decreasing infection in neonatal intensive care units through quality improvement. Arch Dis Child Fetal Neonatal Ed 2016;0:F1-F7. doi: 10.1136/archdischild-2015-310165.
26. Kaplan HC, Lannon C, Walshe M, Donovan EF for the Ohio Perinatal quality collaborative. Ohio statewide quality-improvement collaborative to reduce late-onset sepsis in preterm infants. Pediatrics. 2011;127:427–35.
27. Polin RA, Denson S, Brady MT. The Committee on fetus and newborn and Committee on infectious diseases. Pediatrics. 2012;129:e1085–93.
28. Stoll BJ, Hansen NI, Adams-chapman I, Fanaroff AA, Hintz SR, Vohr B, for the National Institute of Child Health and Development Neonatal Research Network, et al. Neurodevelopmental and growth impairment among extremely low-birth-weight infants with neonatal infection. JAMA. 2004;292: 2357–65.
29. Schlapbach LJ, Aebischer M, Adams M, Natalucci G, Bonhoeffer J, Latzin P, Swiss Neonatal Network and Follow-Up Group, et al. Impact of sepsis on neurodevelopmental outcome in a Swiss National Cohort of extremely premature infants. Pediatrics. 2011;128:e348–57.

25

Risk factors for necrotizing enterocolitis in neonates

Noor Samuels, Rob A. van de Graaf, Rogier C. J. de Jonge, Irwin K. M. Reiss and Marijn J. Vermeulen*

Abstract

Background: Necrotizing enterocolitis (NEC) is a severe multifactorial disease in preterm neonates associated with high morbidity and mortality. Better insight into prognostic values of the many reported factors associated with NEC is needed to enable identification of neonates at risk for NEC. The aim was to systematically review the literature to identify independent risk factors for NEC from the literature.

Methods: Medline, Cochrane, Embase, Pubmed and Google Scholar were searched systematically for cohort studies reporting prognostic factors for NEC in neonates using multivariable analysis. Studies were scored with the Quality In Prognosis Studies tool (QUIPS).

Results: From 5154 initial hits, 14 prognostic studies were included, with various designs. Study quality was rated high in three studies, moderate or low in the 11 others. Significant prognostic factors for NEC reported in at least two studies were: low birth weight, small for gestational age, low gestational age, assisted ventilation, premature rupture of membranes, black ethnicity, sepsis, outborn, hypotension (all increased risk), surfactant therapy (conflicting results) and cesarean section (lower risk). Meta-analysis was considered not feasible.

Conclusion: High quality studies on prognostic factors for NEC are rare. Several prognostic factors, that are not necessarily causal, are associated with NEC. High quality prognostic research is necessary to establish the predictive values of these factors.

Keywords: necrotizing enterocolitis, intestinal perforation, preterm, neonatal intensive care unit, risk factors, prognosis, epidemiology

Background

Necrotizing enterocolitis (NEC) is one of the most severe complications of preterm birth occurring in 5–10% of very low birth weight infants [1, 2]. Although more and more (extremely) preterm infants survive, the number of deaths attributed to NEC has been increasing [3]. Mortality rates ranging from 15% to 30% have been reported [4]. Surgical treatment is often needed, and survivors are at increased risk for poor long-term growth and neurodevelopmental impairment [5]. Despite preventive strategies such as prenatal glucocorticoid administration, breast feeding, use of donor milk and probiotic supplementation, NEC is still relatively common in most neonatal intensive care units (NICUs) [6–10].

NEC is difficult to predict in individual cases. The etiology is complex and multifactorial, including genetic predisposition, intestinal immaturity, imbalance in microvascular tone, abnormal microbial colonization and highly immune-reactive intestinal mucosa [1]. A common inflammatory pathway leads to intestinal ischemia, pneumatosis, necrosis and eventually perforation [11].

Many observational studies have reported clinical and non-clinical risk factors associated with NEC, but the prognostic value usually is unclear. Most of these studies were not designed to answer prognostic questions properly [12]. To identify independent risk factors for a complex disease as NEC, a (preferably prospective) prognostic cohort design with multivariable analysis including multiple co-variates is considered most appropriate [12–14]. The aim of this study was to provide a

* Correspondence: m.j.vermeulen@erasmusmc.nl
Department of Pediatrics, Division of Neonatology, Erasmus MC, Room SH-3005, P.O. Box 20603015, CN, Rotterdam, The Netherlands

systematic review of the literature on prognostic studies reporting on independent risk factors for NEC in neonates.

Methods

Study selection

This systematic review was guided by the PRISMA Statement, a 27 item checklist to improve the reporting of systematic reviews [15]. A search strategy was developed in collaboration with a clinical librarian to search *PubMed, Embase, Medline, Web-of-science, Cochrane* and *Google Scholar*. An initial search was conducted in January 2014 and updated in August 2016, using terms related to *necrotizing enterocolitis, intestinal perforation, neonates, birth weight, gestation, prediction, prognosis, epidemiology* and *risk factors*. The complete search strategy is reported as supplemental material (Additional file 1). References of included studies were checked for additional eligible studies.

- Studies were included for analysis if satisfying all following criteria: (1) full English written publications, (2) with a prospective or retrospective cohort study or nested case-control design (3) identifying (neonatal or non-neonatal) prognostic factors for NEC (primary or secondary outcome), (4) using multivariable data analysis including more than 2 co-variates, (5) in a study population of neonates/newborns, preterm infants, very low birth weight (VLBW) or extremely low birth weight (ELBW) infants. No explicit use of the term *prognostic* was required for inclusion.
- Excluded were studies (1) only reporting on associative models of one or two variables with NEC (also if adjustment for potential confounders was performed), or (2) focusing only on risk factors for other abdominal problems than NEC such as spontaneous focal intestinal perforation, viral enteritis and allergic colitis.

After duplicates had been removed, two independent reviewers (NS, RG) screened titles and abstracts on both inclusion and exclusion criteria. Articles identified as potentially eligible underwent a full text review. Any disagreements between the two reviewers concerning study selection, quality assessment and interpretation of results were discussed and resolved in consensus meetings with all authors.

Quality assessment

The methodological quality of full text reports was independently assessed by the same researchers using the Quality In Prognosis Studies (QUIPS) tool [16]. The QUIPS tool assesses risk of bias in prognostic studies by rating each individual article in six domains: study participation, study attrition, measurement of prognostic factors, measurement of outcomes, measurement of confounding, and statistical analysis and reporting. As prognostic studies are designed to predict a specific outcome based on a combination of possible prognostic factors of equal interest, the domain of confounding was considered irrelevant. Therefore, an adapted QUIPS without items addressing confounding was used [17]. As NEC was assumed to be a short-term outcome in the included studies, items on long-term follow-up in the quality assessment were not included.

Quality points for a total of 17 items in five domains were assigned to each study, adding up to a total score of 75 points maximum. Domain items were scored as high when sufficient information concerning the risk of bias was present and the estimated risk of bias was considered low. Items were scored as moderate when the article provided insufficient information about this domain and low quality when an item was not reported or was not reported clearly or the estimated risk of bias was considered high. The quality of the studies was ranked high if ≥60 points (≥80% of the maximum score); moderate if 45–59 points (≥60% and <80% of the maximum score); and low if <45 points (<60% of maximum score) were given as described previously [17].

Data extraction and reporting

A standardized form was used to guide and document data extraction systematically. The following data were extracted: study characteristics (publication characteristics, study design, method of analysis, number of subjects, type and number of prognostic factors, outcomes of interest); patient characteristics (gestational age, birth weight, gender); and strength of association (relative risks (RR) and odds ratios (OR)). To restrict the data to those of most clinical interest, we only present details on statistically significant prognostic factors ($p < 0.05$) that were reported in at least two studies.

Results

Search and inclusion

The literature search yielded a total of 11,335 studies (Fig. 1). After removing duplicates 5154 articles remained of which titles and abstracts were screened. Full texts of 78 articles were retrieved after assessment for eligibility. A total of 14 articles met the selection criteria and were included in the study. No additional eligible studies were identified through bibliographic review of the included studies.

Study characteristics

The quality assessment results are listed in Table 1. Three of the included studies were of high quality, 11

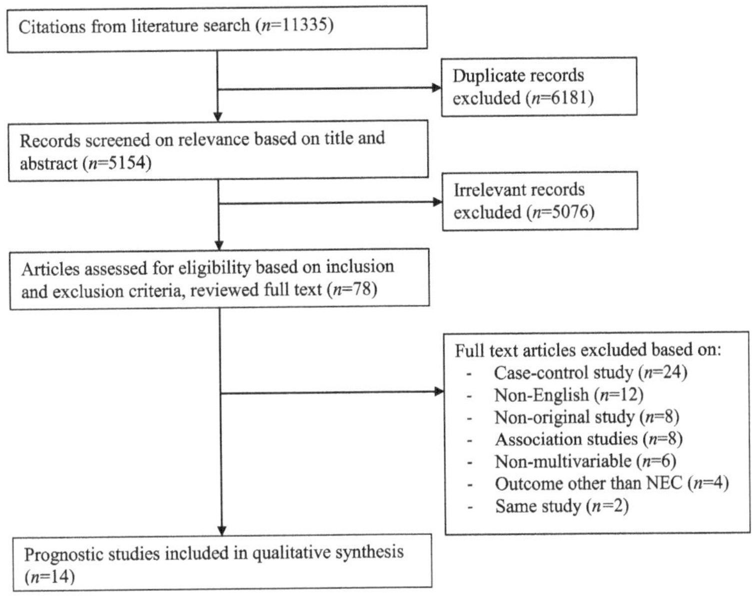

Fig. 1 Flow chart of the systematic literature search

were of moderate quality and none of low quality. Details of the included studies are presented in Table 2. Definitions of study population and outcome varied. Ten studies had a retrospective study design and four studies a prospective study design. In seven studies the study population consisted of VLBW infants, defined by birth weight below 1500 g. One study included neonates with intrauterine growth retardation (IUGR) and two studies neonates admitted to the NICU. In four studies the population was defined by gestational age: below 33 weeks, 23–34, 23–32 and 23–36 weeks. The outcome measure was often not clearly described and included NEC Bell stages I and II in one study, and stages II and III in all others.

Prognostic factors

The 14 included studies described 43 statistically significant risk factors for NEC identified by multivariable analysis. Eleven of these factors were significantly associated with NEC in at least two studies (Table 3). None of the

Table 1 Results of quality assessment of studies on NEC related prognostic factors according to the QUIPS tool [17]

Study	Study participation (max. 15)	Study attrition (max. 15)	Prognostic factor measurement (max. 15)	Outcome measurement (max. 15)	Statistical analysis and reporting (max. 15)	Quality score (max. 75)
Gephart et al. (2014) [18]	15	5	12.5	15	15	62.5
Lee et al. (2016) [38]	15	5	12.5	12.5	15	60
Youn et al. (2015) [30]	15	5	12.5	12.5	15	60
Boo et al. (2012) [21]	15	5	12.5	10	15	57.5
Drenckpohl et al. (2010) [36]	15	5	10	12.5	15	57.5
Guthrie et al. (2003) [23]	15	5	10	12.5	15	57.5
Yee et al. (2012) [27]	15	5	12.5	10	15	57.5
Gagliardi et al. (2008) [28]	15	5	12.5	7.5	15	55
Manogura et al. (2008) [39]	15	5	10	10	15	55
Yamoto et al. (2016) [26]	15	5	10	10	15	55
Faustini et al. (2003) [37]	13.5	5	10	12.5	12.5	53.5
Carter et al. (2008) [22]	15	5	10	10	12.5	52.5
Luig et al. (2004) [25]	15	5	10	7.5	15	52.5
Uauy et al. (1991) [24]	12	5	10	10	12.5	49.5

NEC necrotizing enterocolitis, *QUIPS* quality in prognosis studies

Table 2 Methodologic characteristics of the included prognostic studies on risk factors for NEC

Author	Country (year)	Design	Type of analysis	*N* included	Male (%)	Study population	Outcome	NEC type	Significant prognostic factors from multivariable analysis with $p < 0.05$
Boo et al. (2012) [21]	Malaysia (2007)	Retrospective	Multivariable	3601	52%	VLBW (≤1500 g)	NEC	II, III	Maternal age, BW, surfactant, intrapartum antibiotics, indomethacin, surfactant, congenital pneumonia
Carter et al. (2008) [22]	United States (unknown)	Retrospective	Multivariable	134	54%	GA <35 weeks, BW <1500 g or requiring mechanical ventilation at birth	NEC	II, III	Number of infections, ventilation
Drenckpohl et al. (2010) [36]	United States (2002–2008)	Retrospective	Multivariable	324	54%	GA 23–36 weeks	NEC	II, III	Ethnicity, PROM, sepsis, H2 blockers in TPN
Faustini et al. (2003) [37]	Italy (1999)	Retrospective	Multivariable	221	49%	Live births of the university hospital in Rome	NEC	I, II	Any neonatal pathological condition, first time feeding with formula, any invasive procedure
Gagliardi et al. (2008) [28]	Italy (1999–2002)	Prospective	Multivariable	2035	51%	VLBW (<1500 g), GA 23–37 weeks	NEC-medical, NEC-surgical	II, III	Assisted ventilation, PDA, surfactant, Late-onset sepsis
Gephart et al. (2014) [18]	United States (2007–2011)	Retrospective	Multivariable (Prediction model)	35,013	50%	BW <1500 g and GA < 36 weeks	NEC-surgical, NEC-medical	II, III	GA, outborn, ethnicity, dopamine, dobutamine or milrinone combined with hypotension, metabolic acidosis, probiotics, late sepsis, PRBC transfusion, 2 or more positive cultures (blood, urine, other), human milk at day 7 and 14 of life, unit NEC rate
Guthrie et al. (2003) [23]	United States (1998–2000)	Retrospective	Multivariable	15,072	53%	GA 23–34 weeks	NEC-surgical, NEC-medical	II, III	BW, antenatal glucocorticoids, umbilical vessel catheterization, assisted ventilation, type of delivery, exposed both glucocorticoids and indomethacin during first week of life, Apgar score 5 min.
Lee et al. (2016) [38]	South Korea (2003–2014)	Retrospective	Multivariable	354	53%	GA 23–31(+6) weeks	NEC	II, III	Maternal blood NLR, multiparity, BW, GA
Luig et al. (2004) [25]	Australia (1994–1999)	Retrospective	Multivariable	4649	55%	All NICU admissions	NEC	II, III	Placental abruption, GA (weeks), SGA, year of birth, hyaline membrane disease, hypertensive disease of pregnancy
Manogura et al. (2008) [39]	United States (1997–2006)	Prospective	Multivariable	404	[a]	Neonates with suspected IUGR	NEC	II, III	BW, base deficit
Uauy et al. (1991) [24]	United States (1988–1989)	Prospective	Multivariable	2681	[a]	Infants admitted to one of the network centers <1500 g	NEC	II, III	Center of birth, ethnicity/gender, BW, maternal haemorrhage, duration of ROM, cesarean section
Yamoto et al. (2016) [26]	Japan (2006–2015)	Retrospective	Multivariable	323	53%	BW <1000 g	NEC, FIP, MRI	II, III	Gestational age of <26 weeks, severe cardiac malformations, not received EAP
Yee et al. (2012) [27]	Canada (2003–2008)	Retrospective	Multivariable	16,669	54%	GA <33 weeks	Early-Onset NEC, Late-Onset NEC	II, III	GA, SGA, outborn/inborn, congenital anomalies, narcotic use in <3 days, postnatal glucocorticoids
Youn et al. (2015) [30]	Korea (2013–2014)	Prospective	Multivariable	2326	50%	VLBW (<1500 g)	NEC	II, III	hypotension ≤1 week

BW birth weight, *EPO* erythropoietin, *FIP* focal intestinal perforation, *GA* gestational age, *IVH* intraventricular hemorrhage, *MRI* meconium-related ileus, *NCPAP* nasal continuous positive airway pressure, *NEC* necrotizing enterocolitis, *NICU* neonatal intensive care unit, *NLR* neutrophil-lymphocyte ratio, *PDA* patent ductus arteriosus, *PRBC* packed red blood cell, *(P)ROM* (premature) rupture of membranes, *RDS* respiratory distress syndrome, *SGA* small for gestational age, *SNAP* score for neonatal acute physiology, *TPN* total parental nutrition, *VLBW* very low birth weight
Footnotes: [a] not available

Table 3 Summary of significant prognostic factors for NEC by high, moderate and low quality studies

Prognostic factor	High quality	Moderate quality	Low quality
Birth weight	1×	4×	-
Gestational age (weeks)	1×	3×	-
Sepsis	1×	2×	-
Ethnicity	1×	2×	-
Hypotension	1×	1×	-
Outborn	1×	1×	-
Assisted ventilation	-	3×	-
Cesarean section	-	2×	-
PROM	-	2×	-
Small for gestational age	-	2×	-
Surfactant	-	2×	-

The table shows the statistically significant prognostic factors reported in at least two studies. The quality of the studies was ranked high if ≥60 points (≥80% of the maximum score), moderate if 45–59 points (≥60% and <80% of the maximum score) and low if <45 points (<60% of maximum score) were given. Using the QUIPS tool
NEC necrotizing enterocolitis, *PDA* patent ductus arteriosus, *PROM* premature rupture of membranes, *RDS* respiratory distress syndrome, *QUIPS* quality in prognosis studies

prognostic factors were assessed in all studies. Of the 11 reproducible factors, the following were associated with an increased risk of NEC: small for gestational age, low gestational age, assisted ventilation, sepsis, hypotension, PROM, black ethnicity and outborn status (Table 4). The factor low birth weight was associated differently with NEC in 5 studies. The association with surfactant therapy also showed contrasting directions. Birth by cesarean section was associated with a decreased risk of NEC.

Because of the diversity in study population, definition and incidence of outcome and type of analysis, the measures of associations need to be interpreted in the context of the study characteristics as reported in Table 2. Because of substantial heterogeneity in design, population, prognostic factors and outcomes of the included prognostic studies, it was not feasible to perform a meta-analysis.

Discussion

This is the first systematic review of prognostic studies on risk factors for NEC in neonates. Only three of the 14 included studies scored high for methodological quality; all others scored moderate. This was mostly because of limited information on definition and measurement of the prognostic factor and on the outcome of NEC. Only one report was found on the development of a prediction model for the outcome of NEC [18].

We defined a *prognostic study design* based on several specific criteria suggested in the literature. Aiming to estimate the risk of developing a future clinical outcome (NEC) based on more than one (independent) characteristic, is considered the key feature of a prognostic study design [12–14]. Therefore we only included studies with a defined study population and multivariable analysis of variables of potential equal importance. We did not include trials or studies that focused on the association between NEC and a single risk factor. Although these studies may generate relevant hypotheses, these do not address prognostic questions from a clear prognostic research perspective [12].

Risk factors for NEC

Low birth weight is the most commonly reported significant prognostic factor for NEC among neonates in the current literature, which is in line with large cohort studies describing the highest incidence of NEC among the infants with the lowest birth weights [19, 20]. Interestingly, the clinical relevance of birth weight as an independent prognostic factor for NEC is questionable with odds ratios (ORs) ranging between 0.999–1.001 [21–24]. Presumably, low gestational age or being small for gestational age are clinically more important. However, associations between NEC and these factors were only confirmed by multivariable analysis in four and two of the studies respectively [18, 25–27].

Also of interest, two studies showed a protective effect of cesarean section for developing NEC (OR both 0.60) [23, 24]. The authors suggest that this is due to less stress during delivery, although they point out that selection bias may have occurred. Surfactant therapy proved a positive predictor for NEC in one study but a negative predictor in another [21, 28]. The authors of the latter study explained this by improvement of pulmonary function leading to less gut ischemia. Boo et al. reported that surfactant was administered only to infants with severe respiratory distress syndrome (RDS), suggesting that not surfactant but severe RDS was a significant risk factor for NEC [21]. Kliegman et al. studied RDS and NEC and concluded that neonatal hypoxia is not etiologically related to NEC [29]. They found that mild or no RDS was associated with an increased risk of NEC in contrast to severe RDS, however by performing only univariable analysis. It is unclear whether this can be explained by a protective effect of surfactant in the severe cases or by other factors such as different nutritional or antibiotic treatment. Assisted ventilation was also associated with an increased risk of NEC [22, 23, 28]. The question arises whether this reflects disease severity - as the sickest patients (with the highest risk for NEC) will need ventilation - or the mechanical ventilation itself, as disease severity (other than by birth weight and gestation age) was not adjusted for in all of these studies.

Gephart et al. were the only authors who described the development of a prediction model. Their model

Table 4 Prognostic factors associated with NEC reported in at least two studies

First author:	Boo	Carter	Drenckpohl	Faustini	Gagliardi	Gephart	Guthrie	Lee	Luig	Manogura	Uauy	Yamoto	Yee	Youn
(Low) birth weight[b]	OR 0.999 [0.998,0.999][c]	OR 1.001 [p = 0.164][d,e]	OR 1 [1.000,1.001]	.	.	.	p < 0.001[f]	OR 0.07 [0.01,0.53][g]	.	p < 0.001[f]	OR 0.999 [p < 0.001][c,d,h]	.	.	.
Gestational age (weeks)[b]	.	.	.	.	.	OR 2.37 [1.78,3.16][i]	.	OR 1.14 [0.85,1.54][g]	OR 0.82 [0.77,0.89][g]	.	.	OR 19.32 [3.27,370.43][j]	OR 0.84 [0.81,0.87][g]	.
Sepsis	.	.	OR 4.98 [2.2,11.27][a]	.	OR 5.38 [2.86,10.14][k]	OR 1.49 [1.30,1.72][k]	.	OR 1.41 [0.42,4.67][a]	.	.	.	.	.	OR 1.75 [0.71,2.86][l]
Ethnicity	.	OR 0.571 [p = 0.317][d,m]	OR 0.36 [0.17,0.78][n]	.	.	OR 1.22 [1.09,1.35][m]	.	.	.	.	OR 1.68 [p < 0.001][d,h,m]	.	.	.
Hypotension	.	.	.	.	.	OR 1.51 [1.36,1.69][o]	.	.	.	.	.	.	.	OR 2.00 [1.001,3.999][o]
Outborn	.	.	.	.	.	OR 1.31 [1.17,1.46]	.	.	.	.	.	.	OR 1.55 [1.31,1.83]	.
Assisted ventilation	.	OR 1.053 [p = 0.047][d,a]	.	.	OR 2.71 [1.03,7.15][a]	.	OR 3.5 [2.5,4.7][p]	.	.	.	.	.	.	.
Cesarean section	.	.	.	.	.	.	OR 0.60 [0.50,0.80]	.	.	.	OR 0.60 [p < 0.001][d,h]	.	.	.
PROM	.	.	OR 2.06 [1.02,4.16]	.	.	.	.	.	.	.	OR 1.10 [p < 0.009][d,h]	.	.	.
Small for gestational age[b]	.	.	.	.	.	.	.	.	OR 1.97 [1.19,3.26][a]	.	.	.	OR 1.35 [1.08,1.69][q]	.
Surfactant	OR 1.59 [1.17,2.16]	.	.	.	OR 0.41 [0.19,0.90]	.	.	.	.	.	.	.	.	.

This table shows the strength and the direction of association of prognostic factors, with concomitant confidence intervals if available

NEC necrotizing enterocolitis, *OR* odds ratio, *PROM* premature rupture of membranes

Footnotes: [a] exact definition was lacking; [b] cutt-off values differs between studies; [c] < 1500 g; [d] no CI was given or could be calculated; [e] < 1500 g or requiring mechanical ventilation at birth; [f] OR increased with decreasing weight, no exact ratio was given; [g] calculated for increase of one unit of the continuous variable; [h] calculated by results presented in article; [i] < 28 weeks; [j] < 26 weeks; [k] late-onset sepsis; [l] combination of early- and late-onset sepsis; [m] black ethnicity; [n] white ethnicity; [o] inotropics requirement; [p] mechanical ventilation first day of life; [q] < 10th percentile for the given GA

(GutCheck^{NEC}) included 10 clinical risk factors based on a large neonatal dataset [18]. They found that hypotension requiring inotropic treatment was associated with an increased risk of NEC. Also, Youn et al. considered hypotension within a week of life, as an independent risk factor for NEC [30]. They suggest that the circulatory collapse in the first week of life may assault the gastrointestinal blood flow resulting in higher NEC incidence. Two studies showed neonates who were born outside of the hospital were at greater risk for developing NEC compared to inborn neonates, which was also included in the model of Gephart et al. [18, 27].

The only maternal or perinatal prognostic factors for which evidence in the prognostic literature was found were PROM, cesarean section and being inborn. Interestingly, for commonly assumed clinical neonatal risk factors for NEC such as umbilical lines, red cell transfusions, H2 blockers, and (high osmolar) formula feeding no prognostic evidence was found [20, 31–35]. These factors showed no significant associations in prognostic studies, or have only been reported in studies without a prognostic design.

White ethnicity was associated with a lower risk for NEC compared to black ethnicity in multivariable analyses [18, 24, 36]. However, one study could not confirm these findings, probably due to the overwhelming effects of other factors in the multivariable model [22]. Another finding from two multivariable analyses is an association between diagnosis and treatment of sepsis and NEC, which was defined as blood culture proven late onset sepsis in one study and undefined sepsis prior to NEC in the other [28, 36].

Interpretation of results

When interpreting the results, the following considerations should be taken into account. Firstly, most included studies were of limited quality and heterogeneous. The incidence of NEC stages II-III varied widely, probably due to differences in the selection of the study population and in NEC classification [18, 21–28, 30, 36–39].

Secondly, predictability is not synonymous to causality, although this is often inferred. This is most striking in studies that are unclear on or even ignore the temporality between exposure and onset of outcome. This was nicely pointed out by Patel et al., who studied the association between red blood cell (RBC) transfusions and NEC. They showed that severe anemia but not red blood cell (RBC) transfusion was associated with an increased risk of NEC and suggested that prevention of anemia may be more beneficial than minimizing RBC transfusions [40].

Discriminating etiologic and prognostic study designs is complex, especially because the methodological approaches overlap to some extent. Prognostic research focuses on the probability of a particular state of health whereas etiological research aims to assess the causal relationship between risk factors and outcome. Therefore every causal factor is a predictor but not every predictor is causally related to the outcome [12, 41].

Lastly, the problem of unreported negative findings even within a published report is worth mentioning. Not all studies described the total set of baseline variables included in the multivariable model. Univariable significant factors may have tested non-significant in multivariable models and left out of the final model. By not reporting non-significant factors, it remains impossible to rule out factors that are often assumed to be predictors for NEC. Also, the prognostic factors reported in this review, may have been non-significant in other reports.

Strengths and limitations

Strengths of this review are the broad search strategy, the systematic rating of risk of bias using QUIPS and reporting of data according to PRISMA. Dretzke's key points for the methodological approach for systematic review of prognostic factors were followed [42].

Nevertheless, several limitations may have influenced our study selection and results. Reliable identification of prognostic studies can be difficult especially in case of incomplete reporting and diversity of terminology [42]. Language bias may have occurred by excluding non-English articles. Earlier reported but arbitrarily set cut-off points for low, moderate and high quality in the QUIPS rating were used. Prognostic factors studied once were not summarized in this review but can also be relevant predictors of NEC. This concerned, for example, the only report on multivessel fetal Doppler imaging, by Manogura et al., which still may be relevant [39].

Future perspectives

Well-designed prospective prognostic studies are needed with detailed reporting on definitions, methods and measurement of the prognostic factor and outcome. Special attention should be given to timing of the exposures in relation to the diagnosis of NEC. It would be interesting not only to focus on patient factors but also on maternal factors. Maternal lifestyle factors (such as smoking and obesity), morbidity (such as diabetes, pre-eclampsia, and chorioamnionitis) and prenatal medication (such as antibiotics and corticosteroids) may also be relevant risk factors for NEC [43–48]. A second step is the development and validation of a prediction model to quantify individual risk profiles and identify patients at risk. Until now this has only been performed by Gephart et al. who developed a model based on a large set of retrospective data. Their model still needs external validation in other neonatal populations to evaluate its general clinical usefulness. In our opinion development and validation of prospective prediction models are still necessary for preventive strategies and future reduction of the incidence of NEC.

Conclusion

It is concluded that high quality studies on prognostic factors for NEC are rare. Several prognostic factors are associated with NEC, of which not all are necessarily causal. Ruling out factors is hampered by incomplete reporting. Future high quality prognostic (and predictive) research is necessary to enable clinicians to identify patients at high risk for NEC.

Abbreviations

ELBW: Extremely low birth weight; EPO: Erythropoietin; IVH: Intraventricular hemorrhage; NCPAP: Nasal continuous positive airway pressure; NEC: Necrotizing enterocolitis; NICU: Neonatal intensive care unit; OR: Odds ratio; PDA: Patent ductus arteriosus; PRISMA: Preferred reporting items for systematic reviews and meta-analyses; PROM: Premature rupture of membranes; QUIPS: Quality in prognosis studies; RDS: Respiratory distress syndrome; RR: Relative risk; SNAP: Score for neonatal acute physiology; TPN: Total parenteral nutrition; VLBW: Very low birth weight

Acknowledgements

We gratefully appreciate the support of our biomedical information specialist, Wichor M. Bramer, who contributed to the literature search.

Funding

Not applicable.

Authors' contributions

All authors were involved in the concept and design of the study. NS and RG conducted independent literature searches, quality assessment, and data extraction and wrote the first draft of the manuscript. MJV and RCJ supervised the article selection, quality assessment and data presentation. MJV, RCJ and IKMR critically reviewed and revised the manuscript. All authors have read and approved the final manuscript and agree to be accountable for all aspects of the work. No form of payment was given to anyone to produce the manuscript.

Competing interests

The authors declare that they have no competing interests.

References

1. Neu J, Walker WA. Necrotizing enterocolitis. N Engl J Med. 2011;364(3): 255–64.
2. Thompson AM, Bizzarro MJ. Necrotizing enterocolitis in newborns: pathogenesis, prevention and management. Drugs. 2008;68(9):1227–38.
3. Patel RM, Kandefer S, Walsh MC, Bell EF, Carlo WA, Laptook AR, Sanchez PJ, Shankaran S, Van Meurs KP, Ball MB, et al. Causes and timing of death in extremely premature infants from 2000 through 2011. N Engl J Med. 2015; 372(4):331–40.
4. Lin PW, Stoll BJ. Necrotising enterocolitis. Lancet. 2006;368(9543):1271–83.
5. Schulzke SM, Deshpande GC, Patole SK. Neurodevelopmental outcomes of very low-birth-weight infants with necrotizing enterocolitis: a systematic review of observational studies. Arch Pediatr Adolesc Med. 2007;161(6): 583–90.
6. AlFaleh K, Anabrees J. Probiotics for prevention of necrotizing enterocolitis in preterm infants. Cochrane Database Syst Rev. 2014;4:CD005496.
7. Bury RG, Tudehope D. Enteral antibiotics for preventing necrotizing enterocolitis in low birthweight or preterm infants. Cochrane Database Syst Rev. 2001;1:CD000405.
8. Good M, Sodhi CP, Hackam DJ. Evidence-based feeding strategies before and after the development of necrotizing enterocolitis. Expert Rev Clin Immunol. 2014;10(7):875–84.
9. Halac E, Halac J, Begue EF, Casanas JM, Indiveri DR, Petit JF, Figueroa MJ, Olmas JM, Rodriguez LA, Obregon RJ, et al. Prenatal and postnatal corticosteroid therapy to prevent neonatal necrotizing enterocolitis: a controlled trial. J Pediatr. 1990;117(1 Pt 1):132–8.
10. Deshpande G, Rao S, Patole S, Bulsara M. Updated meta-analysis of probiotics for preventing necrotizing enterocolitis in preterm neonates. Pediatrics. 2010;125(5):921–30.
11. Markel TA, Crisostomo PR, Wairiuko GM, Pitcher J, Tsai BM, Meldrum DR. Cytokines in necrotizing enterocolitis. Shock. 2006;25(4):329–37.
12. Moons KG, Royston P, Vergouwe Y, Grobbee DE, Altman DG. Prognosis and prognostic research: what, why, and how? BMJ. 2009;338:b375.
13. Hemingway H, Croft P, Perel P, Hayden JA, Abrams K, Timmis A, Briggs A, Udumyan R, Moons KG, Steyerberg EW, et al. Prognosis research strategy (PROGRESS) 1: a framework for researching clinical outcomes. BMJ. 2013;346: e5595.
14. Riley RD, Hayden JA, Steyerberg EW, Moons KG, Abrams K, Kyzas PA, Malats N, Briggs A, Schroter S, Altman DG, et al. Prognosis Research Strategy (PROGRESS) 2: prognostic factor research. PLoS Med. 2013;10(2):e1001380.
15. Liberati A, Altman DG, Tetzlaff J, Mulrow C, Gotzsche PC, Ioannidis JP, Clarke M, Devereaux PJ, Kleijnen J, Moher D. The PRISMA statement for reporting systematic reviews and meta-analyses of studies that evaluate health care interventions: explanation and elaboration. PLoS Med. 2009;6(7):e1000100.
16. Hayden JA, van der Windt DA, Cartwright JL, Cote P, Bombardier C. Assessing bias in studies of prognostic factors. Ann Intern Med. 2013;158(4): 280–6.
17. de Jonge RC, van Furth AM, Wassenaar M, Gemke RJ, Terwee CB. Predicting sequelae and death after bacterial meningitis in childhood: a systematic review of prognostic studies. BMC Infect Dis. 2010;10:232.
18. Gephart SM, Spitzer AR, Effken JA, Dodd E, Halpern M, McGrath JM. Discrimination of GutCheck(NEC): a clinical risk index for necrotizing enterocolitis. J Perinatol. 2014;34(6):468–75.
19. Clark RH, Gordon P, Walker WM, Laughon M, Smith PB, Spitzer AR. Characteristics of patients who die of necrotizing enterocolitis. J Perinatol. 2012;32(3):199–204.
20. Llanos AR, Moss ME, Pinzon MC, Dye T, Sinkin RA, Kendig JW. Epidemiology of neonatal necrotising enterocolitis: a population-based study. Paediatr Perinat Epidemiol. 2002;16(4):342–9.
21. Boo NY, Cheah IG. Risk factors associated with necrotising enterocolitis in very low birth weight infants in Malaysian neonatal intensive care units. Singap Med J. 2012;53(12):826–31.
22. Carter BM, Holditch-Davis D. Risk factors for necrotizing enterocolitis in preterm infants: how race, gender, and health status contribute. Adv Neonatal Care. 2008;8(5):285–90.
23. Guthrie SO, Gordon PV, Thomas V, Thorp JA, Peabody J, Clark RH. Necrotizing enterocolitis among neonates in the United States. J Perinatol. 2003;23(4):278–85.
24. Uauy RD, Fanaroff AA, Korones SB, Phillips EA, Phillips JB, Wright LL. Necrotizing enterocolitis in very low birth weight infants: biodemographic and clinical correlates. National Institute of Child Health and Human Development Neonatal Research Network. J Pediatr. 1991;119(4):630–8.

25. Luig M, Lui K. Nsw, Group AN: Epidemiology of necrotizing enterocolitis–Part II: Risks and susceptibility of premature infants during the surfactant era: a regional study. J Paediatr Child Health. 2005;41(4):174–9.
26. Yamoto M, Nakazawa Y, Fukumoto K, Miyake H, Nakajima H, Sekioka A, Nomura A, Ooyama K, Yamada Y, Nogami K, et al. Risk factors and prevention for surgical intestinal disorders in extremely low birth weight infants. Pediatr Surg Int. 2016;32(9):887–93.
27. Yee WH, Soraisham AS, Shah VS, Aziz K, Yoon W, Lee SK, Canadian Neonatal N. Incidence and timing of presentation of necrotizing enterocolitis in preterm infants. Pediatrics. 2012;129(2):e298–304.
28. Gagliardi L, Bellu R, Cardilli V, De Curtis M, Network Neonatale L. Necrotising enterocolitis in very low birth weight infants in Italy: incidence and non-nutritional risk factors. J Pediatr Gastroenterol Nutr. 2008;47(2):206–10.
29. Kliegman RM, Hack M, Jones P, Fanaroff AA. Epidemiologic study of necrotizing enterocolitis among low-birth-weight infants. Absence of identifiable risk factors. J Pediatr. 1982;100(3):440–4.
30. Youn YA, Kim EK, Kim SY. Necrotizing Enterocolitis among Very-Low-Birth-Weight Infants in Korea. J Korean Med Sci. 2015;30(Suppl 1):S75–80.
31. Been JV, Lievense S, Zimmermann LJ, Kramer BW, Wolfs TG. Chorioamnionitis as a risk factor for necrotizing enterocolitis: a systematic review and meta-analysis. J Pediatr. 2013;162(2):236–42. e232.
32. Holman RC, Stoll BJ, Curns AT, Yorita KL, Steiner CA, Schonberger LB. Necrotising enterocolitis hospitalisations among neonates in the United States. Paediatr Perinat Epidemiol. 2006;20(6):498–506.
33. Martinez-Tallo E, Claure N, Bancalari E. Necrotizing enterocolitis in full-term or near-term infants: risk factors. Biol Neonate. 1997;71(5):292–8.
34. Rand T, Weninger M, Kohlhauser C, Bischof S, Heinz-Peer G, Trattnig S, Popow C, Salzer HR. Effects of umbilical arterial catheterization on mesenteric hemodynamics. Pediatr Radiol. 1996;26(7):435–8.
35. Stout G, Lambert DK, Baer VL, Gordon PV, Henry E, Wiedmeier SE, Stoddard RA, Miner CA, Schmutz N, Burnett J, et al. Necrotizing enterocolitis during the first week of life: a multicentered case-control and cohort comparison study. J Perinatol. 2008;28(8):556–60.
36. Drenckpohl D, Knaub L, Schneider C. Risk factors that may predispose premature infants to increased incidence of necrotizing enterocolitis. ICAN: infant, Child, & Adolescent Nutrition 2010;2(1):37–44.
37. Faustini A, Forastiere F, Giorgi Rossi P, Perucci CA. An epidemic of gastroenteritis and mild necrotizing enterocolitis in two neonatal units of a University Hospital in Rome. Italy Epidemiol Infect. 2004;132(3):455–65.
38. Lee JY, Park KH, Kim A, Yang HR, Jung EY, Cho SH. Maternal and Placental Risk Factors for Developing Necrotizing Enterocolitis in Very Preterm Infants. Pediatr. Neonatol 2016;58(1):57–62.
39. Manogura AC, Turan O, Kush ML, Berg C, Bhide A, Turan S, Moyano D, Bower S, Nicolaides KH, Galan HL, et al. Predictors of necrotizing enterocolitis in preterm growth-restricted neonates. Am J Obstet Gynecol. 2008;198(6):638 e631–5.
40. Patel RM, Knezevic A, Shenvi N, Hinkes M, Keene S, Roback JD, Easley KA, Josephson CD. Association of Red Blood Cell Transfusion, Anemia, and Necrotizing Enterocolitis in Very Low-Birth-Weight Infants. JAMA. 2016; 315(9):889–97.
41. Tripepi G, Jager KJ, Dekker FW, Zoccali C. Testing for causality and prognosis: etiological and prognostic models. Kidney Int. 2008;74(12): 1512–5.
42. Dretzke J, Ensor J, Bayliss S, Hodgkinson J, Lordkipanidze M, Riley RD, Fitzmaurice D, Moore D. Methodological issues and recommendations for systematic reviews of prognostic studies: an example from cardiovascular disease. Syst Rev. 2014;3:140.
43. Cetinkaya M, Ozkan H, Koksal N. Maternal preeclampsia is associated with increased risk of necrotizing enterocolitis in preterm infants. Early Hum Dev. 2012;88(11):893–8.
44. Downard CD, Grant SN, Maki AC, Krupski MC, Matheson PJ, Bendon RW, Fallat ME, Garrison RN. Maternal cigarette smoking and the development of necrotizing enterocolitis. Pediatrics. 2012;130(1):78–82.
45. Garcia-Munoz Rodrigo F, Galan Henriquez G, Figueras Aloy J, Garcia-Alix Perez A. Outcomes of very-low-birth-weight infants exposed to maternal clinical chorioamnionitis: a multicentre study. Neonatology. 2014;106(3):229–34.
46. Weintraub AS, Ferrara L, Deluca L, Moshier E, Green RS, Oakman E, Lee MJ, Rand L. Antenatal antibiotic exposure in preterm infants with necrotizing enterocolitis. J Perinatol. 2012;32(9):705–9.
47. Wong D, Abdel-Latif M, Kent A, Network N. Antenatal steroid exposure and outcomes of very premature infants: a regional cohort study. Arch Dis Child Fetal Neonatal Ed. 2014;99(1):F12–20.
48. Grandi C, Tapia JL, Cardoso VC. Impact of maternal diabetes mellitus on mortality and morbidity of very low birth weight infants: a multicenter Latin America study. J Pediatr. 2015;91(3):234–41.

26

Validity of anthropometric equations to estimate infant fat mass at birth and in early infancy

Jennifer S. Cauble, Mira Dewi and Holly R. Hull*

Abstract

Background: In newborns and children, body fat estimation equations are often used at different ages than the age used to develop the equations. Limited validation studies exist for newborn body fat estimation equations at birth or later in infancy. The study purpose was to validate 4 newborn fat mass (FM) estimation equations in comparison to FM measured by air displacement plethysmography (ADP; the Pea Pod) at birth and 3 months.

Methods: Ninety-five newborns (1–3 days) had their body composition measured by ADP and anthropometrics assessed by skinfolds. Sixty-three infants had repeat measures taken (3 months). FM measured by ADP was compared to FM from the skinfold estimation equations (Deierlein, Catalano, Lingwood, and Aris). Paired t-tests assessed mean differences, linear regression assessed accuracy, precision was assessed by R^2 and standard error of the estimate (SEE), and bias was assessed by Bland-Altman plots.

Results: At birth, FM measured by ADP differed from FM estimated by Deierlein, Lingwood and Aris equations, but did not differ from the Catalano equation. At 3 months, FM measured by ADP was different from all equations. At both time points, poor precision and accuracy was detected. Bias was detected in most all equations.

Conclusions: Poor agreement, precision, and accuracy were found between prediction equations and the criterion at birth and 3 months.

Keywords: Prediction equations, Infant, Fat mass, Anthropometrics, ADP, Skinfolds

Background

Body weight for length measures are commonly used to identify those at risk for obesity development. Though widely used, weight for length measures do not differentiate the proportion of body weight that is fat mass (FM) or fat free mass (FFM) and are poor indicators of nutritional status and growth [1, 2]. To assess obesity risk and answer critical questions related to nutritional status and growth, infant body composition measurement is required. A number of techniques are available to measure infant body compositon; however the equipment is expensive, not widely available, impractical to use in large population studies, and often located in research laboratories. To combat these limitations, anthropometric equations have been developed and are commonly used in large epidemiologic or multi-site cohort studies [3–9].

There is a track record for studies to use equations that have been developed in one age group and then validated in another age group [10–12] or equations are used in age groups where they were not developed or validated [9, 13, 14]. Some equations have been validated whereas other equations lack proper validation data suggesting they should not be used. The Dauncey et al. [15] equation was developed in newborns and validated by Kulkarni et al. [10] in infants 6–18 months old, and used in one year old infants [16]. The Slaughter et al. equation [17] was developed in children and youth aged 8–29 years and was validated in infants from birth to four months of age [11, 18] and 6–7 year old children [19], and was used in children aged 3–5 years [13, 14]. The Goran et al. equation [19] was developed in children 4 to 10 years old and validated by Hussain et al. [12] in

* Correspondence: hhull@kumc.edu
Department of Dietetics and Nutrition, School of Health Professions, University of Kansas Medical Center, 3901 Rainbow BLVD, Mail Stop 4013, Kansas City, KS 66160, USA

14 year old children. The Westrate et al. [20] equation was developed in 7 to 10 year old children but used to estimate infant FM [4, 6, 21] even though the equation was reported to result in significant bias when applied to young infants [22]. It is important to use equations that have validation data in the age range they are being applied and have validated results otherwise incorrect conclusions may be drawn from the data.

Recently developed and commonly used infant FM estimation equations include Deierlein et al. [23], Catalano et al. [24], Lingwood et al.[11], and Aris et al. [25]. Limited validation studies have been completed in these equations. The Deierlein et al. equation has never been validated [23], while the Lingwood and Aris equations have not been validated in a population other than what was used to develop the equation [11, 25]. It is important to validate equations in the age group they were developed to verify accuracy, in age groups where equations are used but have not been validated, and in age groups where the equations may be used [26]. Therefore, the aim of this study was to validate the Deierlein et al. [23], Catalano et al. [24], Lingwood et al. [11], and Aris et al. [25] infant anthropometric equations at birth and 3 months in comparison to body fat measured using air displacement plethysmography (ADP).

Methods

Participants

The study analyzed data from 95 infants that participated in the Pregnancy Health Study approved by the Institutional Review Board (#13126 and 12793). For the parent study, women were recruited and followed during pregnancy. Of the 95 infants who completed the first visit (1–3 days after birth), 63 came back for their second visit at 3 months.

Ethnicity was self-selected by the mother using a questionnaire. The mother was asked to self-identify her own ethnicity and the ethnicity of the father of the baby. Next, the mother self-identified the ethnicity of her parents and the parents of the baby's father (grandparents to the infant). The following categories were available for selection: Asian, non- Hispanic Black (African American), non-Hispanic White, and Hispanic. When all selected categories matched for parents and grandparents, the infant was identified by that category. If multiple categories were identified, the infant was classified as "other."

Study procedures

Women with a healthy full term (>37 weeks) pregnancy were recruited at a prenatal visit at the OB clinic. The inclusion criteria were: maternal age 18–40 years, singleton pregnancy, and body mass index (BMI) >18 kg/m^2. Women were excluded if they had a serious pregnancy complication, developed gestational diabetes, pre-eclampia, gestational hypertension, or the infant was born with a congential anomaly known to effect fetal growth. Maternal data were collected at visits to the research laboratory in the first, second and third trimesters. Infant body composition was assessed after discharge from the maternity unit. Informed written consent was obtained before any measurement was completed. Women gave consent on behalf of their infant.

Estimation equations

Four different infant FM estimation equations were validated at birth (1–3 days) and at 3 months. The equations were Deierlein et al. [23], Catalano et al. [24], Lingwood et al. [11], and Aris et al. [25]. The Lingwood equation yielded predicted FFM, therefore FM was calculated by subtracting the predicted FFM from body weight. The details regarding equation predictor variables, reference method used when developing the equation, and details on the sample used to develop the equation are listed in Table 1. Gender, infant age, infant ethnicity, body weight, length and various skinfolds are examples of the variables used in the equations. All equations were developed in newborns ranging in age from 0 to 4 days old. Catalano et al. used total body

Table 1 Anthropometric equations to estimate infant fat mass (kg)

Reference	Equations	Reference method	N subjects	Subject age of range
Deierlein et al. [21]	−0.012 − 0.064*gender(1 = male; 0 = female) + 0.0024*age (days) − 0.150*body weight (kg) + 0.055*body weight^2 (kg)^2 + 0.046*ethnicity (1 = Hispanic; 0 = not Hispanic) + 0.020*sum of 3 skinfolds (triceps, subscapular and thigh)	ADP	128	1-3 days
Catalano et al. [20]	0.54657 + 0.39055 * Birth weight (g) + 0.0453*Flank Skinfold (mm) − 0.03237* Length (cm)	TOBEC	194	1-3 days
Lingwood et al. [11]	FFM = 0.057 + 0.646 * weight (kg) - 0.089 * gender (1 = male; 2 = female) + 0.009 * length (cm) FM = weight - FFM	ADP	77	0-4 days
Aris et al. [22]	−0.022 + 0.307 * weight (kg) - 0.077 * gender (1 = male; 0 = female) - 0.019 * gestational age (week) + 0.028 * subscapular skinfold (mm)	ADP	88	1-3 days

*indicates multiplication in the scientific equation

electrical conductivity (TOBEC) as the reference method to develop the prediction equations while all other equations used ADP as the reference method.

Anthropometric measures

All measurements were collected using standardized procedures to our Laboratory [27] and took place on the same day as the body composition assessment by ADP. All skinfolds were identified by anatomical landmarks and taken on the right side of the body using Lange calipers (Beta Technology, Santa Cruz, CA). Skinfolds were taken in order from head to toe and then repeated in that same order. If two skinfold measurements differed by more than 0.5 mm, a third measurement was repeated. The two measurements within 0.5 mm were averaged and used for the analysis. Biceps and triceps skinfolds were measured at the midline of the anterior and posterior surface of the arm, respectively, on the mid-point between acromial process of the scapula and olecranon process of the ulna. The subscapular skinfold was measured at the lower angle of the scapula. The thigh skinfold was measured at the mid-point between the proximal edge of the patella (knee cap) and inguinal crease at the anterior surface of the thigh. The flank skinfold was measured immediately above the iliac crest at the mid-axillary line. Technicians completed annual anthropometric training and validity statistics were calculated. Three testers were responsible for collecting the anthropometric data. Intraclass correlations (ICC) were calculated for each skinfold site. The range of ICC's for the skinfold sites ranged from 0.83 to 0.96 and the technical error of measurement ranged from 0.23 to 0.34.

Air displacement plethysmography

Air displacement plethysmography (Pea Pod®, Software version 3.5.0, 2015, CosMed, Concord, CA) was used to measure infant body composition. Body weight was measured using the integrated scale and measured to the nearest 0.01 kg. Body composition was determined by measuring body volume and calculating body density. A cap was worn to minimize air trapped in the hair. All clothing and the diaper were removed before the body volume measurement. After the infant body volume was acquired, body density was calculated and converted to percentage body fat (%fat) using gender specific equations by Fomon et al. [28]. Air displacement plethysmography is a valid technique to assess infant body composition and was validated against the gold standard 4 compartment model (4C) [29] and against total body water using deuterium dilution [30]. No differences were found for percentage body fat when compared to the 4C model or total body water [29, 30]. Infant ages in these validation studies ranged from 0.4 to 23 weeks which includes the ages in our sample. Therefore, ADP will be considered the criterion measure in this validation study.

Statistical analyses

Means and standard deviations were calculated for all continuous variables. For these analyses, ADP was considered the criterion. Differences between the criterion measure and each estimation equation were assessed using paired t-tests. Regression analysis was used to assess the accuracy between the criterion and each of the equations. To be considered accurate, the regression line relating the two measurements should have a slope equal to 1.0. A slope that deviates significantly from 1.0 suggests a unit change in the estimation equation does not correspond to a unit change in the criterion. Precision was assessed by R^2 and standard error of the estimate (SEE). A SEE between 2 and 3% of fat mass is desirable and classified as very good whereas a SEE >4.0% is considered poor [31]. In our sample, an SEE value of 3% is 0.015 kg at birth and 0.067 kg at 3 months. An R^2 value should exceed 0.64. A R^2 value <0.64 suggests poor agreement between the two methods and poor predictive value of the equations relative to the criterion. Bland Altman was used to assess agreement between the methods [32]. This analysis involves an assessment of the correlation or the measure of strength for the relationship between the mean of the criterion and each equation (mean infant FM criterion + mean infant FM from each equation/2) correlated to the difference between the equation estimated infant FM and the criterion measured FM. A non-significant correlation suggests no bias in the technique across the range of fatness. This provides insight into how much the equation estimated FM differs and relates to the criterion measured FM. Statistical analyses were conducted using SPSS version 20.0 (IBM, Armonk, NY). Statistical significance was set as $p \leq 0.05$.

Results

Sample descriptive statistics are reported in Table 2. Fat mass assessed by the criterion and calculated for all equations are presented in Table 3. The average FM measured by the criterion was 0.374 kg at birth and 1.664 kg at visit 2.

Fat mass measured at birth

At birth, mean differences were found between all equations ($p < 0.05$) and the criterion except for the Catalano equation (Table 3). Table 4 reports results for accuracy and precision assessed by regression. The slope measured by regression from all equations against the criterion differed from 1 ($p < 0.0001$). Poor agreement and precision was found between methods with low R^2

Table 2 Maternal and infant descriptive statistics for the sample at birth and at 3 months

	Birth ($n = 95$)	3 months ($n = 63$)
Maternal age (years)	28.9 ± 4.8	29.9 ± 4.0
Maternal pre-pregnancy BMI (kg/m^2)	25.8 ± 6.1	25.4 ± 5.6
Maternal gestational weight gain (kg)	15.6 ± 6.0	15.2 ± 5.5
Gestational age (wks)	39.24 ± 2.8	39.20 ± 3.3
Birthweight (g)	3497.5 ± 404.6	3539.0 ± 445.2
Birth length (cm)	50.4 ± 2.1	50.0 ± 4.8
Male (%)	42 (44.2%)	26 (41.3%)
Infant age (days)	2.3 ± 1.3	117.2 ± 23.2
Ethnicity		
White	68 (71.6)	51 (81.0)
African-American	14 (14.7)	5 (7.9)
Hispanic	8 (8.4)	4 (6.3)
Asian	5 (5.3)	3 (4.8)
Body weight at assessment (g)	3272 ± 388.2	6595.1 ± 841.4
Length at assessment (cm)	50.4 ± 2.1	63.9 ± 4.4
Skinfolds		
Triceps (mm)	5.6 ± 1.5	11.1 ± 2.9
Biceps (mm)	4.4 ± 1.2	7.4 ± 2.1
Subscapular (mm)	5.3 ± 1.4	7.9 ± 2.0
Thigh (mm)	7.7 ± 1.9	20.2 ± 4.4
Percentage body fat by criterion (%fat)	11.2 ± 4.3	25.0 ± 5.1
Fat mass by criterion (kg)	0.374 ± 0.17	1.664 ± 0.44
Fat-free mass by criterion (kg)	2.897 ± 0.29	4.93 ± 0.63

Values are mean ± SD.

values ranging from 0.55 to 0.63 and high SEE values ranging from 0.106 to 0.116 kg.

A residual plot analysis of the predictive error (Bland-Altman plot) from the equations against the criterion is reported in Table 4 and Fig. 1. Bias was detected for the Catalano and Lingwood equations. This suggested the Catalano and Lingwood equations ovestimated FM at lower FM values and underestimated FM values at greater FM values. For the Deierlein equation, no bias was detected though the value approached significance ($p = 0.099$). No bias was detected for the Aris equation ($p = 0.140$). Even though no bias was detected in the Aris equation, the 95% limit of agreement was wide.

Table 3 Fat mass assessed by the different methods at birth and 3 months

Method	Fat mass (kg)	
	Birth ($n = 95$)	3 months ($n = 63$)
Criterion	0.374 ± 0.171	1.664 ± 0.433
Deierlein	0.488 ± 0.154*	4.989 ± 0.987*
Catalano	0.362 ± 0.138	1.392 ± 0.301*
Lingwood	0.330 ± 0.137*	1.378 ± 0.261*
Aris	0.340 ± 0.157*	1.433 ± 0.276*

Values are mean ± SD. Criterion method was ADP

* Significant difference from the criterion method $p < 0.05$

Fat mass measured at 3 month

At 3 months, the mean FM for all equations differed from the criterion ($p < 0.0001$) (Table 3). Table 4 reports results for accuracy and precision assessed by regression. The slope measured by regression from all equations against the criterion differed from 1 ($p < 0.0001$). At 3 months, R^2 values were poor ranging from 0.43 to 0.55 and the SEE values were high ranging from 0.095 to 0.303 kg.

Bias was detected for all equations when compared to the criterion ($p < 0.0001$; Table 4 and Fig. 2). The data suggests that the Deierlein equation overestimates FM at all values with the estimations being greater at higher FM values. Conversely, the Catalano, Lingwood, and Aris equations overestimate FM at lower FM values and underestimates FM at higher FM values.

Discussion

This study validated equations to predict infant FM against a validated technique (ADP) in newborns at birth (1 to 3 days) and in infants at 3 months. The equations we chose to validate were all developed in infants aged 0–4 days old [11, 23–25]. We sought to test the validity of the equations not only at birth but also at a later age range (3 months) since research studies have used the Catalano et al. equation at birth [24] and at 4–6 weeks old [9]. Further, it is not uncommon to use prediction equations in other age populations than they were developed.

At birth, mean differences were detected between the criterion and all equations except for Catalano et al. At 3 months, mean differences were detected between the criterion and all equations. The predictive error (SEE) was poor for all equations at birth. The predictive error increased just 3 months later. Poor agreement was found between all equations at birth and 3 months as represented by R^2 values <0.64. At birth, bias was detected for the Catalano and Lingwood equations while at the 3 month visit, bias was detected in all equations.

We wanted to compare the results of our study to other studies that have validated the infant prediction equations we tested. Catalano et al. [5] recently validated the Catalano et al. equation [24] against ADP in sample of newborns not used to develop the equation. They reported a better correlation than was found in this study ($R^2 = 0.69$ vs 0.55). To our knowledge, the Deierlein equation has never been validated and the Aris and Lingwood equations have only been cross validated

Table 4 Results for regression and Bland Altman analysis for comparison of the criterion method and the fat mass estimation equations at birth and 3 months

Comparison	Regression analysis			Bland and Altman				
	Slope	R^2	*p*-value	SEE	Mean bias ± SD	95% limits of agreement	Pearson Correlation (r)	*p*-value*
Birth (*n* = 95)								
Deierlein vs Criterion	−0.87	0.61	<0.0001	0.108	0.114 ± 0.109	−0.010 - 0.328	−0.17	0.099
Catalano vs Criterion	0.92	0.55	<0.0001	0.116	−0.012 ± 0.116	−0.240 - 0.215	−0.31	0.002
Lingwood vs Criterion	0.93	0.55	<0.0001	0.116	−0.045 ± 0.116	−0.272 - 0.183	−0.33	0.001
Aris vs Criterion	0.87	0.62	<0.0001	0.106	−0.034 ± 0.107	−0.245 - 0.176	−0.15	0.140
3 months (*n* = 63)								
Deierlein vs Criterion	0.29	0.42	<0.0001	0.333	3.325 ± 0.784	1.789 - 4.862	0.77	<0.0001
Catalano vs Criterion	1.02	0.50	<0.0001	0.308	−0.271 ± 0.306	−0.871 - 0.328	−0.47	<0.0001
Lingwood vs Criterion	1.24	0.55	<0.0001	0.294	−0.286 ± 0.298	−0.871 - 0.299	−0.63	<0.0001
Aris vs Criterion	1.15	0.52	<0.0001	0.303	−0.230 ± 0.303	−0.824 - 0.363	−0.57	<0.0001

* Significance for the correlation of the strength for the relationship between the mean of the criterion and each equation correlated to the difference between the equation estimated infant fat mass and the criterion measured fat mass. A non-significant correlation suggests no bias in the technique across the range of fatness

using a portion of the sample that was used to develop the equations. Since there are limited data on the equations we validated, we identified the Dauncey et al. equation [15] as another commonly used infant prediction equation to compare precision and accuracy results. We could not validate the Dauncey et al. equation [15] due to missing variables in our dataset. Validation studies [24, 33, 34] found a similar range of poor agreement ($R^2 = 0.40 - 0.61$) as was found in our study ($R^2 = 0.55 - 0.63$). Even though poor agreement was found the equation is used in research studies [35, 36].

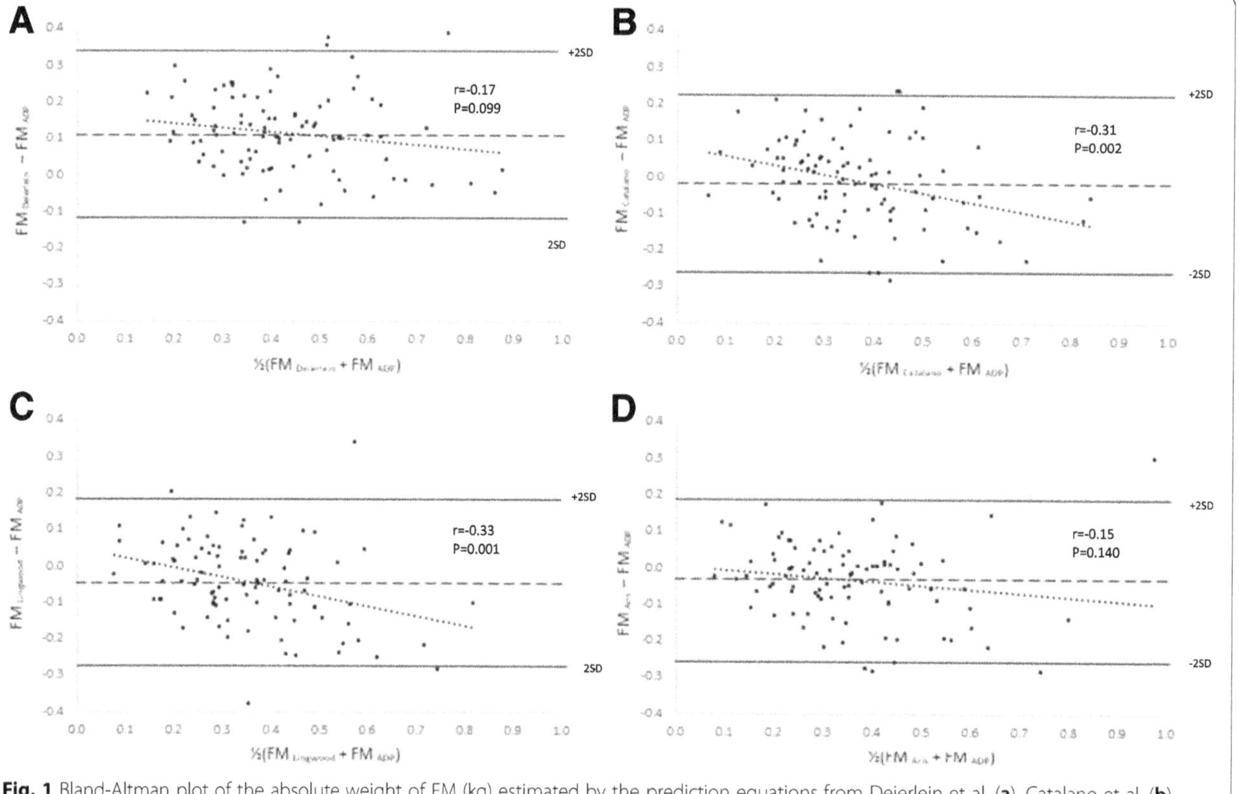

Fig. 1 Bland-Altman plot of the absolute weight of FM (kg) estimated by the prediction equations from Deierlein et al. (**a**), Catalano et al. (**b**), Lingwood et al. (**c**) and Aris et al. (**d**) against the criterion at birth. The *middle dashed line* represents the mean difference between the infant prediction equations and the criterion. The *upper* and *lower solid line* represents ±2SD from the mean

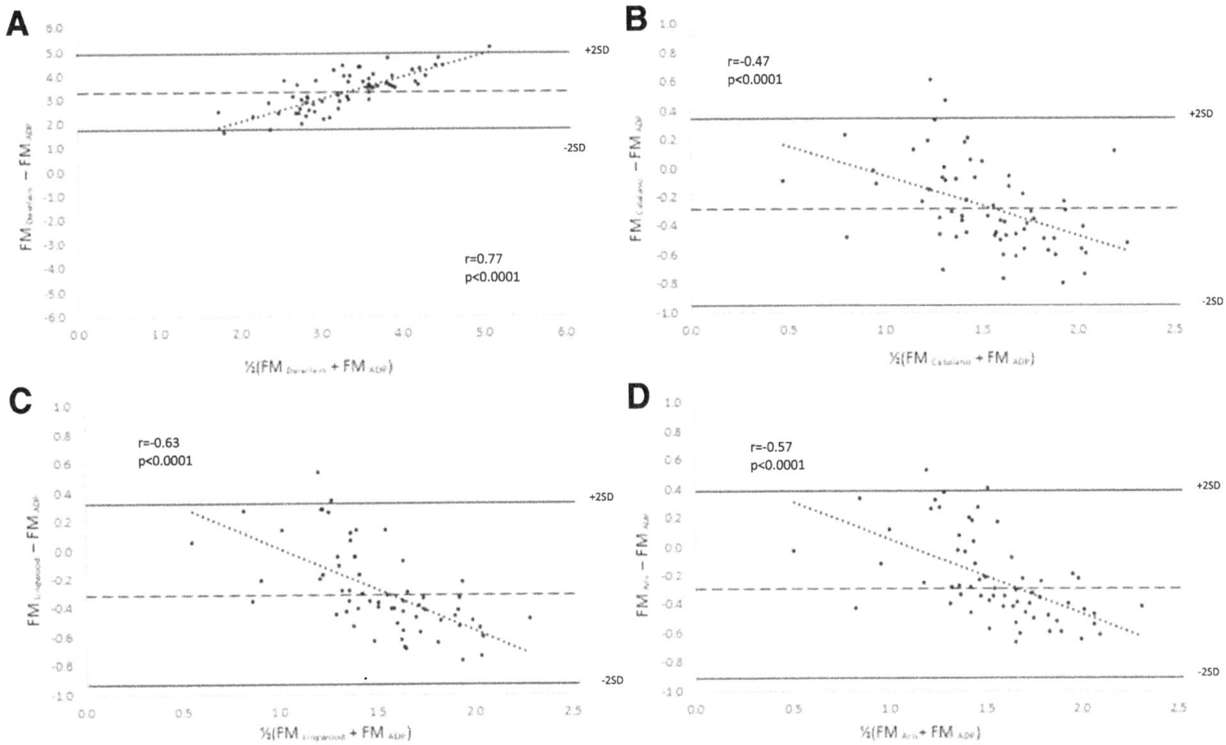

Fig. 2 Bland-Altman plot of the absolute weight of FM (kg) estimated by the prediction equations from Deierlein et al. (**a**), Catalano et al. (**b**), Lingwood et al. (**c**) and Aris et al. (**d**) against the criterion at 3 months. The *middle dashed line* represents the mean difference between the infant prediction equations and the criterion. The *upper* and *lower solid line* represents ± 2SD from the mean

We wanted to explore potential reasons why mean differences and poor agreement and bias have been detected in infant prediction equations. The period of early infancy presents a period of rapid infant growth with a wide range of inter-individual variability. A range of infant growth exists due to gender differences and the infant feeding method (formula vs. breastfeeding) [37]. Differences are especially apparent early from 1–4 months of age where formula fed infants gain more body weight when compared to breast fed infants [38, 39]. Though the growth rate of breast fed infants is slower when compared to formula fed infants, breast fed infants have greater FM from birth to 9 months when compared to formula fed infants [40]. In addition, Shepherd et al. [39] found gender differences in body composition changes in formula fed infants. In the early months, the extra body weight gained in males was detected as FM whereas in females they gained FFM. None of the infant prediction equations validated included feeding method as a predictor variable, likely because they were developed in infants 0–4 days old.

The feeding method may also cause error in assessing infant body composition at birth. Macdonald et al. [41] assessed differences in body weight loss and recovery of birth weight in formula fed and breast fed newborns. The timing of loss was the same between the two groups, but breast fed infants lost 6.6% of their birth weight at day 3 whereas formula fed infants only lost 3.5% of their body weight at day 3. Further, regain to birth weight was slower in breast fed infants (8.3 days) compared to formula fed infants (6.5 days). It is unknown how these differences would impact the prediction of infant body composition but it is plausible the infant feeding method could create error in the prediction of infant body composition at birth.

Further support that rapid infant growth is influencing the accuracy and precision of infant prediction equations can be found in the better performance of prediction equations in children, adolescents, and teenagers. The Slaughter et al. [17] equation is commonly used to predict FM in 8 to 29 year olds. Validation studies in 5 to 19 year olds [12, 23, 42] foundgood agreement and precision ($R^2 = 0.76$-0.81; SEE: 3.73%). As weight gain and body composition becomes more stable in childhood when compared to early infancy, we speculate that prediction equations are more accurate.

Another potential reason poor agreement and bias were detected may be differences in race/ethnicity between the populations. It is well published that there are differences in body composition based on race/ethnicity detected at birth through adulthood [8, 43–46]. If there is a mismatch between the validation population and the population the equations are being applied, errors in estimation may occur. Only the Deirerlein equation included ethnicity as a predictor variable [23]. The race/ethnic breakdown of the Deirerlein pouplation was ~42% Caucasian, 6% African American, 20% Hispanic, 10% Asian, and 22% other. The populations used to develop the other equations were the following: Catalano was primarily Caucasian (64%) and data were collected in the United States [24], the Lingwood equation was developed from an Australian sample that was 89% Caucasian [11], and the Aris sample was an Asian population from Singapore that was comprised of Chinese, Malay, and Indian newborns. Our sample was primarily Caucasian (~71%) and collected in the United States. The Catalano equation included a population similar to ours, however, the other equations were developed with populations that had race/ethnic or location differences. This may contribute to the poor performance of the equations in our sample.

Strength and limitation

One strength of our study is that we compared the estimation equations to ADP, which is a technique that was developed and validated [29, 30] specifically to assess infant body composition. Additionally, our analysis validated and discussed multiple equations that are used to assess infant body composition. A third strength is that we sought to validate this equation at multiple infant ages. Fat mass measurements are needed across infancy and this comparison provides insight into accuracy at time points other than at birth. A potential limitation to our study was the inability to assess the validity of the Dauncey et al. [15] equation. This equation is commonly used and providing a comparison within the context of the other infant prediction equations would have been valuable.

Conclusions

In conclusion, differences were found between the prediction equations and criterion and poor accuracy, agreement and precision was detected. Equipment to measure infant body composition is not widely available and therefore estimation equations are commonly used. The equations we validated performed poorly therefore caution should be used when interpreting data collected with these equations to avoid erroneous conclusions. Development of equations that provide more accurate estimates is desperately needed.

Abbreviations

%fat: Percentage body fat; 4C: 4 compartment model; ADP: Air displacement plethysmography; FFM: Fat free mass; FM: Fat mass; SEE: Standard error of the estimate

Acknowledgements

The authors would like to acknowledge Shengqi Li, the study participants, and the funding agencies for their gracious support.

Funding

Supported by: 5K12HD052027, Thrasher Pediatric Research Foundation.

Authors' contributions

HH conceived the study idea, provided study supervision, participated in data analysis, manuscript writing and editing. JC and MD participated in data analysis, manuscript writing and editing, and data collection. All authors read and approved the final manuscript.

Competing interests

Each author has declared no conflict of financial or personal interests in any company or organization sponsoring this study.

References

1. Daniels SR. The use of BMI in the clinical setting. Pediatrics. 2009;124 Suppl 1:S35–41.
2. Whitlock EP, Williams SB, Gold R, Smith PR, Shipman SA. Screening and interventions for childhood overweight: a summary of evidence for the US Preventive Services Task Force. Pediatrics. 2005;116:e125–44.
3. Aris IM, Soh SE, Tint MT, Liang S, Chinnadurai A, Saw SM, Rajadurai VS, Kwek K, Meaney MJ, Godfrey KM, Gluckman PD, Yap FK, Chong YS, Lee YS. Effect of maternal glycemia on neonatal adiposity in a multiethnic Asian birth cohort. J Clin Endocrinol Metab. 2014;99:240–7.
4. Brunner S, Schmid D, Huttinger K, Much D, Heimberg E, Sedlmeier EM, Bruderl M, Kratzsch J, Bader BL, Amann-Gassner U, Hauner H. Maternal insulin resistance, triglycerides and cord blood insulin in relation to post-natal weight trajectories and body composition in the offspring up to 2 years. Diabet Med. 2013;30:1500–7.
5. Catalano PM, Mele L, Landon MB, Ramin SM, Reddy UM, Casey B, Wapner RJ, Varner MW, Rouse DJ, Thorp Jr JM, Saade G, Sorokin Y, Peaceman AM, Tolosa JE. Inadequate weight gain in overweight and obese pregnant women: what is the effect on fetal growth? Am J Obstet Gynecol. 2014;211:137. e1-7.
6. Hauner H, Much D, Vollhardt C, Brunner S, Schmid D, Sedlmeier EM, Heimberg E, Schuster T, Zimmermann A, Schneider KT, Bader BL, Amann-Gassner U. Effect of reducing the n-6:n-3 long-chain PUFA ratio during pregnancy and lactation on infant adipose tissue growth within the first year of life: an open-label randomized controlled trial. Am J Clin Nutr. 2012;95:383–94.
7. Naf S, Escote X, Ballesteros M, Yanez RE, Simon-Muela I, Gil P, Albaiges G, Vendrell J, Megia A. Serum activin A and follistatin levels in gestational diabetes and the association of the Activin A-Follistatin system with anthropometric parameters in offspring. PLoS One. 2014;9:e92175.
8. Singh KA, Huston-Presley LP, Mencin P, Thomas A, Amini SB, Catalano PM. Birth weight and body composition of neonates born to Caucasian compared with African-American mothers. Obstet Gynecol. 2010;115:998–1002.
9. Badon SE, Dyer AR, Josefson JL, HAPO Study Cooperative Research Group. Gestational weight gain and neonatal adiposity in the Hyperglycemia and Adverse Pregnancy Outcome study-North American region. Obesity (Silver Spring). 2014;22(7):1731–8.
10. Kulkarni B, Mamidi RS, Balakrishna N, Radhakrishna KV. Body composition assessment in infancy and early childhood: comparison of anthropometry with dual-energy X-ray absorptiometry in low-income group children from India. Eur J Clin Nutr. 2014;68:658–63.
11. Lingwood BE, van Leeuwen AMS, Carberry AE, Fitzgerald EC, Callaway LK, Colditz PB, Ward LC. Prediction of fat-free mass and percentage of body fat

in neonates using bioelectrical impedance analysis and anthropometric measures: validation against the PEA POD. Br J Nutr. 2012;107:1545–52.
12. Hussain Z, Jafar T, Zaman MU, Parveen R, Saeed F. Correlations of skin fold thickness and validation of prediction equations using DEXA as the gold standard for estimation of body fat composition in Pakistani children. BMJ Open. 2014;4:e004194.
13. Penalvo JL, Santos-Beneit G, Sotos-Prieto M, Martinez R, Rodriguez C, Franco M, Lopez-Romero P, Pocock S, Redondo J, Fuster V. A cluster randomized trial to evaluate the efficacy of a school-based behavioral intervention for health promotion among children aged 3 to 5. BMC Public Health. 2013;13:656.
14. Rottger K, Grimminger E, Kreuser F, Asslander L, Gollhofer A, Korsten-Reck U. Physical activity in different preschool settings: an exploratory study. J Obes. 2014;2014:321701.
15. Dauncey MJ, Gandy G, Gairdner D. Assessment of total body fat in infancy from skinfold thickness measurements. Arch Dis Child. 1977;52:223–7.
16. Kautz L, Harrison GG. Comparison of body proportions of one-year-old Mexican-American and Anglo children. Am J Public Health. 1981;71:280–2.
17. Slaughter MH, Lohman TG, Boileau RA, Horswill CA, Stillman RJ, Van Loan MD, Bemben DA. Skinfold equations for estimation of body fatness in children and youth. Hum Biol. 1988;60:709–23.
18. Schmelzle HR, Fusch C. Body fat in neonates and young infants: validation of skinfold thickness versus dual-energy X-ray absorptiometry. Am J Clin Nutr. 2002;76:1096–100.
19. Goran MI, Driscoll P, Johnson R, Nagy TR, Hunter G. Cross-calibration of body-composition techniques against dual-energy X-ray absorptiometry in young children. Am J Clin Nutr. 1996;63:299–305.
20. Weststrate JA, Deurenberg P. Body composition in children: proposal for a method for calculating body fat percentage from total body density or skinfold-thickness measurements. Am J Clin Nutr. 1989;50:1104–15.
21. Uebel K, Pusch K, Gedrich K, Schneider KT, Hauner H, Bader BL. Effect of maternal obesity with and without gestational diabetes on offspring subcutaneous and preperitoneal adipose tissue development from birth up to year-1. BMC Pregnancy Childbirth. 2014;14:138.
22. Olhager E, Forsum E. Assessment of total body fat using the skinfold technique in full-term and preterm infants. Acta Paediatr. 2006;95:21–8.
23. Deierlein AL, Thornton J, Hull H, Paley C, Gallagher D. An anthropometric model to estimate neonatal fat mass using air displacement plethysmography. Nutr Metab (Lond). 2012;9.
24. Catalano PM, Thomas AJ, Avallone DA, Amini SB. Anthropometric estimation of neonatal body composition. Am J Obstet Gynecol. 1995;173:1176–81.
25. Aris IM, Soh SE, Tint MT, Liang S, Chinnadurai A, Saw SM, Kwek K, Godfrey KM, Gluckman PD, Chong YS, Yap FK, Lee YS. Body fat in Singaporean infants: development of body fat prediction equations in Asian newborns. Eur J Clin Nutr. 2013;67:922–7.
26. Koo WW. Body composition measurements during infancy. Ann N Y Acad Sci. 2000;904:383–92.
27. Hull HR, Thornton J, Paley C, Navder K, Gallagher D. Maternal obesity influences the relationship between location of neonate fat mass and total fat mass. Pediatr Obes. 2015;10:245–51.
28. Fomon SJ, Haschke F, Ziegler EE, Nelson SE. Body composition of reference children from birth to age 10 years. Am J Clin Nutr. 1982;35:1169–75.
29. Ellis KJ. Evaluation of body composition in neonates and infants. Semin Fetal Neonatal Med. 2007;12:87–91.
30. Ma G, Yao M, Liu Y, Lin A, Zou H, Urlando A, Wong WW, Nommsen-Rivers L, Dewey KG. Validation of a new pediatric air-displacement plethysmograph for assessing body composition in infants. Am J Clin Nutr. 2004;79:653–60.
31. Lohman TG. Advances in body compsoition assessment: current issues in exercise sciences series. Champaign: Human Kinetics; 1992.
32. Bland JM, Altman DG. Statistical methods for assessing agreement between two methods of clinical measurement. Lancet. 1986;1:307–10.
33. Kabir N, Forsum E. Estimation of total body fat and subcutaneous adipose tissue in full-term infants less than 3 months old. Pediatr Res. 1993;34:448–54.
34. de Bruin NC, van Velthoven KA, Stijnen T, Juttmann RE, Degenhart HJ, Visser HK. Body fat and fat-free mass in infants: new and classic anthropometric indexes and prediction equations compared with total-body electrical conductivity. Am J Clin Nutr. 1995;61:1195–205.
35. Luciano A, Bolognani M, Biondani P, Ghizzi C, Zoppi G, Signori E. The influence of maternal passive and light active smoking on intrauterine growth and body composition of the newborn. Eur J Clin Nutr. 1998;52:760–3.
36. McFarland MB, Trylovich CG, Langer O. Anthropometric differences in macrosomic infants of diabetic and nondiabetic mothers. J Matern Fetal Med. 1998;7:292–5.
37. Dewey KG. Growth characteristics of breast-fed compared to formula-fed infants. Biol Neonate. 1998;74:94–105.
38. Nelson SE, Rogers RR, Ziegler EE, Fomon SJ. Gain in weight and length during early infancy. Early Hum Dev. 1989;19:223–39.
39. Shepherd RW, Oxborough DB, Holt TL, Thomas BJ, Thong YH. Longitudinal study of the body composition of weight gain in exclusively breast-fed and intake-measured whey-based formula-fed infants to age 3 months. J Pediatr Gastroenterol Nutr. 1988;7:732–9.
40. Andres A, Casey PH, Cleves MA, Badger TM. Body fat and bone mineral content of infants fed breast milk, cow's milk formula, or soy formula during the first year of life. J Pediatr. 2013;163:49–54.
41. Macdonald PD, Ross SR, Grant L, Young D. Neonatal weight loss in breast and formula fed infants. Arch Dis Child Fetal Neonatal Ed. 2003;88:F472–6.
42. Freedman DS, Horlick M, Berenson GS. A comparison of the Slaughter skinfold-thickness equations and BMI in predicting body fatness and cardiovascular disease risk factor levels in children. Am J Clin Nutr. 2013;98: 1417–24.
43. He Q, Horlick M, Thornton J, Wang J, Pierson Jr RN, Heshka S, Gallagher D. Sex and race differences in fat distribution among Asian, African-American, and Caucasian prepubertal children. J Clin Endocrinol Metab. 2002;87:2164–70.
44. Shaw NJ, Crabtree NJ, Kibirige MS, Fordham JN. Ethnic and gender differences in body fat in British schoolchildren as measured by DXA. Arch Dis Child. 2007;92:872–5.
45. Chumlea WC, Guo SS, Kuczmarski RJ, Flegal KM, Johnson CL, Heymsfield SB, Lukaski HC, Friedl K, Hubbard VS. Body composition estimates from NHANES III bioelectrical impedance data. Int J Obes Relat Metab Disord. 2002;26: 1596–609.
46. Paley C, H Hull, Y Ji, T Toro-Ramos, J Thornton, J Bauer, P Matthews, A Yu, K Navder, K Dorsey, and D Gallagher. Body fat differences by self-reported race/ethnicity in healthy term newborns. Pediatr Obes. 2015. doi: 10.1111/ ijpo.12072. [Epub ahead of print].

Pathogenic bacteria distributions and drug resistance analysis in 96 cases of neonatal sepsis

Huaifu Dong[1], Huiping Cao[2] and Haiyan Zheng[3*]

Abstract

Background: This study aimed to summarize common pathogens and associated drug resistance in neonatal sepsis (NS).

Methods: Blood culture and drug sensitivity results from 96 NS cases treated from January 2010 to August 2014 were retrospectively analyzed.

Results: A total of 97 pathogenic bacteria were detected from these 96 NS cases; Gram-positive cocci accounted for 76.3% of the cases, among which 70.1% involved coagulase-negative staphylococcus (CONS), whereas Gram-negative bacilli and fungi accounted for 19.6% and fungi 4.1% of cases, respectively. Gram-positive cocci exhibited a higher penicillin resistance rate and full vancomycin sensitivity, whereas Gram-negative bacilli exhibited a higher cephalosporin resistance rate, low meropenem resistance rate (6.7%), and no resistance to amikacin.

Conclusions: The main causative pathogens of NS in our hospital were Gram-positive cocci, among which coagulase-negative Staphylococcus spp such as S. epidermidis and S. haemolyticus were the main conditional pathogens; among Gram-negative pathogens, Klebsiella pneumoniae were most frequently isolated and showed widespread resistance to penicillins and cephalosporins.

Keywords: Neonatal sepsis, Pathogen, Drug resistance

Background

Neonatal sepsis (NS) is an inflammation-induced systemic inflammatory response syndrome and an important cause of neonatal deaths [1, 2]; this condition comprises systemic poisoning symptoms caused by a large number of toxins produced by bacteria upon entry into the bloodstream, growth, and reproduction. As the neonatal blood–brain barrier is not completely developed, purulent meningitis is easily contracted and represents a great threat to the life and health of children, particularly preterm children [3]. NS is a serious infectious disease in the neonatal period and is mainly associated with immature neonatal immune functions. Early-onset sepsis (EONS) occurs within 3 days after birth; most pathogens derive from the mother's parturient canal and gastrointestinal tract, Gram-negative bacteria are the most frequently detected pathogens, and symptoms are normally severe. In contrast, late-onset sepsis (LONS) occurs 3 days after birth, with *Staphylococcus* spp. as the most frequently observed pathogens [4].

According to "Practical neonatology" by Shao, NS refers to bacterial and fungal infections, whereas Wang, in the National Teaching Material of Colleges and Universities, defines NS as involving bacterial, fungal, or protozoan pathogens. The present study has accepted the former concept. Despite the prophylactic application of antibiotics, NS currently remains an important cause of neonatal morbidity and mortality both in China and abroad [4].

Because NS has no specific clinical manifestations and blood culture analysis requires a long period of time, the positive blood culture rates among newborns in some developing countries were reported to be as high as 40–50%, whereas in China, Zhang reported a positive

* Correspondence: haiyanzhengcn@163.com
[3]Department of Nursing, the First Affiliated Hospital of Bengbu Medical College, Bengbu 233004, Anhui, China
Full list of author information is available at the end of the article

rate of 10.6%, and Zhang reported a rate of 12.03% [5, 6]. Although peripheral blood analysis can facilitate a diagnosis of sepsis [7, 8], the sensitivity and specificity are low, thus increasing the difficulty associated with clinical diagnosis and treatment; furthermore, NS is likely to be complicated by purulent meningitis, for which the prognosis was poor [9]. All of the above-mentioned factors require clinicians to provide a correct diagnosis and treatment for affected children as soon as possible to avoid unnecessary disability and death, and therefore an understanding of the pathogens and antibiotic resistance associated with the cases of NS admitted at our hospital and in nearby regions would be necessary. This study selected clinical data from 96 NS newborns with positive blood culture results who were treated in our department from January 2010 to August 2014 for a retrospective analysis.

Methods

Study information

Clinical data from a total of 96 NS cases (Neonates, 0–28 days) admitted to the neonatal intensive care unit (NICU) of Bengbu Third People's Hospital from January 1, 2010 to August 31, 2014 because of positive blood culture results were collected. The risk factors for sepsis were trachea cannula, intravenously administered nutrition, and low response. Hematological parameters, pathogen features, major bacteria's resistant organism detection rate, and antimicrobial resistance were reviewed from patients' medical records. Invasive intervention such as endotracheal intubation and central venous catheter insertion were used in the neonates hospitalized.

Diagnostic criteria

A diagnosis was made if patients exhibited clinical manifestations and met any one of the following criteria: (1) positive culture of pathogens from a blood culture or sterile body cavity culture; or (2) in cases with a positive blood culture result for an opportunistic pathogen (such as *coagulase negative staphylococcus aureus, klebsiella pneumoniae* etc.), the same type of bacteria must have been cultivated from another sample collected from the bloodstream, a sterile body cavity, or catheter tip.

Clinical diagnosis

A clinical diagnosis was made if a patient exhibited clinical manifestations and had any of the following criteria: (1) non-specific examination with ≥2 items, including a white blood cell count (WBC) reduction to $<5 \times 10^9$/L; increase in WBC for ≤3 days to $>25 \times 10^9$/L, an increase in WBC for >3 days to $>20 \times 10^9$/L; immature/total neutrophil ratio (I/T) ≥0.16, ≥8 μg/ml, platelet count (PLT) $\leq 100 \times 10^9$/L, and erythrocyte sedimentation rate ≥15 mm/h); or (2) positive pathogen antigen or DNA test results in a blood sample.

Clinical data

Data from a total of 96 NS newborns with positive blood culture results who met the diagnostic criteria for sepsis were obtained from the medical record room and included each patient's name, gender, age at admission, clinical manifestations of onset, laboratory examination findings, blood culture results, and drug sensitivity analysis results.

Blood culture

For blood culture, the BACT/ALERT 3D 240 automatic blood culture system and associated flasks (BioMerieux Co., Lyon, France) were used; detected bacteria were also identified with an ATB Expression bacterial identification/sensitivity analyzer (BioMerieux Co.). WBC and PLT were determined on a Mindray BC-6800 automatic blood cell analyzer (Shenzhen Mindray Medical International Co., Ltd., Shenzhen, China). Serum CRP level was measured on a VITROS 250 automatic dry chemical biochemical analyzer (Johnson & Johnson, Shanghai, China).

Antibiotic sensitivity analysis

Overnight fresh pathogen culture (log-phase broth culture) was flooded onto solid medium plates with the identified strains, and excess culture was removed. The plates were left at 25 °C for 24 h under sterile conditions. The antibiotic discs were placed and the culture plates were incubated at 37 °C for 24–48 h. The plates were examined under a stereo microscope (Leitz) and zones of inhibition were measured in millimeters from the edge of the disc.

Statistical analysis

SPSS21.0 software (SPSS, Inc., Chicago, IL, USA) was used for the statistical analysis. Quantitative data were expressed as percentages or rates, inter-group comparisons were conducted using the χ^2 test and Fisher's exact test with a significance level of $\alpha = 0.05$, and a P-value <0.05 was considered statistically significant.

Results

General information

This study included a total of 96 NS cases and isolated a total of 97 pathogenic strains (two strains were cultured from one sample); the cases included 68 boys (70.8%) and 28 girls (29.2%), for a boy/girl ratio of 2.4:1. Among the cases, 22 involved preterm births (22.9%), 74 involved full-term births (77.1%), and no cases involved post-term birth. The youngest patient at admission was 0.5 h, whereas the oldest was 26 days. Nineteen cases involved low birth-weight children (19.8%), including 12 cases of very low birth-weight children (12.5%), whereas 77 cases involved normal birth-weight children (80.2%). Forty-one cases involved early-onset NS (57.3%), and 55 involved of late-onset NS (42.7%); additionally, 66 cases achieved a complete healing (68.8%), 30 symptom improvement, and no deaths were observed. Lumbar puncture and cerebrospinal fluid (CSF) examination were performed in 23 NS cases, and the CSF findings of 7 cases were abnormal. In the study, there were no statistically significant differences between WBC, lymphocyte count, neutrophil count, and CRP level between EONS and LONS ($P > 0.05$).

Pathogens distribution

Among the 96 cases, 97 pathogenic strains were identified, including 74 strains of Gram-positive cocci, 19 strains of Gram-negative bacteria, and 4 strains of fungi, accounting for 76.3%, 19.6%, and 4.1% of cases, respectively. Among the Gram-positive bacteria, *S. epidermidis* accounted for 44.3% (43/97) of cases, *S. haemolyticus* accounted for 14.4% (14/97), *S. hominis* accounted for 8.2% (8/97), and *S. aureus* accounted for 2.1% (2/97), whereas other bacteria (including *Kocuria varians*, *Listeria monocytogenes*, *Enterococcus faecalis*, *S. equorum*, and *S. bovis*) occurred at low rates. Additionally, among the 97 pathogens, 68 strains of coagulase-negative *Staphylococcus* (CONS) were detected. Among Gram-negative bacteria, *Klebsiella pneumoniae* subspecies accounted for 10.3% of cases (10/97) and *Escherichia coli* accounted for 6.2% (6/97); additionally, 2 strains of *Enterobacter cloacae* were detected along with 1 strain of *Sphingosine monad* and 4 types of fungi (*Candida glabrata*, 2 strains; *C. albicans* and *C. tropicalis*, had 1 strain, each). The specific composition is presented in Table 1.

Table 1 Distributions and constitutions of bacterial strains detected in 97 NS cases

Bacteria	Name	Cases	Percentage
Gram-positive bacteria		74	76.3%
	Kocuria varians	1	1.0%
	S. epidermidis	43	44.3%
	L. Monocytogenes	1	1.0%
	E. faecalis	1	1.0%
	S. aureus	2	2.1%
	S. equorum	1	1.0%
	S. simulans	1	1.0%
	S. bovis	1	1.0%
	S. hominis	8	8.2%
	S. haemolyticus	14	14.4%
	S. warneri	1	1.0%
Gram-negative bacteria		19	19.6%
	E. coli	6	6.2%
	Klebsiella pneumoniae subsp.	10	10.3%
	S. monad	1	1.0%
	E. cloacae	2	2.1%
Fungi		4	4.1%
	C. albicans	1	1.0%
	C. glabrata	2	2.1%
	C. tropicalis	1	1.0%

Drug resistance in pathogens

Among the 74 cases of Gram-positive cocci, 43 strains of *S. epidermidis* were detected, as well as 14 strains of *S. haemolyticus* and 17 other strains. The total resistance rates to the following drugs were high among Gram-positive cocci: penicillin, 93.2%; ampicillin, 90.0%; oxacillin, 84.7%; erythromycin, 81.1%; and SMZ, 63.0%; as well as ciprofloxacin, 50.0%; levofloxacin, 35.0%; teicoplanin, 22.2%; fusidic acid, 18.0%; and rifampicin, 6.8%. No vancomycin-resistant Gram-positive bacteria were detected. Among the 43 strains of *S. epidermis*, the resistance rates were as follows: rifampin, 7.0%; fusidic acid, 10.7%; and teicoplanin, 24.3%. All 14 strains (100%) of *S. haemolyticus* exhibited full resistance to penicillin, erythromycin, and ampicillin, whereas the rates of resistance to oxacillin, levofloxacin, gentamicin, ciproflaxin, teicoplanin, and fusidic acid were 92.9%, 81.8%, 85.7%, 66.7%, 33.3%, and 27.3%, respectively. The remaining 17 strains of Gram-positive cocci were completely resistant to erythromycin and exhibited relatively higher rates of resistance to penicillin, oxacillin, SMZ, and ampicillin of 82.4%, 80%, 62.5%, and 66.7%, respectively; details are shown in Table 2.

Among the 19 Gram-negative bacterial strains, 6 were identified as *E. coli*, 10 were *Klebsiella pneumoniae* subsp., and 3 were other Gram-negative bacteria (2 strains of *E. cloacae* and 1 strain of *S. monad*). The Gram-negative bacterial strains exhibited the following high drug resistance rates: amoxicillin, 93.3%; ticarcillin, 93.3%; piperacillin, 75.0%; cefoxitin, 73.3%; amoxicillin/clavulanate potassium, 73.3%; ticarcillin/clavulanate, 73.3%; piperacillin/tazobactam, 61.1%; cefuroxime, 75.0%; ceftazidime, 73.7%; cefepime, 73.7%; cefalotin, 66.7%; and cefotaxime, 68.8%. In addition, these strains exhibited rates of resistance to gentamicin tobramycin, imipenem, and meropenem of 42.1, 33.3, 21.1, and 6.7%, respectively, whereas no strains were resistant to amikacin. None of the 6 strains of *E. coli* were resistant to meropenem, imipenem, or amikacin, whereas relatively high resistance rates to amoxicillin and SMZ of 83.3% and 66.7%, respectively, were observed; in addition, 33.3% of strains were each resistant to cefoxitin, ceftazidime, and cefepime, whereas 16.7% were resistant to piperacillin/tazobactam. The 10 strains of *K. pneumoniae* subsp. exhibited full resistance (100%) to cefuroxime, cefoxitin, ceftazidime,

Table 2 Drug resistance of Gram-positive bacteria [% (cases)]

	S. epidermidis	S. haemolyticus	Other 17 strains	Sum
Penicillin	95.3 (41/43)	100.0 (14/14)	82.4 (14/17)	93.2 (69/74)
Oxacillin	83.7 (36/43)	92.9 (13/14)	80.0 (12/15)[a]	84.7 (61/72)
Erythromycin	67.4 (29/43)	100.0 (14/14)	100.0 (17/17)	81.1 (60/74)
Levofloxacin	28.6 (10/35)[a]	81.8 (9/11)[a]	14.3 (2/14)[a]	35.0 (21/60)
Vancomycin	0.0 (0/43)	0.0 (0/14)	0 (0/17)	0.0 (0/74)
Rifampicin	7.0 (3/43)	7.1 (1/14)	5.9 (1/17)	6.8 (5/74)
Teicoplanin	24.3 (9/37)[a]	33.3 (4/12)[a]	7.1 (1/14)[a]	22.2 (14/63)
Ampicillin	100.0 (5/5)	100.0 (2/2)[a]	66.7 (2/3)[a]	90.0 (9/10)
Gentamicin	37.2 (16/43)	85.7 (12/14)	56.2 (9/16)[a]	50.7 (37/73)
SMZ	60.5 (26/43)	57.1 (8/14)	62.5 (10/16)[a]	60.3 (44/73)
Fusidic acid	10.7 (3/28)[a]	27.3 (3/11)[a]	27.3 (3/11)[a]	18.0 (9/50)
Ciprofloxacin	44.4 (4/9)[a]	66.7 (2/3)[a]	50.0 (2/4)[a]	50.0 (8/16)

Note: 1. [a]: partial strains were not tested sensitivity to this drug, the denominator inside parentheses was the actual bacterial strains tested sensitivity to this drug. 2. The drug-resistant strains in this study referred to those with drug resistance (R) and interim strain (I)

cefepime, amoxicillin/clavulanate, cefotaxime, amoxicillin, and piperacillin, a 70.0% cephalothin resistance rate, and no resistance to meropenem, amikacin, or netilmicin. The other 3 Gram-negative bacterial strains (2 strains of *E. cloacae* and 1 strain of *S. monad*) exhibited total resistance to amoxicillin, piperacillin/tazobactam, cefoxitin, amoxicillin/clavulanate, cephalothin, and tobramycin, but full sensitivity to amikacin (Table 3).

Furthermore, 4 strains of fungi (2 strains of *C. glabrata*, 1 strain of French *C. albicans*, and 1 strain of *C. tropicalis*) were detected. All 4 strains were sensitive to 5-fluorocytosine and amphotericin B, whereas only 2 strains (1 strain each of *C. glabrata* and *C. tropicalis*) were resistant to fluconazole. Only 1 strain of *C. glabrata* was sensitive to itraconazole, whereas the remaining 3 strains were resistant; additionally, only the *C. tropicalis* strain was resistant to voriconazole, whereas the other 3 strains were sensitive.

Discussion

Sepsis is a severe illness during the neonatal period and remains among the main causes of neonatal death. Children admitted to the NICU are normally in a serious condition or premature; the prevalence of sepsis among long-term hospitalized children may be as high as 30%, with a mortality rate as high as 50%, and survivors experience serious sequelae [8–10]. Given the concentrated spectra of pathogens, foreign countries often classify NS cases according to the age of onset as either EONS or LONS in order to inform the clinical selection of antibiotics and assess prognosis [11]. EONS mainly emphasizes that the infection occurred in utero or during birth and that the pathogens mainly originated in the maternal birth canal, whereas LONS normally occurs after birth. In China, there is current disagreement about the distinction between EONS and LONS, and this study accordingly did not distinguish cases using this classification. The main pathogens of NS reported among cases in China are Gram-positive bacteria, particularly *Staphylococcus* spp. [12]. Certain evidence has proven an increasing trend of *S. epidermidis* infection [13]. Among the 97 strains of bacteria, 68 strains of CONS were detected, accounting for 70.1% of the cases. Among Gram-negative bacteria, *K. pneumoniae* subsp. accounted for the highest proportion, 10.3% (10/97), followed by *E. coli* (6.2%, 6/97) and *E. cloacae*, whereas the overall detection rate was low and basically consistent with that reported by Tang, suggesting that the NS-causative pathogens detected in our department remained mainly Gram-positive cocci, especially coagulase-negative *S. epidermidis* and *S. haemolyticus*, followed by *K. pneumoniae* subsp., whereas the proportions of coagulase-positive *S. aureus* and *Streptococcus* were relatively lower; in contrast, *S. haemolyticus* B is the main pathogen in foreign countries [14], which might be related to geographical differences.

Currently, although the extensive application of antibiotics could quickly control infections or prevent NS to a limited extent and scope, it could also easily induce highly drug-resistant strains [13]. Therefore, when antimicrobial drugs are clinically applied, the principles of antibiotic application and issues related to antibiotic resistance should be strictly controlled, and drugs should be selected according to individual sensitivity to reduce bacterial resistance to antimicrobial drugs and improve drug efficacies. The supplementary issue of the Performance Standards for Antimicrobial Testing, 23rd edition mentioned that in addition to cephalosporins, which exhibit novel anti-MRSA activities, oxacillin-resistant *Staphylococcus* spp. also exhibited resistance

Table 3 Drug resistance of gram-negative bacilli [% (cases)]

	E. coli	Klebsiella pneumoniae subsp.	Others	Sum
Gentamicin	33.3 (2/6)	40.0 (4/10)	66.7 (2/3)	42.1 (8/19)
SMZ	66.7 (4/6)	50.0 (5/10)	33.3 (1/3)	52.6 (10/19)
Amoxicillin	83.3 (5/6)	100.0 (7/7)	100.0 (2/2)	93.3 (14/15)
Piperacillin	50.0 (3/6)	100.0 (7/7)[a]	66.7 (2/3)	75.0 (12/16)
Piperacillin/Tazobactam	16.7 (1/6)	80.0 (8/10)	100.0 (2/2)[a]	61.1 (11/18)
Cefoxitin	33.3 (2/6)	100.0 (7/7)[a]	100.0 (2/2)[a]	73.3 (11/15)
Ceftazidime	33.3 (2/6)	100.0 (10/10)	66.7 (2/3)	73.7 (14/19)
Cefepime	33.3 (2/6)	100.0 (10/10)	66.7 (2/3)	73.7 (14/19)
Cefuroxime	50.0 (3/6)	100.0 (7/7)	66.7 (2/3)	75.0 (12/16)
Meropenem	0.0 (0/6)	0.0 (0/7)[a]	50.0 (1/2)[a]	6.7 (1/15)
Imipenem	0.0 (0/6)	30.0 (3/10)	33.3 (1/3)	21.1 (4/19)
Amikacin	0.0 (0/6)	0.0 (0/10)	0.0 (0/3)	0.0 (0/19)
Amoxicillin/clavulanate	33.3 (2/6)	100.0 (7/7)[a]	100.0 (2/2)[a]	73.3 (11/15)
Cefalotin	50.0 (3/6)	70.0 (7/10)	100.0 (2/2)[a]	66.7 (12/18)
Cefotaxime	33.3 (2/6)	100.0 (7/7)[a]	66.7 (2/3)	68.8 (11/16)
Tobramycin	50.0 (3/6)	10.0 (1/10)	100.0 (2/2)	33.3 (6/18)

Note: 1. [a]: partial strains were not tested sensitivity to this drug, the denominator inside parentheses was the actual bacterial strains tested sensitivity to this drug. 2. The drug-resistant strains in this study referred to those with drug resistance (R) and interim strain (I)

to all β-lactam enzyme-type drugs [15]. The data in the present study revealed that 74 strains of Gram-positive cocci exhibited higher resistance rates to penicillin, ampicillin, oxacillin, and erythromycin while remaining fully sensitive to vancomycin. Common CONS such as *S. epidermidis* and *S. haemolyticus* exhibited penicillin and erythromycin resistance rates as high as 100%. Nineteen strains of Gram-negative bacilli exhibited amoxicillin resistance rates as high as 93.3% and resistance rates higher than 60% to commonly used antibiotics such as piperacillin, cefuroxime, ceftazidime, cefepime, and amoxicillin/clavulanate; in contrast, lower resistance to imipenem and meropenem was observed, and amikacin was the most efficacious drug. The most common strain, *Klebsiella pneumoniae,* was completely resistant to commonly used drugs such as penicillin and cephalosporins, exhibited the highest sensitivity rates to meropenem and amikacin, indicating that previously used penicillins, erythromycin, and cephalosporins could not be used as preferred medications for NS. Vancomycin was the most effective antibiotic against neonatal Gram-positive bacterial infections; although amikacin is completely effective against (the isolated) Gram-negative bacteria, it can induce severe ear and kidney toxicities and therefore has been rarely used for neonatal infection. The rates of resistance to carbapenems such as imipenem and meropenem were low and as these drugs rarely caused adverse reactions, they could be used as a first-line treatment for the prevention or treatment of neonatal Gram-negative bacillus infections. In recent years, given the widespread application of imipenem, vancomycin, and other antibiotics, as well as the continuous development of invasive procedures such as endotracheal intubation and central venous catheter insertion, reports about multi-resistant strains, such as those exhibiting anti-carbapenem and anti-vancomycin characteristics, have continually increased in China and abroad [16]. Although the resistance rates to imipenem, meropenem, and other carbapenems in this study were low, they could not be ignored. Therefore, clinicians should strictly control the conditions under which antibiotics are applied, minimize the use of invasive procedures, and replace antibiotics as necessary and in a timely manner according to the situation to reduce the incidence of drug resistance. Better medical decisions, particularly those for appropriate detection methods and initial antimicrobial therapies, can be made by understanding the different clinical features and causative pathogens in both EONS and LONS. The limitations of this study are the single medical center-restricted data and small sample size.

Conclusion

The main causative pathogens of NS in our hospital were Gram-positive cocci, among which coagulase-negative Staphylococcus spp such as S. epidermidis and S. haemolyticus were the main conditional pathogens; among Gram-negative pathogens, Klebsiella pneumoniae were most frequently isolated and showed widespread resistance to penicillins and cephalosporins.

Abbreviations
CONS: Coagulase-negative staphylococcus; EONS: Early-onset sepsis; LONS: Late-onset sepsis; NICU: Neonatal intensive care unit; NS: Neonatal sepsis; PLT: Platelet count; WBC: White blood cell count

Acknowledgements
We thanked selfless contributions of paediatricians and nurses in the First Affiliated Hospital of Bengbu Medical College, including pathogens and collection of specimen. We also thanked support of Scientific Research Office in Bengbu Medical College that ensured the smooth implementation of this study.

Funding
This study was supported by scientific researching fund projects in Bengbu Medical College in 2015 (No. jyxm1546).

Authors' contributions
HF Dong performed statistical analysis and wrote the manuscript, HP Cao collected samples, and HY Zheng supervised the whole study. All authors read and approved the final manuscript.

Competing interests
The authors declare that they have no competing interests.

Author details
[1]Department of Pediatrics, the First Affiliated Hospital of Bengbu Medical College, Bengbu 233004, Anhui, China. [2]Department of Pediatrics, the Third People's Hospital of Bengbu, Bengbu 233000, Anhui, China. [3]Department of Nursing, the First Affiliated Hospital of Bengbu Medical College, Bengbu 233004, Anhui, China.

References

1. Weston EJ, Pondo T, Lewis MM, Martell-Cleary P, Morin C, Jewell B, et al. The burden of invasive early-onset neonatal sepsis in the United States, 2005–2008. Pediatr Infect Dis J. 2011;30:937–41.
2. Chiabi A, Djoupomb M, Mah E, Nguefack S, Mbuagbaw L, Zafack J, et al. The clinical and bacteriogical spectrum of neonatal sepsis in a tertiary hospital in Yaounde. Cameroon Iran J Pediatr. 2011;21:441–8.
3. Kayange N, Kamugisha E, Mwizamholya DL, Jeremiah S, Mshana SE. Predictors of positive blood culture and deaths among neonates with suspected neonatal sepsis in a tertiary hospital. Mwanza-Tanzania BMC Pediatr. 2010;10:39.
4. Shah BA, Padbury JF. Neonatal sepsis: an old problem with new insights. Virulence. 2014;5:170–8.
5. Viswanathan R, Singh AK, Ghosh C, Dasgupta S, Mukherjee S, Basu S. Profile of neonatal septicemia at adistrict level sick newborn care unit. J Health Popul Nutr. 2012;30:41–8.
6. Zhang G. 160 cases of neonatal blood culture positive result analysis. China's Tradit Chin Med. 2011;3:296–6.
7. Makkar M, Gupta C, Pathak R, Garg S, Mahajan NC. Performance evaluation of hematologic scoring system in early diagnosis of neonatal sepsis. J Clin Neonatol. 2013;2:25–9.
8. Ahmad MS, Waheed A. Platelet counts, MPV and PDW in culture proven and probable neonatal sepsis and association of platelet counts with mortality rate. J Coll Physicians Surg Pak. 2014;24:340–4.
9. Levent F, Baker CJ, Rench MA, Edwards MS. Early outcomes of group B streptococcal meningitis in the 21st century. Pediatr Infect Dis J. 2010;29:1009–12.
10. Tripathi N, Cotten CM, Smith PB. Antibiotic use and misuse in the neonatal intensive care unit. Clin Perinatol. 2012;39:61–8.
11. Hill PC, Onyeama CO, Ikumapayi UN, Secka O, Ameyaw S, Simmonds N, et al. Bacteraemia in patients admitted to an urban hospital in West Africa. BMC Infect Dis. 2007;7:2.
12. Havey TC, Fowler RA, Daneman N. Duration of antibiotic therapy for bacteremia: a systematic review and meta-analysis. Crit Care. 2011;15:R267.
13. Stoll BJ, Hansen NI, Sánchez PJ, Faix RG, Poindexter BB, Van Meurs KP, et al. Early onset neonatal sepsis: the burden of group B Streptococcal and E. coli disease continue. Pediatrics. 2011;127:817–26.
14. Zhou L, Ma X, Gao W, Yao KH, Shen AD, Yu SJ, et al. Molecular characteristics of erythromycin-resistant Streptococcus pneumoniae from pediatric patients younger than five years in Beijing, 2010. BMC Microbiol. 2012;12:228.
15. Marchant EA, Boyce GK, Sadarangani M, Lavoie PM. Neonatl sepsis due to coagulase-negatve Staphylococci. Clin Dev Immunol. 2013;2013:586076.
16. Camacho-Gonzalez A, Spearman PW, Stoll BJ. Neonatal infectious diseases: evaluation of neonatal sepsis. Pediatr Clin North Am. 2013;60:367–89.

Bifidobacterium adolescentis protects against necrotizing enterocolitis and upregulates TOLLIP and SIGIRR in premature neonatal rats

Wenshen Wu[1], Yanli Wang[1], Jingjing Zou[1], Fang Long[1], Huiheng Yan[1], Lijuan Zeng[2] and Yunbin Chen[1*]

Abstract

Background: Necrotizing enterocolitis (NEC) is a serious gastrointestinal disorder that is often seen in premature infants. Probiotics decrease the risk of NEC; however, the mechanism by which probiotics work is not clear. The goal of this study was to evaluate the preventive effect of *Bifidobacterium adolescentis* in an NEC rat model.

Methods: Sprague-Dawley neonatal rats were obtained by caesarean section after 20-21 d gestation and randomly divided into the following 3 groups: dam fed (DF), formula fed (FF), and formula + *B. adolescentis* (FB). Those in the FF and FB groups developed NEC after exposure to asphyxia and cold stress. All rats were sacrificed 72 h after birth and intestinal injury and mRNA expression of TLR4, TOLLIP and SIGIRR were assessed.

Results: *B. adolescentis* significantly increased the 72-h survival rate from 56.3% in the FF group to 86.7% in the FB group. *B. adolescentis* significantly reduced the histological score from a median of 3.0 in the FF group to a median of 1.0 in the FB group,and significantly decreased the rate of NEC-like intestinal injury from 77.8% in the FF group to 23.1% in the FB group. The mRNA expression of TLR4 increased 3.6 fold in the FF group but decreased by 2 fold from *B. adolescentis* treatment. mRNA expression of TOLLIP and SIGIRR decreased 4.3 and 3.7 fold, respectively, in the FF group. *B. adolescentis* significantly increased mRNA expression of TOLLIP and SIGIRR by 3.7 fold and 2.6 fold, respectively.

Conclusions: This study demonstrated *B. adolescentis* prevents NEC in preterm neonatal rats and that the mechanism for this action might be associated with the alteration of TLR4, TOLLIP, and SIGIRR expression.

Keywords: Necrotizing enterocolitis, Toll-like receptor 4, Toll interacting protein, single Ig IL-1-Related receptor

Background

Necrotizing enterocolitis (NEC) is a serious gastrointestinal disorder that frequently affects premature newborns and results in high morbidity and mortality, especially in very low-birth weight (VLBW) infants [1, 2]. NEC affects approximately 7.0% of all VLBW infants [1] and the death rate associated with the disease is >20%, [1, 3] and nearly one-half of NEC infants need surgery [4]. Premature newborns often must receive long-term parenteral nutrition. These infants often develop NEC and are subsequently at increased risk for short bowel syndrome and cholestatic liver disease [4]. In addition, the premature infants with NEC who need surgery are at increased risk for neurodevelopmental disorders, such as microcephaly and cerebral palsy [5]; therefore, it is important to identify a preventive strategy that will reduce the risk of developing NEC.

Although much research has found that NEC might be a multifactor disease with genetic susceptibility, prematurity, formula feeding and abnormal microbial colonization as risk factors, the exact pathophysiology of the disease remains unknown [1, 6]. NEC pathogenesis is characterized by intestinal inflammation [7] and it was recently suggested that the disease is actually caused by excessive

* Correspondence: 1225990082@qq.com
[1]Department of Neonatal Intensive Care Unit, Guangdong Province Maternal and Children's Hospital, Guangzhou Medical University, 13, Guangyuanxi Road, Guangzhou, China
Full list of author information is available at the end of the article

intestinal inflammation, which is associated with an immature innate immune response, such as that in premature infants [8]. Toll-like receptors (TLRs) are a large family of molecules that play a key role in the innate immune response [9]. The ligand of one such TLR, TLR4, is a lipopolysaccharide (LPS), a component of the cell wall of Gram-negative bacteria [9]. TLR4 plays a role in the intestinal immune response; it maintains low levels in mature intestinal epithelium [10] but is overexpressed in human fetal enterocytes [11], which predisposes immature intestinal epithelium to excessive intestinal inflammation when exposed to LPS. The results of a recent study that used an experimental rat model in which NEC was induced by a combination of formula feeding and hypoxia demonstrated that TLR4 mutant mice were more protected from NEC development compared to wild-type mice [10]. It was also reported that intestinal epithelial TLR4 inhibits enterocyte proliferation and migration [12], and that endothelial TLR4 impairs intestinal microcirculatory perfusion [13], suggesting that TLR4 plays an important role in NEC pathogenesis.

TOLLIP and SIGIRR proteins are negative regulators of TLR4 signaling and play an inhibitory role in the TLR-mediated pathway [14, 15]. It was recently reported that they also play an important role in intestinal inflammation [16, 17]. These negative regulators inhibit the signal from TLR4 to downstream pathways by suppressing the activity of interleukin (IL)-1 receptor-associated kinase (IRAK), which is a crucial molecule in the TLR4 signaling pathway [14]. After exposure to dextran sulfate sodium (DSS) for 5.0 d, TOLLIP-deficient mice showed increased severity of intestinal symptoms and greater expression of proinflammatory cytokines compared with wild-type mice [16]. In addition, the level of SIGIRR decreased in ulcerative colitis patients and in the experimental colitis mouse model [17]. There is less TOLLIP and SIGIRR mRNA in immature enterocytes and even less in NEC enterocytes compared with that in mature enterocytes [4]. These results suggest that both TLR4 and its negative regulators may play a critical role in the development of NEC.

Bifidobacterium is one type of probiotic, which are live, beneficial microorganisms that predominate in the intestinal flora of breast-fed infants [18]. Recent clinical studies have shown that oral administration of *B. infantis* and *B. bifidum* could prevent NEC development in premature infants [19, 20]. It is not entirely clear how *Bifidobacterium* species protect the neonatal intestine against NEC, but recent reports show that *B. infantis* exerts an anti-inflammatory effect by decreasing TLR4 mRNA and increasing TOLLIP and SIGIRR mRNA levels in immature human intestinal xenografts and NEC intestinal epithelial cells [4]. It is unknown whether *B. adolescentis* has the same effect in the NEC rat model; therefore, the aim of this study was to determine whether *B. adolescentis* could protect against NEC and whether TLR4, TOLLIP and SIGIRR expression could be influenced by *B. adolescentis.*

Methods

Animal model

All animal experiments were reviewed and approved by the Animal Care and Welfare Committee of Guangzhou Medical University (Guangzhou, China). All animal experiments were performed in accordance with the U.S. National Institutes of Health's "Guide for the Care and Use of Laboratory Animals" (NIH Publications No. 80-23 revised 1996). Every effort was made to minimize the number of animals used and reduce suffering. Adult Sprague-Dawley (SD) rats were purchased from Guangdong Medical Laboratory Animal Center (Foshan, China). They were housed at the Guangzhou Medical University Laboratory Animal Center and kept in a room at 22 °C, with a 12-h light-dark cycle [21]. Premature pups were delivered from time-dated pregnant SD rats by Cesarean section 20-21 d of gestation and were reared in incubators at 37 °C [10].

Forty five premature pups were randomly divided into the following three groups: dam fed (DF, $n = 14$), formula fed (FF, $n = 16$), and formula + *B. adolescentis* (FB, $n = 15$). Pups in the DF group were fed by surrogate mothers, and the newborn rats in the FF and FB groups were fed 2.0 h after birth with Esbilac puppy formula (PetAg, Inc., Hampshire, IL, USA). Feeding started with 0.15 mL every 4.0 h and advanced, as tolerated, to a maximum of 0.20 mL per feeding after 24 h of life through a homemade orogastric feeding catheter. Premature newborn rats from the FB group were treated with 1.0×10^8 CFU live *B. adolescentis* per day, (Livzon, Zhuhai, China) diluted in formula.

NEC protocol was followed in the FF and FB groups after the first feeding. Experimental NEC was induced by 90 s of 100% nitrogen exposure and subsequent 10 min cold exposure (4.0 °C) twice daily for 72 h. Rats in the DF group were fed by surrogate mothers and not exposed to asphyxia or cold stress [18].

Sample collection and tissue processing

After termination, all premature rats were euthanized by neck dislocation and laparotomies were performed. A 2.0-cm piece of distal ileum was removed and stained with hematoxylin and eosin (H&E) and used for RNA extraction. One-half of each intestinal specimen was fixed in 4.0% paraformaldehyde, paraffin embedded, cut into 4.0-μm sections, and stained with H&E to observe the histological changes under an optical microscope. The remaining one-half of each intestinal tissue was washed with cold normal saline (4.0 °C) and stored in liquid nitrogen for subsequent RNA analysis.

Histological changes in the ileum were evaluated by a blinded assessor using the following NEC scoring criteria [18]: 0 (normal), no damage; 1 (mild), slight submucosal and/or lamina propria separation; 2 (moderate), moderate separation of submucosa and/or lamina propria, and/or edema in submucosal and muscular layers; 3 (severe), severe separation of submucosa and/or lamina propria, and/or severe edema in submucosa and muscular layers, regional villi sloughing; 4 (necrosis), loss of villi and necrosis. Scores ≥2 represented NEC-like intestinal damage.

RNA extraction and quantitative polymerase chain reaction

The mRNA expressions of TLR4, TOLLIP, and SIGIRR were evaluated using GAPDH as the endogenous gene control by real-time quantitative polymerase chain reaction (RT-qPCR). Total RNA was extracted from frozen ileal tissue using the HiPure Total RNA Mini Kit (Magen, Guangzhou, China) and following the manufacturer's instructions. RNA integrity was verified by agarose gel electrophoresis. The purity and concentration of RNA were quantified using the Nanodrop ND-1000 UV Spectrophotometer (Thermo Fisher Scientific, Waltham, MA, USA).

Reference Sequence Database access codes were as follows: NM_019178 (TLR4), NM_001109668 (TOLLIP), NM_001024887 (SIGIRR), and NM_017008.4 (GAPDH). TLR4 upstream primers were 5′-TATCCAGAGCCGTT GGTGTATT-3′ and the downstream primers were 5′-AATGAAGATGATGCCAGAGCG-3′. The length of the PCR product was 85 base pairs (bp). TOLLIP upstream primers were 5′-CCAAGTGGAGGACGAGTGGTAT -3′ and the downstream primers were 5′-GCTTCAAG-CACAGAACGGATT-3′. The length of the PCR product was 330 bp. SIGIRR upstream primers were 5′-TGGTGAACCTGAGTCGCTGTC -3′ and the downstream primers were 5′-CCCTCCACGGGTCTCTAT TG-3′. The length of the PCR product was 310 bp. GAPDH upstream primers were 5′-TTCCTACCCC-CAATGTATCCG-3′ and the downstream primers were 5′-CATGAGGTCCACCACCCTGTT-3′. The length of the PCR product was 281 bp. PCR primers were designed using the Primer-BLAST tool (NCBI, Bethesda, MD, USA) and synthesized by Goodbio Technology Company (Wuhan, China). cDNA was synthesized using the PrimeScript™ RT Reagent Kit (TaTaRa, Dalian, China) and following the manufacturer's instructions.

mRNA levels were detected in triplicate using SYBR Premix Ex Taq™ Kit (Takara, Dalian, China) on a Mx3000P (Stratagene, California, La Jolla, CA, USA) with a 20-μL RT-qPCR reaction mixture. The amplification reaction was started at 95 °C for 60 s for initial denaturation, followed by 40 consecutive PCR cycles at 95 °C for 5.0 s, and 60 °C for 30 s. The fold changes in specific gene expression were calculated using the ##CT method [22].

Statistical analyses

The statistical analyses were conducted using SPSS13.0 software (Armonk, NY, USA). mRNA expression of TLR4, TOLLIP and SIGIRR are presented as the mean ± SE. The difference in expression among DF, FF, and FB groups was analyzed using one-way analysis of variance followed by the Student–Newman–Keul multiple comparisons test. The Mann–Whitney test was used to compare different pathological ileum scores between the FF and FB groups. Survival time was analyzed using Kaplan–Meier analysis (with the log-rank test). The incidence of NEC-like intestinal injury was evaluated using the Fisher's exact test. $P < 0.05$ was considered statistically significant. All analyses were two-tailed tests.

Results

General status

There were no statistically significant differences in birth weight among the three groups: Throughout the entire experiment, the premature rats in the DF group increased their weight. The rats in the FB group maintained their body weight but those in the FF group gradually lost body weight, one symptom of the disease. The mean body weight of rats in the DF, FF group and FB groups was 7.90 ± 0.50 g, 5.58 ± 0.73 g and 6.40 ± 0.67 g, respectively, with a statistically significant difference at the end of the 72 h ($P < 0.001$). The other NEC-like symptoms appeared between 48 and 72 h; these were abdominal distension and diarrhea, which were similar to those described in a previous study [23]. The mean survival time was 64.8 h (64.8 ± 2.3) in the FF group and 71.3 h (71.3 ± 0.5) in the FB group. The 72-h survival rates in the FF, FB and DF groups were 56.3 (9/16), 86.7 (13/15) and 100% (14/14), respectively. Rats in the FB group had a significantly better survival rate than those in the FF group ($P = 0.005$, Fig. 1).

Effects of *B. adolescentis* on the incidence and severity of NEC-like injury in neonatal rats

The ileal histological score was lower in the FB group (median, 1.0) than in the FF group (median, 3.0) ($P = 0.013$). Administration of *B. adolescentis* significantly decreased the rate of NEC-like intestinal injury from 77.8% (7/9) in the FF group to 23.1% (3/13) in the FB group ($P = 0.027$). In the DF group, the incidence of NEC-like intestinal injury was 0% (0/14) and the median histological score was 0 (Fig. 2). Representative images from each group are shown in Fig. 3a, b and c.

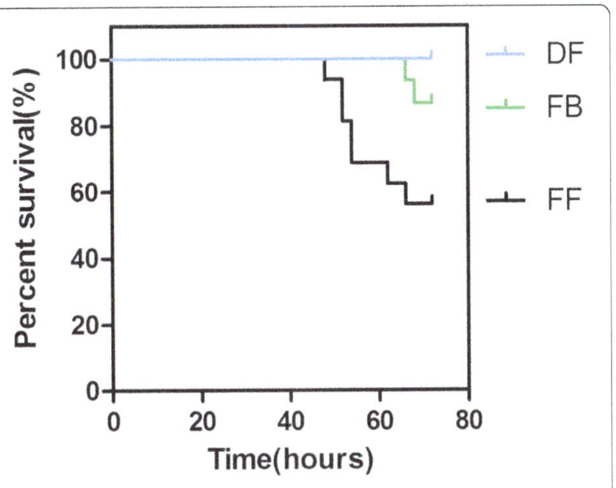

Fig. 1 Kaplan–Meier survival analysis. The mean survival time was 64.8 h (64.8 ± 2.3) in the formula fed (FF) group and 71.3 h (71.3 ± 0.5) in the formula + *Bifidobacterium adolescentis* (FB) group. Rats in the FB group had a significantly better 72-h survival rate than in the FF group ($P < 0.05$)

Evaluation of mRNA expression of TLR4, TOLLIP, and SIGIRR in the ileum tissues

The ileum mRNA expression of TLR4 increased by 3.6 fold in the FF group compared with that in the DF group ($P < 0.05$), while the expression of TLR4 mRNA decreased by 2.0 fold as a result of *B. adolescentis* treatment ($P < 0.05$) (Fig. 4a). In contrast, the mRNA expression of TOLLIP and SIGIRR decreased 4.3 and 3.7 fold in the FF group, respectively compared with those in the DF group ($P < 0.05$) (Fig. 4b and c). Administration of *B. adolescentis* significantly increased mRNA expression of TOLLIP and SIGIRR by 3.7 and 2.6 fold, respectively ($P < 0.05$) (Fig. 4b and c). There was no statistical difference in mRNA expression of TLR4, TOLLIP, or SIGIRR between the FB and DF groups ($P > 0.05$).

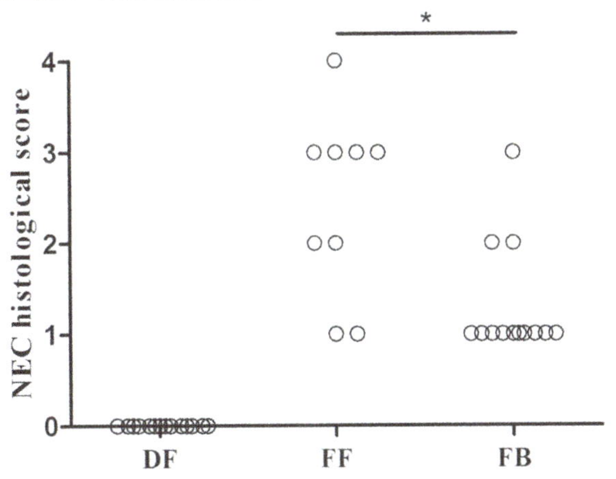

Fig. 2 Necrotizing enterocolitis (NEC) histological score of ileum in each group. Histological scoring of the terminal ileum of premature newborn rats in dam-fed (DF), formula-fed (FF), and formula + *Bifidobacterium adolescentis* (FB) groups (DF, $n = 14$; FF, $n = 9$; FB, $n = 13$). NEC-like intestinal damage was defined as scores ≥ 2. *indicates $P < 0.05$

Discussion

The model used is a well-established NEC model [24] that is based on the induction of intestinal injury using formula feeding and hypoxia-hypothermia treatment as two critical instigating factors on premature rats [24]. Previous studies [23, 25] suggested that all dam-fed pups or pups without exposure to hypoxia-hypothermia showed normal intestinal histology or less intestinal injury. We recognize that NEC development in human infants is more complex, thus the pathophysiology of a rat model might be different from that seen in humans; however, we used this model to explore the protective effect of *B. adolescentis* on pathophysiologic mechanisms associated with NEC.

In this study, prophylactic *B. adolescentis* significantly alleviated ileum damage in the NEC rat model, and also inhibited the increase in TLR4 expression and the decrease in TOLLIP and SIGIRR expression in the intestine. These results indicated that *B. adolescentis* protects premature rats from intestinal injury from hypoxia and cold stress, the mechanism of which might be by reducing the expression of TLR4 and increasing the expression of TOLLIP and SIGIRR.

Although the pathogenesis of NEC is not entirely known [1],the theory that inappropriate microbial colonization in the intestine induces the immature intestine to mount an excessive inflammatory response that results in tissue injury and necrosis is a consideration [1]. IL-8 increases in response to inflammatory stimuli in immature enterocytes compared with mature enterocytes [26]. It was reported that the same effect is seen in animal models, intestinal explants, and xenografts [27]. Clinical observation has shown that patients with NEC, especially infants who need surgery, have much higher levels of proinflammatory cytokines [28].

TLR4 is activated by LPS, a Gram-negative bacteria in the cell wall and the main ligand for TLR4, then signal through MyD88 to promote the production and release of proinflammatory cytokines though NF-κB [7]. Myd88 is a TLR4 adaptor molecule that is recruited to TLR4 and subsequently recruits IRAK [7]. TOLLIP and SIGIRR impair signaling from TLR4 by suppressing IRAK, which results in reducing the synthesis of proinflammatory cytokines [14]. TOLLIP binds to IRAK and inhibits IRAK phosphorylation [16] to downregulate the TLR4 signal. SIGIRR impairs TLR4 signaling that leads to NF-κB activation by competing with MyD88 and IRAK recruitment at the Toll-IL-1-receptor (TIR) domain [29], which participates in the interaction of SIGIRR with TLR4 [30]. Nanthakumar [8] suggested that

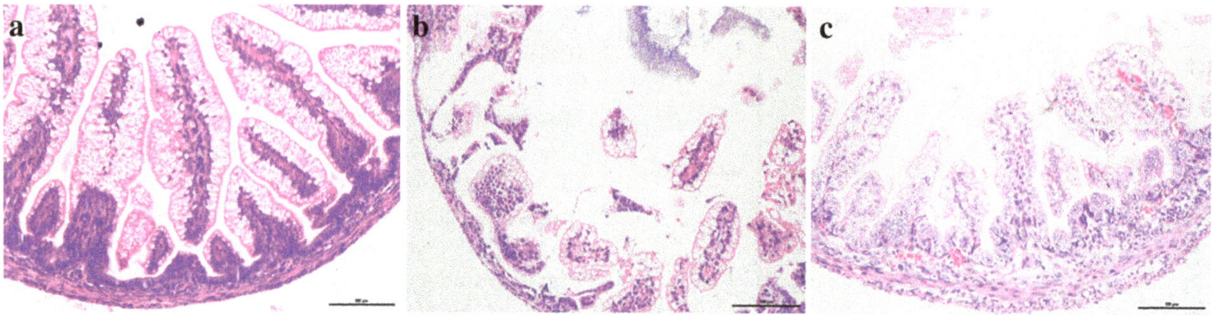

Fig. 3 Histological changes of ileum in premature newborn rats. The representative images from each group are presented. (**a**) The structure of intestinal mucosa is intact in the dam-fed (DF) group; (**b**) the structure of ileum villus was broken and even lost in the formula-fed (FF) group; (**c**) the ileum of premature rats in formula + *Bifidobacterium adolescentis* (FB)group had less necrotic ilea and lost villi. Scale bar represents 100 μm. Original magnification: 200 ×

the inappropriate inflammatory response in the immature intestine is a result of the imbalance between TLR4 and its negative regulators. TLR4 and chemokine expression is greater in both fetal and NEC enterocytes than that in mature human enterocytes [8]. SIGIRR and TOLLIP expression, which inhibits the inflammatory reaction, is lesser in both immature and NEC enterocytes than that in mature enterocyte [8]. In this study, we demonstrated that the level of TLR4 increases while the level of negative effector molecules decreases. Accordingly, it is reasonable to speculate that NEC is related to TLR4 and its negative regulators.

Many treatments have been proposed to prevent NEC but few have proved promising [1]. The most recently reported multicenter trial suggested that prophylactic probiotic treatment decreases the incidence of NEC [19, 31, 32]. *Bifidobacterium* is one type of Gram-positive probiotic that quantitatively colonizes in the intestine more than Gram-negative pathogenic bacteria [19, 31, 32]. Bergmann et al. [33] reported that the administration of *B. infantis* inhibits an increase in intestinal permeability and reduces NEC incidence in the NEC neonatal mouse model. B. *longum subsp. infantis* decreases the level of proinflammatory cytokines, which are important in NEC pathogenesis [34]. It was also reported that probiotics attenuates TLR4 expression in the NEC rat model at the protein level [34]. Recently, Ganguli et al. [4] reported that TOLLIP and SIGIRR mRNA levels increase and TLR4 mRNA level decreasese when immature human intestinal xenografts incubate with conditioned media of *B. infantis*, and that TOLLIP and SIGIRR mRNA expressions also increase in NEC intestinal epithelial cells. In this study, we demonstrated that *B. adolescentis* confers significant protection against intestinal injury in the NEC premature rat model and alter the expression of TLR4, TOLLIP and SIGIRR, all factors in the NF-κB signaling pathway; therefore, we speculate that *B. adolescentis* modulates the NF-κB signaling pathway by upregulateing TOLLIP and SIGIRR, and decreasing TLR4 to protect against intestinal injury.

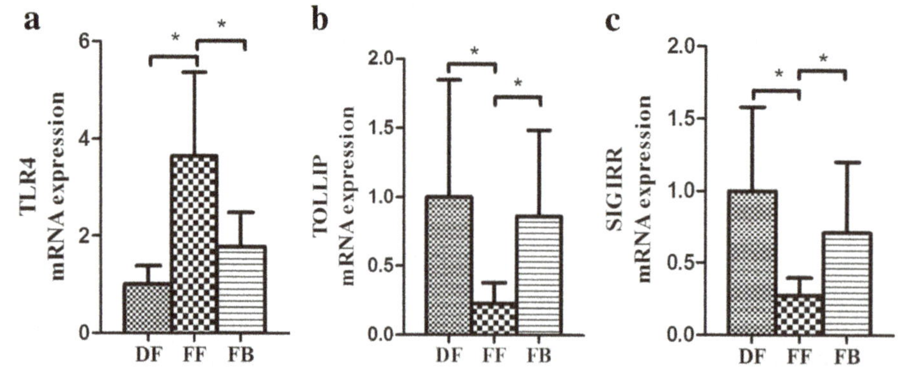

Fig. 4 Fold changes in the relative mRNA expression of TLR4, TOLLIP, and SIGIRR of the ileum of premature neonatal rats in dam-fed (DF), formula-fed (FF), and formula + *Bifidobacterium adolescentis* (FB) groups. The mRNA expression of TLR4 (**a**), TOLLIP (**b**), and (**c**) SIGIRR(B) in DF, FF, and FB groups (DF, $n = 14$; FF, $n = 9$; FB, $n = 13$) is shown. The mRNA expression for the DF group is set a value of 1.0, and mRNA levels for the FF and FB groups are determined relative to this number. Values are presented as the mean ± SE. *indicates $P < 0.05$

Probiotics exert their anti-inflammatory effects to reduce the incidence of NEC, but the mechanism is not known. These effects might be mediated by products secreted by probiotic bacteria. Probiotic conditioned media contain secreted products, free of intact bacteria, and it was recently reported that this media reduces NEC-like intestinal damage in an animal model [35]. Probiotic conditioned media inhibites the NF-κB signaling pathway and its proinflammatory cytokine production [36], which contributes to attenuating the intestinal inflammatory response [36]. It was also reported that *Bifidobacterium*-conditioned media reduces the level of TLR2 and TLR4 in xenograft epithelium and increases the level of SIGIRR and TOLLIP [4]; therefore, it is reasonable to speculate that *Bifidobacterium* species might alleviate intestinal injury through their secreted products, although what the probiotic conditioned media contains is not clear. Ganguli [4] suggested that a protein or nucleic acid from 5.0 to 10 kDa, might be in the media; however, Shiou [35] suggested that it is not a protein. This controversy will require further experiments, which is beyond the scope of the current study.

Another possible bioactive effector that protects premature rats from NEC might be some component of killed bacteria [37]. It was recently reported that heat-killed probiotics are as effective as live probiotics in maintaining the intestinal barrier [38] and that they can alleviate intestinal inflammation [39]. Both TOLLIP and SIGIRR are closely related to the intestinal barrier. Intestinal permeability in TOLLIP-deficient [16] and SIGIRR-deficient mice [40] treated with DSS increases compared with that in wild-type controls. It was also reported that the heat-killed probiotics alleviate intestinal inflammation through the downstream TLR4 pathway [41]. Dead *Lactobacillus*, which were isolated from newborn infant feces and breast milk, as well as live bacteria, activate TLR4-associated negative regulators, including TOLLIP, SOCS1, SOCS3 and IκBα [41]. It appears that the protective effect of *B. adolescentis* on NEC might be the result of upregulating SIGIRR and TOLLIP using some component of dead *B. adolescentis*.

Conclusions

We believe that prophylactic *B. adolescentis* protects against intestinal injury in a well-established premature newborn rat model, and inhibits the increase in intestinal TLR4 and the decrease in TOLLIP and SIGIRR expression. These results help to gather insight into the mechanisms behind the protective effects of probiotics in the intestine; however, in this study the increases in the expression of both SIGIRR and TOLLIP were demonstrated only in the NEC rat model, further studies are required to better determine the mechanisms underlying the beneficial effects of probiotics.

Abbreviations

DF: Dam fed group; DSS: Dextran sodium sulfate; FB: Formula + *Bifidobacterium adolescentis* group; FF: Formula Fed group; GAPDH: Glyceraldehyde-3-phosphate dehydrogenase; IL: Interleukin; IRAK: IL-1 receptor-associated kinase; NEC: Necrotizing enterocolitis; qPCR: Quantitative polymerase chain reaction; RNA: Ribonucleic acid; SD: Sprague-dawley; SIGIRR: Single Ig IL-1-Related Receptor; TIR: Toll-IL-1-receptor; TLR: Toll-like receptor; TOLLIP: Toll Interacting Protein; VLBW: Very low birth weight

Acknowledgements

We acknowledge Yuejun Huang from the Transforming Medical Center, Second Affiliated Hospital of Shantou University Medical College, China, for her assistance with revising the manuscript. We thank Luning Zhao from the Experimental Medicine Research Center, Guangzhou Medical University, for supporting the RT-qPCR procedure. We also thank Li Huang from the Guangzhou Medical University Laboratory Animal Center for supporting the animal experiments. A scientific writer was not used in the production of this manuscript.

Funding

Not applicable.

Authors' contributions

WW and YC conceived and designed the study. WW performed the animal experiments, carried out the RT-qPCR procedures, performed the statistical analyses, and drafted and submitted the manuscript. YC helped draft and revise the manuscript. YW and JZ helped establish the experimental animal model and analyzed the data. HY and FL procured the reagents that were used in the experiments. LZ helped to perform the statistical analyses. All authors read and approved the final manuscript.

Competing interests

The authors declare that they have no competing interests.

Author details

[1]Department of Neonatal Intensive Care Unit, Guangdong Province Maternal and Children's Hospital, Guangzhou Medical University, 13, Guangyuanxi Road, Guangzhou, China. [2]Department of Pediatrics, Guangdong Province Maternal and Children's Hospital, Guangzhou Medical University, 13, Guangyuanxi Road, Guangzhou, China.

References

1. Neu J, Walker WA. Necrotizing enterocolitis. N Engl J Med. 2011;364(3):255–64.
2. Hull MA, Fisher JG, Gutierrez IM, Jones BA, Kang KH, Kenny M, Zurakowski D, Modi BP, Horbar JD, Jaksic T. Mortality and management of surgical necrotizing enterocolitis in very low birth weight neonates: a prospective cohort study. J Am Coll Surg. 2014;218(6):1148–55.
3. Wang Q, Dong J, Zhu Y. Probiotic supplement reduces risk of necrotizing enterocolitis and mortality in preterm very low-birth-weight infants: an updated meta-analysis of 20 randomized, controlled trials. J Pediatr Surg. 2012;47(1):241–8.
4. Ganguli K, Meng D, Rautava S, Lu L, Walker WA, Nanthakumar N. Probiotics prevent necrotizing enterocolitis by modulating enterocyte genes that regulate innate immune-mediated inflammation. Am J Physiol Gastrointest Liver Physiol. 2013;304(2):G132–41.

5. Martin CR, Dammann O, Allred EN, Patel S, O'Shea TM, Kuban KC, Leviton A. Neurodevelopment of extremely preterm infants who had necrotizing enterocolitis with or without late bacteremia. J Pediatr. 2010;157(5):751–6.
6. Gephart SM, McGrath JM, Effken JA, Halpern MD. Necrotizing enterocolitis risk: state of the science. Adv Neonatal Care. 2012;12(2):77–87. 88-89.
7. Frost BL, Jilling T, Caplan MS. The importance of pro-inflammatory signaling in neonatal necrotizing enterocolitis. Semin Perinatol. 2008;32(2):100–6.
8. Nanthakumar N, Meng D, Goldstein AM, Zhu W, Lu L, Uauy R, Llanos A, Claud EC, Walker WA. The mechanism of excessive intestinal inflammation in necrotizing enterocolitis: an immature innate immune response. PLoS One. 2011;6(3):e17776.
9. Lu P, Sodhi CP, Hackam DJ. Toll-like receptor regulation of intestinal development and inflammation in the pathogenesis of necrotizing enterocolitis. Pathophysiology. 2014;21(1):81–93.
10. Jilling T, Simon D, Lu J, Meng FJ, Li D, Schy R, Thomson RB, Soliman A, Arditi M, Caplan MS. The roles of bacteria and TLR4 in rat and murine models of necrotizing enterocolitis. J Immunol. 2006;177(5):3273–82.
11. Fusunyan RD, Nanthakumar NN, Baldeon ME, Walker WA. Evidence for an innate immune response in the immature human intestine: toll-like receptors on fetal enterocytes. Pediatr Res. 2001;49(4):589–93.
12. Leaphart CL, Cavallo J, Gribar SC, Cetin S, Li J, Branca MF, Dubowski TD, Sodhi CP, Hackam DJ. A critical role for TLR4 in the pathogenesis of necrotizing enterocolitis by modulating intestinal injury and repair. J Immunol. 2007;179(7):4808–20.
13. Yazji I, Sodhi CP, Lee EK, Good M, Egan CE, Afrazi A, Neal MD, Jia H, Lin J, Ma C, et al. Endothelial TLR4 activation impairs intestinal microcirculatory perfusion in necrotizing enterocolitis via eNOS-NO-nitrite signaling. Proc Natl Acad Sci U S A. 2013;110(23):9451–6.
14. Zhang G, Ghosh S. Negative regulation of toll-like receptor-mediated signaling by Tollip. J Biol Chem. 2002;277(9):7059–65.
15. Wald D, Qin J, Zhao Z, Qian Y, Naramura M, Tian L, Towne J, Sims JE, Stark GR, Li X. SIGIRR, a negative regulator of Toll-like receptor-interleukin 1 receptor signaling. Nat Immunol. 2003;4(9):920–7.
16. Maillard MH, Bega H, Uhlig HH, Barnich N, Grandjean T, Chamaillard M, Michetti P, Velin D. Toll-interacting protein modulates colitis susceptibility in mice. Inflamm Bowel Dis. 2014;20(4):660–70.
17. Kadota C, Ishihara S, Aziz MM, Rumi MA, Oshima N, Mishima Y, Moriyama I, Yuki T, Amano Y, Kinoshita Y. Down-regulation of single immunoglobulin interleukin-1R-related molecule (SIGIRR)/TIR8 expression in intestinal epithelial cells during inflammation. Clin Exp Immunol. 2010;162(2):348–61.
18. Khailova L, Dvorak K, Arganbright KM, Halpern MD, Kinouchi T, Yajima M, Dvorak B. Bifidobacterium bifidum improves intestinal integrity in a rat model of necrotizing enterocolitis. Am J Physiol Gastrointest Liver Physiol. 2009;297(5):G940–9.
19. Garland SM, Tobin JM, Pirotta M, Tabrizi SN, Opie G, Donath S, Tang ML, Morley CJ, Hickey L, Ung L, et al. The ProPrems trial: investigating the effects of probiotics on late onset sepsis in very preterm infants. BMC Infect Dis. 2011;11:210.
20. Lin HC, Hsu CH, Chen HL, Chung MY, Hsu JF, Lien RI, Tsao LY, Chen CH, Su BH. Oral probiotics prevent necrotizing enterocolitis in very low birth weight preterm infants: a multicenter, randomized, controlled trial. Pediatrics. 2008;122(4):693–700.
21. Hogberg N, Stenback A, Carlsson PO, Wanders A, Lilja HE. Genes regulating tight junctions and cell adhesion are altered in early experimental necrotizing enterocolitis. J Pediatr Surg. 2013;48(11):2308–12.
22. Schmittgen TD, Livak KJ. Analyzing real-time PCR data by the comparative C(T) method. Nat Protoc. 2008;3(6):1101–8.
23. Caplan MS, Hedlund E, Adler L, Hsueh W. Role of asphyxia and feeding in a neonatal rat model of necrotizing enterocolitis. Pediatr Pathol. 1994;14(6): 1017–28.
24. Lu P, Sodhi CP, Jia H, Shaffiey S, Good M, Branca MF, Hackam DJ. Animal models of gastrointestinal and liver diseases. Animal models of necrotizing enterocolitis: pathophysiology, translational relevance, and challenges. Am J Physiol Gastrointest Liver Physiol. 2014;306(11):G917–28.
25. Le Mandat SA, Bonnard A, Barreau F, Aigrain Y, Pierre-Louis C, Berrebi D, Peuchmaur M. Expression of TLR-2, TLR-4, NOD2 and pNF-kappaB in a neonatal rat model of necrotizing enterocolitis. PLoS One. 2007;2(10):e1102.
26. Nanthakumar NN, Fusunyan RD, Sanderson I, Walker WA. Inflammation in the developing human intestine: A possible pathophysiologic contribution to necrotizing enterocolitis. Proc Natl Acad Sci U S A. 2000;97(11):6043–8.
27. Buisine MP, Aubert JP, Walker WA, Savidge TC. Developmental patterns of mucin gene expression in human fetal small intestinal xenografts maintained in severe-combined immunodeficient mice. Pediatr Res. 2003; 53(6):898–904.
28. Bhatia AM, Stoll BJ, Cismowski MJ, Hamrick SE. Cytokine levels in the preterm infant with neonatal intestinal injury. Am J Perinatol. 2014;31(6):489–96.
29. Garlanda C, Riva F, Bonavita E, Mantovani A. Negative regulatory receptors of the IL-1 family. Semin Immunol. 2013;25(6):408–15.
30. Kawasaki T, Kawai T. Toll-like receptor signaling pathways. Front Immunol. 2014;5:461.
31. Manzoni P, Rinaldi M, Cattani S, Pugni L, Romeo MG, Messner H, Stolfi I, Decembrino L, Laforgia N, Vagnarelli F, et al. Bovine lactoferrin supplementation for prevention of late-onset sepsis in very low-birth-weight neonates: a randomized trial. JAMA. 2009;302(13):1421–8.
32. Samanta M, Sarkar M, Ghosh P, Ghosh J, Sinha M, Chatterjee S. Prophylactic probiotics for prevention of necrotizing enterocolitis in very low birth weight newborns. J Trop Pediatr. 2009;55(2):128–31.
33. Bergmann KR, Liu SX, Tian R, Kushnir A, Turner JR, Li HL, Chou PM, Weber CR, De Plaen IG. Bifidobacteria stabilize claudins at tight junctions and prevent intestinal barrier dysfunction in mouse necrotizing enterocolitis. Am J Pathol. 2013;182(5):1595–606.
34. Underwood MA, Arriola J, Gerber CW, Kaveti A, Kalanetra KM, Kananurak A, Bevins CL, Mills DA, Dvorak B. Bifidobacterium longum subsp. infantis in experimental necrotizing enterocolitis: alterations in inflammation, innate immune response, and the microbiota. Pediatr Res. 2014;76(4):326–33.
35. Shiou SR, Yu Y, Guo Y, He SM, Mziray-Andrew CH, Hoenig J, Sun J, Petrof EO, Claud EC. Synergistic protection of combined probiotic conditioned media against neonatal necrotizing enterocolitis-like intestinal injury. PLoS One. 2013;8(5):e65108.
36. Petrof EO, Claud EC, Sun J, Abramova T, Guo Y, Waypa TS, He SM, Nakagawa Y, Chang EB. Bacteria-free solution derived from Lactobacillus plantarum inhibits multiple NF-kappaB pathways and inhibits proteasome function. Inflamm Bowel Dis. 2009;15(10):1537–47.
37. Patel RM, Myers LS, Kurundkar AR, Maheshwari A, Nusrat A, Lin PW. Probiotic bacteria induce maturation of intestinal claudin 3 expression and barrier function. Am J Pathol. 2012;180(2):626–35.
38. Chang B, Sang L, Wang Y, Tong J, Zhang D, Wang B. The protective effect of VSL#3 on intestinal permeability in a rat model of alcoholic intestinal injury. BMC Gastroenterol. 2013;13:151.
39. Li N, Russell WM, Douglas-escobar M, Hauser N, Lopez M, Neu J. Live and heat-killed Lactobacillus rhamnosus GG: effects on proinflammatory and anti-inflammatory cytokines/chemokines in gastrostomy-fed infant rats. Pediatr Res. 2009;66(2):203–7.
40. Garlanda C, Riva F, Veliz T, Polentarutti N, Pasqualini F, Radaelli E, Sironi M, Nebuloni M, Zorini EO, Scanziani E, et al. Increased susceptibility to colitis-associated cancer of mice lacking TIR8, an inhibitory member of the interleukin-1 receptor family. Cancer Res. 2007;67(13):6017–21.
41. Chiu YH, Lu YC, Ou CC, Lin SL, Tsai CC, Huang CT, Lin MY. Lactobacillus plantarum MYL26 induces endotoxin tolerance phenotype in Caco-2 cells. BMC Microbiol. 2013;13:190.

Permissions

All chapters in this book were first published in PEDIATRICS, by BioMed Central; hereby published with permission under the Creative Commons Attribution License or equivalent. Every chapter published in this book has been scrutinized by our experts. Their significance has been extensively debated. The topics covered herein carry significant findings which will fuel the growth of the discipline. They may even be implemented as practical applications or may be referred to as a beginning point for another development.

The contributors of this book come from diverse backgrounds, making this book a truly international effort. This book will bring forth new frontiers with its revolutionizing research information and detailed analysis of the nascent developments around the world.

We would like to thank all the contributing authors for lending their expertise to make the book truly unique. They have played a crucial role in the development of this book. Without their invaluable contributions this book wouldn't have been possible. They have made vital efforts to compile up to date information on the varied aspects of this subject to make this book a valuable addition to the collection of many professionals and students.

This book was conceptualized with the vision of imparting up-to-date information and advanced data in this field. To ensure the same, a matchless editorial board was set up. Every individual on the board went through rigorous rounds of assessment to prove their worth. After which they invested a large part of their time researching and compiling the most relevant data for our readers.

The editorial board has been involved in producing this book since its inception. They have spent rigorous hours researching and exploring the diverse topics which have resulted in the successful publishing of this book. They have passed on their knowledge of decades through this book. To expedite this challenging task, the publisher supported the team at every step. A small team of assistant editors was also appointed to further simplify the editing procedure and attain best results for the readers.

Apart from the editorial board, the designing team has also invested a significant amount of their time in understanding the subject and creating the most relevant covers. They scrutinized every image to scout for the most suitable representation of the subject and create an appropriate cover for the book.

The publishing team has been an ardent support to the editorial, designing and production team. Their endless efforts to recruit the best for this project, has resulted in the accomplishment of this book. They are a veteran in the field of academics and their pool of knowledge is as vast as their experience in printing. Their expertise and guidance has proved useful at every step. Their uncompromising quality standards have made this book an exceptional effort. Their encouragement from time to time has been an inspiration for everyone.

The publisher and the editorial board hope that this book will prove to be a valuable piece of knowledge for researchers, students, practitioners and scholars across the globe.

List of Contributors

Marta Yemane Hadush and Amanuel Hadgu Berhe
School of Medicine, Mekelle Univesity, College of Health Sciences, Mekelle, Ethiopia

Araya Abrha Medhanyie
School of Public Health, Mekelle University, College of Health Sciences, Mekelle, Ethiopia

Tsehaynesh G/eyesus
Amhara Regional Health Bureau, South Gondar Zonal Health Bureau, Debre Tabor, Ethiopia

Feleke Moges, Setegn Eshetie and Ebba Abate
Department of Medical Microbiology, School of Biomedical and Laboratory Sciences, College of Medicine and Health Sciences, University of Gondar, Gondar, Ethiopia

Biruk Yeshitela
Armauer Hansen Research Institute (AHRI), Addis Ababa, Ethiopia

Saif AlSaif, Ma. Bella Ponferrada, Ibrahim Ahmed, Mohammed Khawaji, Khalid AlHathlol and Beverly Baylon
Division of Neonatology, Department of Pediatrics, King Abdulaziz Medical City, Ministry of National Guard Health Affairs, Riyadh 11426, Kingdom of Saudi Arabia

Khalil AlTawil
Division of Neonatology, Department of Pediatrics, Prince Mohammad bin Abdulaziz Hospital, Ministry of National Guard Health Affairs, Al Madinah, Al Medina 41511, Kingdom of Saudi Arabia

Adel Sallam
Division of Neonatology, Department of Pediatrics, King Abdulaziz Medical City, Ministry of National Guard Health Affairs, Jeddah 21423, Kingdom of Saudi Arabia

Khalid AlKhairy, Ahmed AlSuhaibani and Mohammed AlBalwi
Department of Pathology and Laboratory Medicine, King Abdulaziz Medical City, Ministry of National Guard Health Affairs, Riyadh 11426, Kingdom of Saudi Arabia

Mohammed AlBalwi
Medical Genomics Research Department, King Abdullah International Medical Research Center, Ministry of National Guard Health Affairs, Riyadh 11426, Kingdom of Saudi Arabia

Ahmed AlSuhaibani and Mohammed AlBalwi
College of Medicine, King Saud bin Abdulaziz University for Health Sciences, Riyadh 11481, Kingdom of Saudi Arabia

Abadi Kidanemariam Berhe
Adigrat University, College of Medicine and Health Sciences, Adigrat, Ethiopia

Fitiwi Tinsaes
Department of Nursing, College of Medicine and Health Sciences, Adigrat University, Adigrat, Ethiopia

Gebremedhin Gebreegziabher
Department of Midwifery, College of Medicine and Health Sciences, Adigrat University, Adigrat, Ethiopia

Susan Kerr, Caroline King and Kerri McPherson
School of Health & Life Sciences, Glasgow Caledonian University, Cowcaddens Road, Glasgow G4 OBA, Scotland

Rhona Hogg
National Health Service (NHS) Greater Glasgow & Clyde, West House, Gartnavel Royal Hospital, 1055 Greater Western Road, Glasgow G12 0YN, Scotland

Janet Hanley
School of Health and Social Care, Edinburgh Napier University, Sighthill Campus, Sighthill Court, Edinburgh EH11 4BN, Scotland

Maggie Brierton and Sean Ainsworth
Victoria Hospital, NHS Fife, Hayfield Road, Kirkcaldy KY2 5AH, Scotland

Zhen-hua Gong
Department of general surgery, Shanghai Children's Hospital, Shanghai Jiao Tong University, road, West Lane 1400, number 24. Shanghai, Beijing 200040, China

Guo-li Tian, Yan-min Wang and Hong-ping Xu
Neonatal screening center, Shanghai Children's Hospital, Shanghai Jiao Tong University, Shanghai, China

Qi-wei Huang
Department of neonatology, Shanghai Children's Hospital, Shanghai Jiao Tong University, Shanghai, China

Kelsey D. J. Jones, Arati Rao and Narendra Aladangady
Neonatal Unit, Homerton University Hospital NHS Foundation Trust, London, UK

Kelsey D. J. Jones
Department of Paediatrics, Imperial College, London, UK

S E. Grossman, Dharshini Kumaranayakam, Arati Rao and Narendra Aladangady
Barts and the London School of Medicine & Dentistry, Queen Mary, University of London, London, UK

Greg Fegan
Swansea Trials Unit, School of Medicine, Swansea University, Swansea, UK

Maria Lorella Gianni, Paola Roggero and Fabio Mosca
Neonatal Intensive Care Unit (NICU), Department of Clinical Science and Community Health, Fondazione IRCCS "Ca' Granda" Ospedale Maggiore Policlinico, University of Milan, Milan, Italy

Charlotte Baudry and Pascale le Ruyet
Nutrition Department, Lactalis R&D, Retiers, France

Catherine Fressange-Mazda
Lactalis Nutrition Europe, Torcé, France

Claudio Galli
University of Milan, Milan, Italy

Carlo Agostoni
Pediatric Intermediate Care Unit, Department of Clinical Science and Community Health, Fondazione IRCCS "Ca' Granda" Ospedale Maggiore Policlinico, University of Milan, Milan, Italy

Shigeo Iijima
Department of Neonatology, Toho University Medical Center, Tokyo, Japan

Mahama Saaka, Fusena Ali and Felicia Vuu
University for Development Studies, School of Allied Health Sciences, Tamale, Ghana

Yan-ping Xu and Li-ping Shi
NICU, Children's Hospital, Zhejiang University School of Medicine, Hangzhou 310053, China

Jiajun Zhu
Department of Neonatology, Women's Hospital, Zhejiang University School of Medicine, Hangzhou 310006, China

Tamorah Lewis and Ashley Sherman
Department of Pediatrics, Children's Mercy Hospital, University of Missouri Kansas City School of Medicine, 2401 Gillham Rd, Kansas City, MO 64108, USA

Simisola Kuye
School of Medicine, University of Missouri Kansas City, Kansas City, MO, USA

Y. Amare
Consultancy for Social Development, Addis Ababa, Ethiopia

S. Paul
Nell Hodgson Woodruff School of Nursing, Emory University, 1520 Clifton Road NE, 30322 Atlanta, Georgia

L. M. Sibley
Nell Hodgson Woodruff School of Nursing and Rollins School of Public Health, Emory University, 1520 Clifton Road NE, 30322 Atlanta, Georgia

Brennan Vail and Melissa C. Morgan
Department of Pediatrics, University of California San Francisco, 550 16th Street, 4th Floor, San Francisco, CA 94158, USA

Melissa C. Morgan
Maternal, Adolescent, Reproductive, and Child Health Centre, London School of Hygiene and Tropical Medicine, Keppel Street, London WC1E 7HT, UK

Melissa C. Morgan, Hilary Spindler and Dilys M. Walker
Institute for Global Health Sciences, University of California San Francisco, 550 16th Street, San Francisco, CA 94158, USA

Amelia Christmas
PRONTO International, State RMNCH+A Unit, C-16 Krishi Nagar, A.G. Colony, Patna, Bihar 80002, India

Susanna R. Cohen
College of Nursing, University of Utah, 10 South 2000 East, Salt Lake City, UT 84112, USA

Dilys M. Walker
Department of Obstetrics and Gynecology and Reproductive Services, University of California San Francisco, 1001 Potrero Ave, SanFrancisco, CA 94110, USA
PRONTO International, 1820 E. Thomas Street APT 16, Seattle, WA 98112, USA

Irene Plaza Pinto, Claudio Carlos da Silva and Aparecido Divino da Cruz
Biotechnology and Biodiversity PhD Program, Federal University of Goias, Rede Centro Oeste de Pós-Graduação de Pesquisa e Inovação, Rua 235, n. 40, Setor Leste Universitário, Goiânia, GO 74605-050, Brazil

Irene Plaza Pinto and Lysa Bernardes Minasi
Replicon Research Group, Department of Biology, Pontifical Catholic University of Goias, Rua 235, n. 40, Setor Leste Universitário, Goiânia, GO 74605-050, Brazil

Lysa Bernardes Minasi, Claudio Carlos da Silva and Aparecido Divino da Cruz
Genetics Master's Program, Pontifical Catholic University of Goias, Rua 235, n. 40, Setor Leste Universitário, Goiânia, GO 74605-050, Brazil

Raphael Steckelberg
Maternity Hospital Amparo, Av T-12 n° 280 Setor Bueno, Goiânia, GO, Brazil

Dr Henrique Santillo Rehabilitation and Readjustment Center, Av. Ver. José Monteiro, 1655, Setor Negrão de Lima, Goiânia, GO, Brazil

Claudio Carlos da Silva and Aparecido Divino da Cruz
Human Cytogenetics and Molecular Genetics Laboratory, Secretary of Goias State for Public Health, Goiânia, GO, Brazil

Claudio Carlos da Silva
State University of Goias, Eseffego, Goiânia, Goiás, Brazil

Wen-Yuan Liu and Hai-Yan Qiu
Key laboratory of maternal-fetal medicine, Ningbo Women and Children's Hospital, Ningbo 315012, China

Zhe-Bin Yu, Jian-Bing Wang, Xue-Yu Chen and Kun Chen
Department of Epidemiology and Biostatistics, School of Public Health, Zhejiang University, Hangzhou 310058, China

Zhe-Bin Yu, Jian-Bing Wang and Kun Chen
Research Center for Air Pollution and Health, Zhejiang University, Hangzhou 310058, China

Rinawati Rohsiswatmo, Hanifah Oswari, Hikari Ambara Sjakti, Endang Windiastuti, Rosalina Dewi Roeslani and Indrayady Barchia
Department of Child Health, Faculty of Medicine, Universitas Indonesia - Cipto Mangunkusumo Hospital, Jl Pangeran Diponegoro No. 71, Salemba, Kenari, Senen, Jakarta Pusat, DKI Jakarta 10430, Indonesia

Rinawati Rohsiswatmo and Radhian Amandito
Neonatal Intensive Care Unit, Pondok Indah General Hospital, Jl Metro Duta Kav UE, Pondok Indah, Pondok Pinang, Kebayoran Lama, Jakarta Selatan, DKI Jakarta 12310, Indonesia

Tammy E. Corr and Ian M. Paul
Penn State College of Medicine, Department of Pediatrics, 500 University Drive, Hershey, PA 17033-0850, USA

Eric W. Schaefer and Ian M. Paul
Penn State College of Medicine, Department of Public Health Sciences, Hershey, PA, USA

Camille Brotelande, Christophe Milési and Gilles Cambonie
Department of Neonatology and Paediatric Intensive Care Unit, Arnaud de Villeneuve Hospital, Montpellier University Hospital, 371 Avenue du Doyen Gaston Giraud, 34295 Montpellier, Cedex 5, France

Nicolas Leboucq
Department of Paediatric Radiology, Arnaud de Villeneuve Hospital, Montpellier University Hospital, Montpellier, France

Mohamed Akkari and Michel Mondain
Department of Otorhinolaryngology, Gui-de-Chauliac Hospital, Montpellier University Hospital, Montpellier, France

Thomas Roujeau
Department of Neurosurgery, Gui-de-Chauliac Hospital, Montpellier University Hospital, Montpellier, France

Massimo Di Maio
Neonatal Intensive Care Unit, Carémeau Hospital, Nîmes University Hospital, Nîmes, France

Charles Raybaud
Division of Neuroradiology, Hospital for Sick Children, University of Toronto, 555 University Avenue, Toronto, ON M5G1X8, Canada

Mucheye Gizachew, Moges Tiruneh, Feleke Moges and Belay Tessema
Department of Medical Microbiology, School of Biomedical and Laboratory Sciences, College of Medicine and Health Sciences, University of Gondar, Gondar, Ethiopia

Mulat Adefris
Department of Gynecology and Obstetrics, School of Medicine, College of Medicine and Health Sciences, University of Gondar, Gondar, Ethiopia

Zemene Tigabu
Department of Pediatrics, School of Medicine, College of Medicine and Health Sciences, University of Gondar, Gondar, Ethiopia

Nu Ri Hwang and Jin Kyu Kim
Department of Pediatrics, Chonbuk National University Medical School, 20, Geonjiro Deokjin-gu, Jeonju-si, Jeollabuk-do 54907, South Korea

Jin Kyu Kim
Research Institute of Clinical Medicine of Chonbuk National University- Biomedical Research Institute of Chonbuk National University Hospital, Jeonju, Korea

Jonathan P. Sturgeon, Beatrice Zanetti and Dwight Lindo
Department of Paediatrics, Kingston Hospital, Kingston, London KT2 7QB, UK

Eleanor Jones, Beck Taylor, Gavin Rudge, Christine MacArthur and Carole Cummins
Institute of Applied Health Research, University of Birmingham, Edgbaston, Birmingham B15 2TH, England

Deepthi Jyothish
Birmingham Women's and Children's NHS Foundation Trust, Steelhouse Lane, Birmingham B4 6NH, England

Doug Simkiss
Division of Mental Health and Wellbeing, Warwick Medical School, University of Warwick, Coventry, UK

Gary Alcock, Helen G. Liley, Lucy Cooke and Peter H. Gray
Newborn Services, Mater Mothers' Hospital, Raymond Tce, South Brisbane, QLD 4101, Australia

Helen G. Liley and Peter H. Gray
Mater Research Institute-The University of Queensland, South Brisbane, QLD, Australia

Gary Alcock
The Townsville Hospital, 100 Angus Smith Drive, Douglas 4814, Australia

Noor Samuels, Rob A. van de Graaf, Rogier C. J. de Jonge, Irwin K. M. Reiss and Marijn J. Vermeulen
Department of Pediatrics, Division of Neonatology, Erasmus MC, Room SH-3005, CN, Rotterdam, The Netherlands

Jennifer S. Cauble, Mira Dewi and Holly R. Hull
Department of Dietetics and Nutrition, School of Health Professions, University of Kansas Medical Center, 3901 Rainbow BLVD, Mail Stop 4013, Kansas City, KS 66160, USA

Huaifu Dong
Department of Pediatrics, the First Affiliated Hospital of Bengbu Medical College, Bengbu 233004, Anhui, China

Huiping Cao
Department of Pediatrics, the Third People's Hospital of Bengbu, Bengbu 233000, Anhui, China

Haiyan Zheng
Department of Nursing, the First Affiliated Hospital of Bengbu Medical College, Bengbu 233004, Anhui, China

Wenshen Wu, Yanli Wang, Jingjing Zou, Fang Long, Huiheng Yan and Yunbin Chen
Department of Neonatal Intensive Care Unit, Guangdong Province Maternal and Children's Hospital, Guangzhou Medical University, 13, Guangyuanxi Road, Guangzhou, China

Lijuan Zeng
Department of Pediatrics, Guangdong Province Maternal and Children's Hospital, Guangzhou Medical University, 13, Guangyuanxi Road, Guangzhou, China

Index

www.ingramcontent.com/pod-product-compliance
Lightning Source LLC
Chambersburg PA
CBHW081214180926
51613CB00003B/236

* 9 7 8 1 6 3 9 2 7 4 3 1 4 *